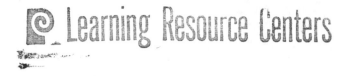
HARD LABOR

HARD LABOR

SUSAN L. DIAMOND,
B.S.N., R.N.

FORGE®

A Tom Doherty Associates Book ‖ *New York*

HARD LABOR

Copyright © 1996, 1998 by Susan L. Diamond

All rights reserved, including the right to reproduce this book,
or portions thereof, in any form.

This book is printed on acid-free paper.

A Forge Book
Published by Tom Doherty Associates, Inc.
175 Fifth Avenue
New York, NY 10010

Forge® is a registered trademark of Tom Doherty Associates, Inc.

Design by Sara Stemen

Library of Congress Cataloging-in-Publication Data

Diamond, Susan L.
    Hard labor / by Susan L. Diamond.
        p.   cm.
    "A Tom Doherty Associates book."
    ISBN 0-312-85308-4
    1. Childbirth—Popular works.   2. Maternity nursing.
    3. Diamond, Susan L.
    I. Title.
    RG652.D496   1996
    618.4—dc20   96-1555
                                                         CIP

First Hardcover Edition: October 1996

First Trade Paperback Edition: October 1998

Printed in the United States of America

0   9   8   7   6   5   4   3   2   1

For D . . . 1343, always and all ways,
and
Rebecca and Michael, who started it all—
I love you two!

AUTHOR'S NOTE

Hard Labor consists of chapters that trace my personal evolution as a clinical nurse and chapters that focus on specific aspects of the birth process as I have witnessed them. Reflections on obstetrical practices and procedures, hospital policies and regulations, physician and nurse behaviors and techniques are mine, and mine alone, and do not represent or claim to be those of any institution or organization. Interpretation of events or medical theory are also mine and reflect both my professional knowledge and my unwitting ignorance.

While many of the stories come from the earlier years of my career as a labor and delivery nurse, I have attempted to convey my increasing disillusionment in the narratives about my later work years. Where possible, I have tried to anchor each narrative in chronological time so the reader will generally know where I was on the journey from naïveté to cynicism.

Because Hard Labor is about my work experience, it is imperative that the reader understand that the stories in this book are drawn from my memories alone. I have reported events as I remember them, without contributions from anyone else who may have been present. Although presented in quotes, conversations with and remarks by participants in the stories are all reconstructed from memory and do not purport in any way to be verbatim conversations. To change the identities of people and hospitals in this book, I have altered names, changing gender in some cases, manufacturing physical descriptions, and modifying or combining some medical details about specific cases. I sincerely hope that readers who may think they recognize themselves will realize that the portraits I've painted are altered and the events I've described arise out of such common and/or universal experiences, and consequently, those portraits and events are not necessarily their own.

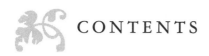

CONTENTS

ACKNOWLEDGMENTS

Hard Labor represents more than fourteen years of work: four years of nursing school and eight years of active employment as a L&D nurse, along with a couple more years of writing. It would be impossible to pay tribute to all the people over all those years who contributed to the making of this book. I know I'm leaving out a whole bunch of good folks—the mothers and babies and their families, instructors and students, doctors and nurses, relatives and friends—but I need to mention at least a few names and beg forgiveness from any and all who aren't specifically mentioned here.

Doris Budner "discovered" me: she read sample chapters of *Hard Labor* and insisted that her publisher husband, Stanley, "do something with this book." Did he ever! Acting informally as my agent, Stan found a publisher for me and has advised and encouraged me long-distance for several years now. The gods blessed me when they connected me to the Budners.

Everyone at Tom Doherty Associates has been wonderfully helpful and supportive. It has been an absolute joy and delight to work with my editor, Melissa Ann Singer. Her enthusiasm about *Hard Labor* and her insights and editorial gifts are more than any writer could ever want. Having her share news of her own pregnancy with me, long-distance, has been an added pleasure in our working relationship.

In nursing school, Steven Borecky gave me the best college course I ever had. Clare Hopkins guided me through the swamps of sophomore summer and gave me the kind of guidance every student needs and should be fortunate enough to receive. Without Edie Robinson-Stone, my beloved friend and cohort, I simply would not have survived nursing school (or any of the years that have followed). I am forever indebted to Linda Dempster for teaching me so much about nursing and being my good friend. Myra Wesley-King— my therapist, mentor, surrogate mother, and Ideal Woman—made me do much of the writing under threat of dire consequences if I didn't perform to her satisfaction! Simon and Rosalie Auster helped me through a particularly difficult period with medical care and a critique of my writing. Simon's kind assessment provided a much needed boost just when I was getting fed up with the idea of writing any more of this book.

Not surprisingly, the people who had the most impact on me as a nurse were other nurses. Along with others unnamed, through their daily efforts, these people demonstrated qualities and ethics that affected my education and practice in such profound and unique ways that I will always hold them dear in my heart. So thank you Dennis Dupuis, Susan DeLucia, Dalilah Lopez, Emma Jackson, Libby Broadhurst, Debbie Merkel, Lynn Cooler, Sue McHugh, Mildred Davis, Rachel Partin, Joan Loughney, and Jan Burkhead.

Mimi Harris taught me what courage, fortitude, and maternal devotion really are, and her daughter, Andrea, has demonstrated, every day of her life, how to overcome adversity and live life to the fullest. Rick and Julie Staelin and Robin and John Gallagher offered encouragement, editorial and financial assistance at another crucial time. My dear friends, Carole and Bill Wadlin, have been steadfast and constant through some very difficult years, finding me work, listening to me obsess and cry, and always, always helping me see the basic absurdity and humor in life, filling my heart with laughter and the wonder of their loving friendship.

Naturally, my extended family, including my sisters-in-law, nieces, and nephews, has been my rock. How do I ever express enough gratitude for my mother's love and faith in me, along with the fact that she kept a roof over my head during the last year of writing *Hard Labor*? My siblings have never stopped giving to me. Dan helped pay for nursing school, cosigned my mortgage, and remains a doctor I respect and admire. Katy listened to all the stories in this book as they happened, laughed and cried over them with me, shared a home with me, and helped raise my kids. Jessie has held my hand, literally, and kept me from falling into an abyss of despair; she is directly responsible for my continuing existence. Dave's knees are almost worn out from all the praying he's done for me; he also rescued me from complete insanity by providing me with his computer and laser printer! Stan wrapped me in great bear hugs exactly when I needed them and just listened, without commentary or his own agenda, a truly rare ability; Stan's my gentle giant, my psychic protector. My "first" baby, long-lost twin Jed, has redeemed me too many times to count; the bonds we forged during his infancy only grow stronger and the love deeper with each passing year. And DeeDee, a paragon of motherhood, has been a soulmate since we discovered each other.

Finally, my children. Rebecca and Michael have never disappointed me; the significance of their love and support during the long years of my work cannot be measured. Without you, my glorious, beautiful children, my life simply would not be.

PREFACE

H*ard Labor* is a book about work. It is about my work as an obstetrical nurse. It is about the work of doctors and nurses who provide obstetrical care. And it is about the momentous work women do to become mothers.

Hard Labor is, first and foremost, an account of my transformation from a wife and mother, unemployed outside of my home, to a clinically accomplished, reasonably well-paid, professional nurse. While this account is uniquely my story, it is also a detailed insider's view of the education, training, and clinical activities of nurses, particularly nurses who care for obstetrical patients. In tracing my odyssey from the home to the hospital, my story mirrors those of countless American women who have left behind the mythical, traditional hearth and home for outside employment; women who struggle daily with the burdens of work and family and the desire for self-fulfillment and meaning in their lives.

I became involved with childbirth out of a naïve enthusiasm over the process of birth after I delivered my own two children. In addition to that enthusiasm, I was suffering from a vague dis-ease, a feeling of emptiness after the birth of my second and last child. At the age of thirty, I was suddenly face to face with the reality that my life's reproductive activities were completed—that it was extremely unlikely I would ever be pregnant or give birth again. The imagined loss of that potential (I was young enough to bear more children, but my marriage did not include the possibility of more than two children), along with the nature of my two pregnancies and deliveries, impelled me into the work I have embraced for the last twelve years.

I was born in the late forties, the third child and second daughter of a physician father and a college-educated mother. During the course of my childhood, my family grew by four more siblings—another sister and three more brothers. We lived in five different states, thanks to my father's peregrinations with the military service and his advanced surgical training. I attended seven different schools, the last three of them Catholic schools.

We were a close-knit family as a result of all our relocations and even more so after my parents divorced when I was fourteen. We had little money, no television, and we rarely went to movies. Reading was big in our household, along with board games and endless hours of pretend play, usually out in the woods around whatever house we occupied. We all had chores, and the older children were responsible for the younger ones. After our family became Roman Catholic, we participated in many church activities. It was a pleasant childhood, filled with the comings and goings of seven active children, marred only by all the moves and the divorce of our parents. We all helped our mother after Dad left, but they both instilled in us a sense of obligation to help others.

At eighteen, I left home, then in the deep South, for Boston University, where I earned a bachelor's degree in English literature. I was married the same year I graduated, at the end of the sixties. After my husband finished graduate school, we migrated from New England to the Midwest, where he began a career in academia and I planned on pregnancy. Four years into my marriage, I gave birth to my first child, Rebecca. Four years later, my marriage foundering, I gave birth to my second child, Michael. It was after Michael's birth that I began the journey this book narrates.

My desire to continue to participate in the fascinating, complex process of birth led me first to become a prepared childbirth instructor. My classes with expectant couples were wonderfully gratifying and a lot of fun. I loved sharing their anticipation, helping them prepare for this life-changing event, and admiring them and their babies after the births. Over a period of four years, teaching classes and reading numerous books on childbirth, I became more sophisticated in my understanding of how women give birth in most hospitals in this country. I knew there were problems inherent in the system, but I was still one step removed from the actual event. I wanted to be on the scene, helping to enhance the births of other people's babies. Nursing school was the next step, but I was already aware that what I really dreamed of being was a midwife. First I would get my nursing degree and then do a graduate program in nurse-midwifery. Eventually, as the fantasy went, I would be able to actually deliver babies myself. How much more involved in the birth process could I get?

I started nursing school four years after Michael's birth. At the same time, my husband and I separated. After four years of study, I received a bachelor's degree in nursing, moved to another city, and began work as a labor and delivery nurse in a large military hospital on the East Coast. I spent four years there (amazing, these increments of four years), learning my craft. My next job, as an assistant nurse manager, lasted a year. After that I worked for a nursing agency, hiring out at various hospitals while I labored over the beginnings of this book. After a year and a half as an agency nurse, I moved to a southern state to work as a staff nurse again, in a family birthing center. By then my daughter was seventeen and in college, and my son was thirteen, living with his father and stepmother in another state. I worked in the birthing center for a year and a half, until I quit to complete this book. Somehow it doesn't surprise me that my employment record reiterates somewhat the several moves of my childhood.

Many aspects of hospital childbirth are positive—even miraculous. Who can deny the pride an obstetrical team feels when a potential miscarriage is averted; when a premature baby is protected and guided through the terror-filled maze of an intensive-care beginning; when a woman suffering a life-threatening disease of pregnancy is treated and enabled to carry her baby to term successfully; when a distressed infant is delivered by cesarean section before it dies in its mother's womb? And there are all the "normal" deliveries I've been a part of, rejoicing with the family over the arrival of another human being into their lives. Those stories are in this book; I hope they are as uplifting to the reader as they were to me when I experienced them.

But as I progressed in my work, I lost my housewife's innocence. I learned what really happens in the hospital during childbirth. With that privileged knowledge came disillusionment and ultimately anger over the abuses within the obstetrical health-care system. Out of all the experiences narrated in this book came the realization that I feel terribly conflicted about working in this system. I have enormous difficulty participating in care that all too often dehumanizes the woman, ignores or mistreats the family of the baby, and fails to promote and facilitate a propitious beginning for the new family and new little person. When I am part of a team that actually brutalizes a woman under the guise of medical care—that strips her of her dignity, her rights to choose how she will be cared for, her integrity as a human being undergoing a perfectly normal physiological process—I am tormented by my own culpability. I want to holler at the world, "Look at this! This is terrible! This shouldn't be happening! Why are we doing these things to this mother? Why is she letting us?"

Childbirth shouldn't be a nightmare. Having a baby should be an experience more of joy and pride than of agony and torment. Obstetrical teams have an extremely significant opportunity to shape in a positive, life-affirming way, the beginning of a person's sojourn on this earth. It is a heavy responsibility, fraught with danger and threatened by the high-tech nature of medicine today. Medicine's potential is diminished by the crush of work and chronic fatigue, and care is reduced to numbers and data by hours of paperwork and the stifling routine of procedures at all hours of the day and night.

But this responsibility is also a precious privilege for obstetrical workers. We are the first people this new child is exposed to, other than its family. I remain convinced that this is too crucial a responsibility and too special a privilege to take lightheartedly. I have tried to illustrate this conviction through the chapters of *Hard Labor*, to show how wondrous it is to be the nurse touching a newborn child fresh from its mother.

Hard Labor documents my evolution from an insulated, trusting, unsuspicious housewife to a cynical, assertive, hypercritical, exhausted professional nurse. I have written about some of the conflicts I experienced as I moved through nursing school: my fears of incompetence, my struggle to behave professionally with patients when my emotions were in turmoil. I have shown how I was forced to learn to compromise, to realize that sometimes the patient might have to suffer, whether I like it or not; that sometimes I have to close my eyes to the negligence of medical people if I'm going to keep my job and pay my mortgage. Through various cases, I have attempted to illustrate some of the critical issues of hospital obstetrical practice and the manner in which the theories behind this practice can interfere with the patient's best interests.

In telling my story, I have tried to reveal how hard the medical care system is on doctors and nurses, as well as patients, and why so many health-care providers lose their dedication to their work. There are stories within these pages about doctors and nurses who taught me how to do my work and shared my passion for the intricacies of giving birth. There are also stories that illustrate the dismay I felt on learning that there are many people in obstetrics who simply do not give a damn about their patients, who see patients and their families as "the enemy," to be thwarted at every opportunity. This book may help to explain how the conflicts between doctors and nurses, which arise out of bias, misunderstanding, and power grabbing, diminish both parties' ability to provide the best service to their patients. There are a few examples of the continued domination of physicians over nurses, which results in a perception of powerlessness among nurses and causes many (myself included) to sabotage themselves on a regular basis, rendering their efforts meaningless and reducing them to shrill complainers and bitter cynics.

Because of my anguish over the abuses in the system, it may seem as if this book is nothing but a condemnation of hospital obstetrical practice. I hope, however, that it is seen less as a condemnation and more as an apologia for that practice. If this book expresses outrage at the wrongs in the system, it also expresses sympathy for the people working within it. Most of them are extraordinary people, working killer hours, making difficult decisions, struggling to get along with one another and the strangers who have placed their health and well-being into their hands. They are people who still get a lift from a newborn's first wails, who can still laugh at their own mistakes and be patient with those among their colleagues, who are working to make the experience of birth a positive one for everyone involved.

Finally, *Hard Labor* is about my fascination with the work of the mothers themselves. In the universal act of giving birth may be found the complete range of human emotions. There is so much to be learned about human behavior while observing the inevitable physiological events of labor and delivery—how women respond to the demands of their bodies and the pain of bearing a child; how they actually do the work of giving birth; how their personalities, families, education, and upbringing affect this work; how the presence of a helpless newborn changes them; how the death of a newborn alters their world. There are sad stories in this book, stories that convey my inner conflicts, and there are happy stories. The joy I feel when I place an infant in his mother's arms, the wonder I experience as I watch a small body begin life on its own, the magic I watch as a man, a woman, and a baby become a family before my eyes—these are the underlying motivations and rewards of the work I do. More than my anguish, more than my disenchantment with the obstetrical system, it is these emotions that I hope will shine through in this book. These are the qualities that give depth and meaning and substance to my work, to the work of my fellow doctors and nurses, and to the work of women giving birth.

HARD LABOR

Chapter One

THE BEGINNING

Twenty-odd years ago, I had my first baby. I was twenty-six years old. I attended Lamaze classes with my husband, went into labor, used the techniques I'd been taught, and successfully delivered a daughter in a large, midwestern urban hospital without benefit of medication or medical intervention. That task, performed by untold millions of other women, was to be a pivotal one for me. My daughter's birth was the first of a series of events that would shape the middle years of my life.

My labor was short, by usual reckoning for primiparas, or first-time mothers. Three weeks past my due date, I finally experienced real, timeable contractions that increased in frequency and intensity. During the days before, I had watched endless hours of Watergate hearings with my mother, stroking my huge belly and timing false contractions that would tease me for several hours and then cease. I visited the obstetricians weekly and was told "it could happen any day now," only to return a week later, frustrated and heavy with my child.

The evening of July 8, my husband, Frank, and I had hamburgers for dinner. Ravenous as usual, I ate two and was watching TV when uterine contractions began to assert themselves. My eyes were on the clock when the phone rang. It was an old college friend, who asked casually, "What are you doing?"

"I'm timing contractions," I said, with a laugh.

"Are you serious? You sound so calm!" he sputtered.

"They don't hurt, Mark," I answered, "but they're about four minutes apart. It may be the real thing, but this has been going on for weeks now, so I don't know." I surrendered the phone to Frank and walked around for a while, watching the clock, wondering over the inscrutable activity of my body.

At eleven that night, as I sat down on the bed, preparing for sleep, I was gripped by a contraction that startled me with its strength. I couldn't catch my breath. The flavor of the contraction reminded me of bad menstrual cramps. It felt like a dim purple warmth deep down in my pelvis, under my pubic bone, that flared suddenly into a bright red flame as the contraction peaked. Belatedly, I deep-breathed, calling out to Frank as it subsided, "That one wasn't kidding!" After two more similar contractions, I suggested we call the doctor.

Less than an hour later we were driving under a full moon to the hospital. Frank was nervous, I was afraid it was false labor, and we were both elated. I was separated from Frank at the emergency room counter and wheeled off in a chair to the maternity unit. The inexorable routine began then: remove your clothes, give a urine sample, give an oral history, describe the contractions, get an enema, lose your identity, become a "patient in labor." It's relatively vague in my memory now, except for the feeling of being stripped of my identity, of feeling forlorn and alone in the business-like atmosphere of the hospital. Where was the excitement, the anticipatory thrill of a new life on its way? Where was my husband?

I was using slow, deep-chest breathing with each contraction when Frank appeared, looking worried and flustered. A resident—a physician in specialty training—with large hands checked my cervix and announced that I was two centimeters dilated. I remonstrated with him, "Dr. Russell said I was three centimeters the last two times he checked me!" Dilation being what it is, a subjective call by feel only, it wasn't surprising that this man's big fingers felt less of an opening, but I wasn't giving up a single centimeter! Dr. Russell was in the obstetrical group practice providing my prenatal care and was one of the three physicians I saw on alternating visits. Although Dr. Russell had examined me the most recently, which of the doctors would deliver me depended entirely on their call schedule: the doctor on call when I was ready to deliver would catch the baby. I had no say in the matter.

The night passed. Frank ate a sandwich from the Lamaze goody bag, politely offering to share with a nurse who stood over me, as I huffed and puffed. I remember being furious that he could be so casual, talking about food as I struggled with each contraction. He couldn't use the techniques we had practiced: my contractions were so irregular in frequency and length he had no way of anticipating their beginning. I would just start breathing and he'd time the contraction and write down the times. There was no electronic fetal monitoring and I have absolutely no memory of anyone listening to the fetal heartbeat during my entire labor.

Not long after I had settled into the bed and begun the serious work of dealing with these sensations, a nurse came in and told me I was breathing too fast—I was panting at that point—that I wasn't far enough along and needed to slow down or I'd wear out. She held my hand and breathed with me, slow, deep-chest respirations again. I calmed down and moved into a rhythm. The room grew smaller; I could talk to Frank, become aware of his discomfort. He needed to go to the bathroom; we hadn't packed any aspirin and he had a terrible headache; his ulcer was killing him. I made suggestions and voiced my concern, but with each contraction, he faded into the periphery, outside of this powerful force that gripped me.

I lay in the bed and felt the muscles in my lower back start to tighten. The tightness migrated around to my front, my belly surging upward, becoming rock-hard as I breathed, breathed, breathed. In and out, in and out, in and out. *Now it's waning, in and out, belly softens, relax. . . .* I turned on my side twice, only to experience a strong urge to urinate, mistaking it for the urge to push. Nurses were duly called, my cervix duly checked, "No, you're just five centimeters, just seven . . ."

The power within me, this incredible muscular flexing, stunned me. Never had I experienced anything like this. My body had taken over: all I could do was go with it, breathe and attempt to stay on top of the pain. It was unlike any pain I'd ever known. It wasn't that it burned or ached or fired within me: it was just strong and profoundly powerful. My world shrank to become my body, my breathing and my uterus: contracting, thrusting upward, pulling itself open, squeezing, as though a giant's arms were wrapped around my belly, hugging me, forcing my breath out, threatening to pop me like an overripe seedpod. Time expanded: I had no concept of minutes or hours of the day or day of the week. Light changed: the room became gray, gray as the feel of this power within. I lost all peripheral vision, could see only a fog around me.

The panting wasn't working anymore. I began to have difficulty maintaining a breathing pattern through the contraction, wanting to thrash in the bed, wanting to get out of my body and leave it behind to struggle without my consciousness. Frank and I had practiced breathing in fifteen-second intervals, so I searched for fifteen-letter words to spell to myself with each pant. Both names we had chosen worked: I spelled them monotonously with each breath. *Go on, see if you can spell this whole name, evenly, regularly. Concentrate on the next letter, focus on the whole name, keep going, spell, spell.* Then, oddly, I asked Frank how many letters there were in "anti-depressant." Puzzled, he counted fifteen, with the hyphen. I spelled anti-depressant hundreds of times that night, alternating with the children's names. It was the only way I could maintain control through the contractions. (Why did I pick that word? Why did it seem so right? What did my subconscious mean, giving me that word? A message from my future?)

Finally, Dr. Samuels, one of my obstetricians, came in to check me, to my disappointment. I had hoped my favorite, the easy-going, handsome Dr. Russell, would be on call for my delivery. I had no particular feeling for this doctor; he was somewhat cold, and his apparent indifference during my prenatal office visits had turned me off. As he bent to check my cervix, I watched his face: lean, middle-aged, almost ascetic. He announced that I was completely dilated and could begin to push. Aha! Second stage of labor! According to Lamaze class, the fun time! Second wind! Active involvement in the process!

Except it wasn't true. I had no second wind. It wasn't fun, and worst of all, I had absolutely no urge to push. (For many women this is a ferocious impulse, undeniable and almost impossible to control.) But I pushed anyway. Did I ever push! *Scrunch up the body, grab the legs, pull them back, and bear down! Bear down! Into my butt, into my ass, push, push, push! Feel the contraction start. Take two deep cleansing breaths, hold the third, and PUSH, goddammit!* I pushed for more than two hours. I worked harder, physically, than I ever had before, straining with every muscle in my body to expel this baby. I could feel the mass of her within me, down deep, like a watermelon in my pelvis. I could feel her move, grudgingly, centimeter by centimeter, in the latter half of each push, as though all the effort in the first half was for nought. But I kept pushing.

She, this unknown baby, moved down, slowly, slowly, and never ceased to let me know she was there (as if I could ignore a watermelon in my rectum!). She kicked all the way out. After two hours of pushing every four to five minutes for the duration of the contractions, some of which were two minutes long, I got angry. A nurse was tapping my perineum, shouting "Push here! Push here!" *Where do you think I'm pushing, you bitch?* I screamed at her in my mind. An unidentified man came into the room, stood at the foot of my bed and watched me silently as I pushed. He was another resident, I supposed, since he was dressed in green scrubs. He didn't identify himself or say anything at all to me, just stood there inspecting my exposed genitals. That made me truly angry. *What is this, some goddamned sideshow?* I fumed as I grunted with effort. Then I overheard him telling Frank that he didn't think I'd be able to deliver vaginally. The baby was posterior (facing up instead of down toward my tailbone), making for a longer second stage since she had to be rotated with the pushing efforts in addition to being forced down the vaginal canal. Even though I was pushing well, I was wearing out, so he thought I probably wouldn't make it.

Unknowingly, that unidentified man provided me with just enough furious motivation—*Oh yeah? I'm wearing out, huh? I can't keep this up, huh? Just watch me, you bastard!* I worked with renewed determination. And then, suddenly it seemed, it was time to go to the delivery room. The baby was crowning, I was almost there! The move to the delivery room was horrible; I felt tossed and tumbled somehow, rolling down the hall on a gurney with my knees bent and sprawled open, this urgent weight on my bowels. As I was transferred to the delivery table, Dr. Russell entered the room to do the delivery. Garbed in traditional scrubs, his feet slapping the floor in thongs, his beard barely covered by the paper mask and cap—I was delighted to see him.

Feet in stirrups, genitals exposed to the lights, I pushed a final time and felt the baby's head emerge, then the slippery slide of her body leaving mine, with several final kicks as she swam away from my body into the air and Dr. Russell's hands. The sensation of the umbilical cord trailing after that huge mass was almost orgasmic. *A girl, a daughter!* "Oh, Rebecca, I'm so glad it's you! I didn't like 'Matthew' at all!" Dr. Russell held her upside down by the feet, just like in all the movies, and I watched her take her very first breath of air, her bluish torso shuddering, ribcage expanding, a pink tinge moving outward from her chest. Oh, it was magical to see her breathe!

She looked just like her paternal grandfather. I laughed with amazement that recognizable features were there, that this child was so apparently an offspring of her father's father! She had dark hair, too, something totally unexpected, since her father and I are both blond and fair. I always thought I'd have a blond, baldish, Diamond-looking baby. The process of claiming, recognizing, and imprinting this new being began instantaneously, as I lay there on the table, waiting for the placenta.

It wouldn't come out. Dr. Russell massaged my belly so fiercely I thought he would puncture my abdomen. While pushing, I had popped the IV right out of my arm and now I thought I would pop myself. But then, there it came—plop! into a basin. Dr. Russell held it up for my inspection, announcing that it looked "about three weeks old." Frank was at the warmer, watching the nurse with the baby. I could see her tiny hands waving. Then he was at my side, holding her, grinning and talking nonstop about the whole experience. I was glad he was the first to touch her, to hold her. I hoped it would help him bond to her. I was also absurdly pleased with myself. I had done it! I had gone through labor and delivery without any medications, without any interference, and wow, it felt fantastic! I was so proud of myself! I wanted to get off the table and dance around the room! I wanted to shout out to everyone, "I had a baby! I had a baby!" I could hardly think of the baby, I was so filled with myself. I had never gone through any experience so rigorous, so demanding; I had never felt such an extraordinary sense of accomplishment.

My mother had delivered five of her seven children without benefit of an-algesics or anesthesia. She was my role model. Her ability to give birth with such apparent ease was the one attribute for which I ever heard my father openly praise her. When I'd told him I was planning a natural childbirth, he snorted and said I'd never be able to do it, that I didn't have my mother's strength. Now I had proved him wrong. My elation was indescribable.

Rebecca was born at 8:54 A.M. I breast-fed her for the first time in the recovery room, still ebullient, engorged with pride in myself. That evening, when my mother arrived to visit, I was out of bed, bustling around the room, filled with energy. Visibly startled to see me up, Mom laughingly told me of her first experience after delivering my oldest brother in 1944. They hadn't allowed her to sit up or get out of bed for nine days; when she finally did, her legs were too weak to stand on! I was not only standing; I was walking, flying on the ceiling! Such self-delight, what a high! When I called my father the next day, I cried as I received his gruff praise.

Four years later I was once again heavy with child. Frank and I had attended Lamaze classes again, but I had difficulty getting him to practice with me. He scoffed at the need to do so, saying I had done so well the first time it seemed kind of ridiculous. This pregnancy hadn't been as much fun, though. I couldn't sleep whenever I wanted to, as I had during the first, since I had an active four-year-old. The child within felt heavier and kicked me so violently I had a permanent bruise, quite tender to the touch, just under my diaphragm.

The final three weeks took on the aura of a nightmare as I shared the agony of my best friend's delivery of a handicapped infant. I had frequent nightmares during which I dreamed of being in bed, surrounded by unknown people clad in white coats, who stared solemnly at me. Performance anxiety dreams, I think. *How would I do this time? Now I had an idea of what to expect. Would I be able to do as well? And what if something is wrong with my baby?* None of these thoughts had entered my mind during the first pregnancy. I was blissfully ignorant then. Now I knew better.

Each night before falling asleep, Frank and I would talk about my friend's baby, our fear almost palpable in the quiet, dark air-conditioned bedroom. I would silently reach for his hand, gripping it tightly until I slipped into sleep. I worried about how I would cope with another child; whether I could ever love another child as I loved my daughter; and I wondered how another child could possibly hold my heart as my glorious little girl had done for the past four years.

The night my labor started, there was no doubt in my mind. A contraction greeted me with a ferocity that caught my undivided attention. It was one day before my due date; there had been some false labor, but nothing like with Rebecca. When it was time to go to the hospital, the contractions were four minutes apart and the gray-edged pain of them was familiar. I sat on the bed, dressing, realizing that I'd forgotten precisely how true labor pains felt until this moment. *Ah yes, I remember this. How could it have ever faded from my mind?*

It was raining hard outside at 11:00 P.M. when Frank preceded me down the stairs with a sleeping child in his arms, off to the neighbors for the night. I walked down those stairs more slowly than I ever had before, wearing my favorite blue maternity dress, stroking my abdomen, staring at the bannister, trailing my hand along the wall, feeling a great sadness sweep over me. *Go slow. This is the last night you'll ever be pregnant.* My reluctance to leave the stairs, to walk out of the house, surprised me. It was as though all the months of pregnancy had passed too swiftly; I felt distinctly unprepared and unwilling to give up this inner being.

There was a full moon again, its glow visible in spite of the rain, and the same routines at the hospital. My cervix was just three centimeters dilated. I continued to have contractions every three minutes, but they weren't painful; I didn't need to use controlled breathing. Frank and I sat bored and restless through the small hours of the night, growing sleepier and crankier as the hours passed. At some point I asked if we could go home, but the nurses said no, that I needed to be checked by the doctor first. They neglected to explain that meant waiting until the morning when the doctor came in to the hospital; the nurses were letting him sleep because I wasn't in active labor.

At 6:15 A.M., Dr. Mauller sailed into the room. Frank and I had been awake since early morning the day before, but this guy was fresh and well rested. His skin shone pink from his morning shower. Aftershave perfumed our dark, tile-walled little labor room. With a brusque "hello," he sat on my bed and thrust his fingers into my vagina. With those fingers buried inside me, he asked for a "hook," announcing my cervix was unchanged. Before I knew what was happening, he was rupturing the amniotic membranes. A flood of warm fluid poured out of me and I knew I was committed to delivery now. I hadn't seen Dr. Mauller, the third obstetrician in my group of doctors, in any recent prenatal visits, so I asked him if we could review what I hoped to have happen if my labor progressed normally.

He sat silently as I told him how I would like to approximate a Leboyer birth, if possible, by limiting the number of personnel in the delivery room, by dimming the lights, and by allowing me to touch the baby as soon as possible. He was brusque and noncommittal, looking aggravated by my requests. He stood at the end of the bed, chatting with Frank, as my contractions suddenly increased in intensity and frequency. I was flabbergasted to see him light up a cigarette and casually puff away while I lay there, trapped in the bed, huffing with effort as contractions clamped me in their grip. I found it increasingly difficult to concentrate on my breathing as the contractions seemed to be coming back to back and yet the two men carried on their conversation without a thought about me. Timidly, I asked them to be quiet or leave the room. Dr. Mauller snorted rudely and said, "This is what you wanted, right? Natural childbirth, okay?"

As he continued his conversation with Frank, who was oblivious to my travail, I struggled on. It was as if I had been tossed into a maelstrom; my body heaved upward off the bed with the massive squeezing of the contractions. I fought to stay in control, counting, spelling, panting. In the brief breaks between these powerful sensations, I fought my panic: *Dear God, these are hard; how can I go on without screaming, what can I do? The breathing isn't working. Oh God, here comes another one.* Panting with each second, I tried to focus on the wall clock opposite my bed. But the clock refused to remain stationary; it wavered around on the wall and made me dizzy. I spelled "s-m-i-l-e" repeatedly, but couldn't convince myself there was anything to smile about. The only thing that worked was a tremendous mental effort to recite the alphabet backward, a pant per letter.

This labor was completely unlike my first. The way in which my body attempted to open itself for this infant seemed almost vicious. There was a savage urgency in the uterine surges: *Get this baby out, get this baby out, get this baby out!* The gray fog returned; I couldn't see or hear anything outside the silent roaring of my body, like ocean waves building and cresting and sweeping me along and then crashing me down, breathless, frantically trying to prepare for the next wave. It wasn't pain, per se, it was force, powerful and overwhelming, eliminating all consciousness of anything but itself.

Someone spoke: "Let me check your cervix. She's nine, let's get her to the delivery room." It was Dr. Samuels, the quiet, nondescript partner of my obstetrical group. *Oh, Dr. Samuels, I'm so glad to see you.* His hands felt so comforting to me. But then they moved me to the delivery room, down the hall, the bed shaking me, each tremor like a scourge to my exhausted body. I started cursing, my knees up and askew, the sheets tumbled helter-skelter over my sweaty self. *Oh God, goddamn it, it hurts, slow down, oh hurry, oh another contraction, shit, fuck, oh God, fuck!*

In the delivery room, Dr. Mauller, the smoker, was putting on a gown. "Get on the delivery table," he commanded me.

"I can't, I can't move."

He turned to me, "Do you want to have your baby in the labor bed?"

"Yes! Yes, I do!"

"Well, you can't. Now get your butt on that table!"

Shaken by his hostility, I slid onto the table. A faceless nurse lifted my legs into the stirrups. I cried out, "They're too far apart, they're too high, I can feel myself tearing, oh, oh, they're too far apart!" My legs were stretched open so far I couldn't push. Dr. Mauller argued with me and then gruffly told the nurse to adjust the legs. Then he told me to push. I pushed: again it felt like a watermelon, of immense proportions this time, moving through my core. *Oh fuck, this hurts!* Embarrassed, Frank told me to stop cursing and I felt enraged at him. The second time I pushed I realized all the effort was going down my arms into my hands, which gripped metal handles on the table edge. Outrageous grunts came out of my mouth as I gathered every ounce of energy I possessed and bore down.

Then it was as if I stepped outside of myself. I thought quite clearly and calmly, *You have to do this. You're going to tear open but you have no choice, you have to get this mass out of yourself.* I pushed again, into my bottom and felt the baby move. As he moved, I felt him tearing me open. I could feel the inner tissues, the meat and muscle of the vaginal canal ripping; I could feel the color, fiery red and hot; I could see the torn edges of myself and I strained to finish it, a long, sustained animal growl squeezing between my clenched jaws and teeth. The doctor was snip-snipping with scissors as I pushed, but I could tell an episiotomy was too late; I was ripping my own door open for this child.

The head popped out, then the shoulders in a final tearing sensation and glory be, my son was born! Dr. Mauller cut the cord and slapped the baby onto my belly, less than two hours after my membranes had been ruptured. *Oh my God, a boy, a boy! Look at you, oh to touch you, to feel you hot from my body, oh how fast and hard you came to me!* I placed my hands on this little body with eagerness. What a joy to be able to touch him so fresh from inside me, so new! He was a sticky, mucky, marvelous little cone-headed baby, warm and wet on my belly. Frank took pictures as I stroked him, overcome with a mix of emotions. I felt grief that I hadn't been allowed to touch Rebecca this way; pride that it was over and I had managed to survive it with a modicum of dignity; sheer delight in this little boy; and anger at the doctor: so many feelings, including the realization that the act of childbirth was over for me, forever, even as I caressed the naked child on my belly.

The nurse took him from me and Dr. Mauller repaired my episiotomy. I began to shake all over, uncontrollably and violently. He kept telling me to be still; I kept telling him I was sorry, I couldn't help it. He insisted I had been wrong about the positioning of my legs. I kept quiet about that and shook. While he stitched, Frank paced back and forth, talking to me and looking with horror at my bottom. Years later, after seeing for myself what a woman's bottom looks like after a fourth-degree laceration, I understood Frank's horror. The door I ripped for this baby was a tear through the vaginal and rectal walls right into the rectum. Before such damage is repaired, the genital area looks like raw hamburger.

Finally the repair was over: I cradled my son in my arms as we were moved to the recovery room. I breast-fed him and laughed over his cone head with Frank, but felt somehow strangely detached, emotionally uninvolved with the baby. When the nurses took him away I collapsed back in the bed, exhausted. Over the next four hours, I dozed intermittently, only peripherally aware of being moved around the room as other mothers were brought in. One after another they rolled in, the nurses frantic for space and time to care for all these women. At one point, there were fourteen of us in the room and I was the only nonmedicated, "natural" mother present. Women were moaning, crying, or out cold. The last to arrive was a twelve-year-old girl, who had had a cesarean section and was whimpering in pain.

I kept asking when I could go to my room. The nurses kept saying, soon, there were no beds available yet. I sat on a bedpan and urinated copiously. When the nurse came to remove the pan, I was crying.

"What's wrong?"

I sobbed, "I want to see my baby, I want to be with my baby, I'll wait in the hallway, but I've got to be with my baby, please!" I felt bereft, lost in a madhouse of strangers, the child of my body torn from me, being handled by strangers.

The days in the hospital passed in a blur. I was tired, whipped. I cared for my son with confidence and experimented with different names for him. Frank came and went in a flurry, bringing my in-laws, my mother, and Rebecca to visit. Rebecca was manic, jumping on and off the bed, trying my patience with her exuberance. She seemed so large to me, her skin so rough, her limbs so long, now that I had this new little one to touch and stroke. Unnamed until my last hospital day, the baby was ugly, almost bald, with swollen eyes and a fat face. I loved holding him close to me as I nursed him and enjoyed the afternoon feedings the most, sitting in the armchair, feeling his mouth tug at my breast, quiet and peaceful together.

Dr. Swenson, the youngest and newest member of my obstetrical group, made rounds the second day of my hospitalization. I talked to him about my delivery. He told me about my fourth-degree laceration: his description made me even more furious with Dr. Mauller. The second morning I went early to the nursery to get my son, only to have the nurses tell me I couldn't have him until they had taken his vital signs. I stood in the hall, looking at him through the glass, and wept. I felt bereaved, powerless, unable to claim my own flesh and blood. I moved through the days in a fog of sadness. It was all so different from the euphoria of Rebecca's first days. I didn't understand it, I didn't like it, yet I tried to hide my feelings from everyone.

Years later I realized that the entire experience had been colored by my unconscious fear that something would be wrong with the baby. If it could happen to my friend, then why should I be immune? I started the labor feeling angry; the doctor had behaved abominably toward me; the labor had been very brief but wretchedly difficult; and all my expectations of a repeat performance of the joy of Rebecca's birth had gone unfulfilled.

My feelings of sadness didn't transfer to the baby. I was overjoyed that now I had a child of each sex. I reveled in his newness, the smoothness of his skin, the pleasure of nursing him, his lovely smell. His *bris* (circumcision) was a ceremony of unparalleled joy: as I read a blessing over him, my heart contracted with love and the sense of family and tradition evoked by this gathering. My hopes for and pleasure in this baby were boundless. But I was still burdened with a puzzling sense of grief.

My marriage was in trouble, even though Frank and I hadn't really admitted it yet. I was tired and older, of course, than when I had cared for my first newborn. It wasn't easy juggling the needs of an infant and an active four-year-old, who suddenly had to share her mama. But there was something deeper, unacknowledged but very real. I was grieving. I knew Frank didn't want any more kids; he hadn't really wanted a second one. It wasn't clear that our marriage would survive a second child. Deep within, I was grieving over the loss of my reproductive role. Pregnancy had been so easy for me, in spite of the usual fatigue and physical complaints. I blossomed when I was pregnant. I felt healthier and more integrated, physically and emotionally, than I had at any other time in my adult life.

My body glowed as it grew. I carried my huge belly and lovely large breasts with such pride! I loved having people touch my stomach; I enjoyed the way their eyes softened when they looked at me. Total strangers would smile at me. The policeman directing traffic outside the grocery store would stop the cars and escort me grandly across the street, both of us grinning like imbeciles. I felt fulfilled; my body was harboring a new human being, feeding it, growing it, protecting it with my very flesh and bones.

Throughout both pregnancies I had a physical, visceral awareness, even before I felt the babies move, of the life within me. I would stand in front of my full-length mirror and study my ripe, full body with exhilaration. I made Frank take pictures of me naked and nine months gone. I wanted to be able to look at them and remember. I was a vessel, an enchanted being, somehow purified and consecrated, moving through the days with a private, unvoiced sense of holiness about myself. To make new life! To be able to produce a child! To help people my world, to add another person to my family. To carry this seed to its fruition. I was filled with love for myself, for my husband, for the process, for the chance to experience it. Those two pregnancies were the only time in my life, after the confusion of puberty, that I felt truly whole, and the first year of each child's life continued this feeling of well-being: I absolutely adored having those two little babies to care for.

But even as I rejoiced in this little boy baby, inside there was pain. *Could it really be over for me? I'm only thirty years old. I always wanted to have five babies. Why can't I do this again?* I went through the months of Michael's first year with a thick lump just under my diaphragm, a lump of sadness over what was finished, not to be experienced again. And I began to look for a way to displace the sadness, to cough up the lump. I had inquired about becoming a Lamaze instructor during our classes before Michael's birth. The teacher informed me her organization had only just begun to accept nonnurses into their teaching group. Seven months after Michael's delivery, I signed up for the training.

Chapter Two

BIRTHING BABIES

There is nothing more captivating—to me, at least—than watching a new baby begin his or her life. All babies are born the same way: they either emerge from their mothers' birth canals or are lifted out of their mothers' abdomens by the hands of the birth attendant. But even while the process is much the same, each birth is unique. A baby must leave behind the safe walls of its mother's womb and function on its own. No longer are there secure uterine walls to enfold and warm amniotic fluid in which to bathe. No longer do nutrients and wastes get processed by its mother's body. The soothing rhythm of its mother's heartbeat will no longer lullaby it through sleep cycles. At birth, its body must function independently, or it will be subjected to the machines, medicines, and rhythms of a neonatal intensive care unit.

Before it does anything else, this little body has to breathe. Oxygen, heretofore provided by the mother via placenta and umbilical cord, now has to be obtained through the neonate's own respiratory efforts. Pulling in those first breaths, oxygenating lungs that previously were not required to work at anything other than growth, sending bright-red blood throughout the vascular system: this is the first critical activity. Brain, heart, and lungs must work in tandem. Without their efforts, muscles won't function, food can't be digested, wastes can't be excreted, the world can't be learned, life can't be lived.

To witness a newborn begin this complicated biological function is electrifying. No matter how often I watch a baby emerge from its mother's vagina, there is always an instant, however brief, of incredulity that flashes through my mind: *Good God, there's a person right there! Squeezing out of an impossibly small space! A head! A skull, filled with brain matter, covered with scalp and hair, attached to a live body—arms, legs, torso, buttocks, internal organs, a beating heart, blood coursing through veins, neural synapses firing. . . . Good God! Who ever thought up such an preposterous idea? WOW!* Even though I know, intellectually and experientially, how the process delivers this little form into the light, the metaphysical wonder of it staggers me.

After the cervix—the opening of the uterus—has dilated, the expulsive factors begin their work. The uterus itself heaves with contractions, constricting and pushing down against the mass it holds. Almost always, an irresistible urge to bear down assails the mother, who tightens her abdominal muscles and presses her diaphragm down, applying pressure on the uterus. These combined forces slowly maneuver the infant body past the pelvic bones and down the elastic, spongy vaginal channel. Initially, I can only feel with my fingers the firm sphere of skull, far up that passage. With continued expulsive efforts, the head becomes visible. Not infrequently, the scalp is folded or wrinkled and feels lumpy, almost mushy under my fingers. This folding occurs as the skull bones underneath the flesh are briefly molded by the narrow space through which they pass. The articulations or divisions between the bones, called sutures, are soft and pliable so the bone plates can overlap, reducing the size of the head as it goes through the canal. The corrugation of the scalp reminds me of how I looked when, as a small child, I tried to pull off a too-small T-shirt. The skin of my face was stretched, pulling my eyes into slits, flaring my nostrils and jerking my mouth into a thin sneer. All my skin had gone up to the top of my head!

Not surprisingly, hair amount and color are key concerns of the prospective parents, as the process of claiming the baby as their own biological offspring begins, even before birth. They always want to know if I can see the head and ask me to describe the hair amount and color. Sometimes, when the effort of pushing has become such a serious, solemn task that the parents' spirits are flagging, I will tease them about the baby's hair. To a straight-haired, blond couple I might announce that the baby has black, curly hair; to a black couple I'll talk about blondness. The reactions to my joking are usually positive ones: once I laughed and assured them I'm just trying to get them to lighten up, the shocked expressions dissolve into giggles. But on occasion, such kidding can be dangerous: if there is any question in the father's mind about the baby's paternity, I'm in trouble. After making this mistake a couple of times, I learned to keep my mouth shut unless I'm sure about the couple's sense of humor!

When the baby finally crowns, its head is pressed against the widening vaginal orifice. The labia stretch and expand, thinning out until the tissue is almost bloodlessly white. Massage of these tissues or a surgical cut, the episiotomy, by the obstetrician or midwife, helps ease the circle open until the head begins to emerge. In most cases, the baby is facing its mother's tailbone, so it is the top and back of the head that is first seen. Stooping down, I can watch the forehead, then eyebrows, then eyes, then nose and cheeks, then mouth and chin slide free of the surrounding maternal tissues.

The mother has accomplished the most difficult aspect of her pushing efforts: the largest, hardest part of the baby's body is now delivered from her enclosing body. Quite often, a baby will take its first breath right then, squalling and gasping before he's even out. I have seen obstetricians lift the head of a baby out of a cesarean incision, only to have that head scream with indignation at being pulled thus from its mother's body. It is a sight to behold: surrounded by green-gowned, masked surgeons and techs is a draped mound. In the center of the mound is a gory knife wound. An infant's head fills this bleeding slit, wide-open mouth hollering to beat the band, body still submerged, like a child buried in sand at the beach!

The birth attendant works quickly to suction mucus and amniotic fluid from the baby's mouth and nostrils, to prevent the infant from inhaling muck along with air. As this suctioning is being performed during a vaginal delivery, the infant's body is rotating inside the mother in order for the shoulders to be delivered. Until this moment, the baby has been tunneling out on its belly, butting its head against its confinement. Now, with the rotation, the baby is assuming a sidelying position. This rotation can be observed as the head turns from facing the mother's rectum to the mother's leg. It is quite remarkable to watch this turning of the head, caused by the unseen expulsive force of the uterus: it looks like the baby is doing it all by itself, sort of casually turning its head to check out what's beside its face! Then, with a little downward tug by the attendant—or without help—some babies don't wait, they just squirt on out—the top shoulder frees itself by pivoting under the pubic bone, followed by the bottom shoulder. The rest of the wet, slippery body follows easily, slithering out without much ado, trailing the blue-gray umbilical cord behind it. Piece of cake!

In less common presentations, another part of the body may emerge from the vagina first. I have been charmed by babies whose hand or hands appear alongside their faces, fingers spread against the nose or cheek. Sometimes the baby comes out facing up, away from his mother's tailbone. Such "sunny-side-up" babies are usually a surprise to the attendant, provoking hilarity in everyone present. A breech presentation, in which one or both feet, knees or buttocks emerge, is an infrequent sight nowadays. Current obstetrical practice is to deliver breech babies by cesarean section, since there is added risk of injury to the baby when the head is the last part of the body to be delivered. No one wants to be faced with a head too large to go through the bony pelvic opening: if the head won't come out, you can't really stuff the baby back inside and turn it around! But I have observed several vaginal breech deliveries, performed almost always by older doctors. The sight of a baby's body, all out except for the head, is unnerving.

One such delivery was accomplished by an old hand, Dr. Markham. I didn't know this doctor: I was new to this particular hospital and Dr. Markham rarely admitted his patients to our unit. However, my fellow nurses gave me a general idea of what to expect. According to them, he was conservative, aloof, somewhat stern, and expected nurses to toe the line. *Oh nuts, one of those, probably, a prima donna,* I thought, unfairly jumping to conclusions before I even met the man. *Oh well, I can handle it.* But my guard went up as I called him to the hospital, steeling myself against any potential difficulties.

Dr. Markham's patient, Mrs. Weston, was carrying twins who were embracing each other's legs inside the womb. The first baby, lower down and nearer the cervix, was in the normal, head-down position with his feet in the second baby's face. The second baby's head was up under his mother's diaphragm, so that he was standing up, so to speak, inside his mom.

The obstetrician arrived, a short, dignified man with thirty-some years' experience. He listened to my report without comment and examined the mother, with both fingers and ultrasound, to verify the fetal positions. He informed me that he hoped to to turn the second infant around inside the uterus after the first baby was born, and gave instructions for a double set-up: the obstetrical team, myself included, set up an operating room for both vaginal and cesarean deliveries, just in case we had to do an emergency cesarean to deliver the second baby. Two infant warmers with all the requisite resuscitative equipment and a team of pediatricians were crowded into the room, along with several nurses to assist with supplies, machines, and instruments. As a private attending physician, Dr. Markham was not required to include any obstetrical residents in his deliveries. Nonetheless, anticipating a possible breech delivery of the second twin, he invited two residents to observe and possibly assist him with the delivery. Because of the rarity of vaginal breech births, this was an uncommon and invaluable opportunity for the residents. Even a simple twin delivery is usually accomplished via surgery, so the residents were being offered a unique learning experience with this case.

All of us were keyed up, looking forward to whatever was going to happen with just enough concern over the potential risks to get our adrenaline flowing. Dr. Markham's quiet air of confidence, as though twins and a breech delivery were ordinary events, had a calming effect on everyone. Except for the mother, everyone in the room was gowned, gloved, and masked in blue surgical paraphernalia, bustling around the white-tiled, inhospitable room. Mrs. Weston lay ensconced on a high steel table, draped with sterile cloths, her husband standing close by her shoulder at the head of the table. Fetal monitors tick-ticketed, the rhythmic rapid drumming of two babies' hearts the most prominent sound, flickering in and around soft-spoken exchanges between nurses and doctors and the rustle and clatter of instruments and equipment. Whatever the activity, as we worked quickly but efficiently, every ear in that room was attuned to the sound of those heartbeats, reassured by their rate and regularity.

The first twin was delivered without effort, head and body sliding into the obstetrician's waiting hands, parents heaving a sigh of relief and pleasure over the task half completed. Dr. Markham handed the baby over to the pediatricians and then slipped his entire gloved hand inside the mother, feeling around the interior of the uterus to determine the second baby's position.

"It's still breech, feet first, legs extended, a complete breech. I don't think he's going to curl up, he's a good size, but I don't know if I can turn him, either," Dr. Markham informed us.

"Oh, may as well give it a try!" he added.

His arm went in further, up to his elbow, disappearing inside the mother. I watched his face grow red, beads of perspiration glistening in the harsh surgical light, as his buried hand and arm fumbled for purchase on the unseen fetal body within. We all stood silently, on the alert, fingers crossed as he exerted himself for several minutes, the baby's heartbeat still audible and reassuring in the background.

Finally, he removed his hand, shaking his head: "Nope, it's just too tight in there. I can't turn him around without the risk of hurting him. So . . ."

He took a deep breath and wiped his forehead, still calm and dignified. "I need clean gloves and a couple of sterile towels." Two sturdy green towels were handed over by the scrub tech. Fresh sterile gloves were snapped onto his hands.

"Now, you stand right here beside me," he instructed the third-year resident. "I'll tell you what to do when it's time." Looking up at the mother, he asked her to push.

"Still contracting, Mrs. Weston? Good. I want you to push again, with the next contraction. While you push, I'm going to pull and between us, we'll get this baby out, okay?"

As Mrs. Weston pushed, Dr. Markham reached inside her body again. Before the contraction was over, I could see his hand emerging, two tiny feet grasped in his fingers.

"Push a little more, please," he asked as he gently extracted the baby's body from the vagina. Supporting the body with both hands, the baby's head still invisible, hooked by the pubic bone, Dr. Markham instructed the resident: "Step in here now. Wrap those towels around the torso. Like that, right. Now grab on tight to the towel ends and lift up gently when I tell you to." The blue body of the baby was quickly swaddled in towels from the armpits to the knees, held up and out straight from the vaginal orifice. Dr. Markham felt with his fingers around the head and then commanded:

"Okay, now gently, lift up. Gently, gently, nope. Wait. Lower it down straight again. Let me try again." Fumble, grope, feel. "Lift again. Gently, gently . . . Stop. Put it down level again, carefully now. Hand me those forceps, please."

It seemed like we were all holding our breath. I was right behind the physician and the resident, with a direct view of the action, bouncing up on my toes with anxiety. *Oh, get him out! Get him out! What if he's trying to breathe in there, sucking in all that muck? Get him out! Now! Time's awasting, Doc, come on! Come on!* I was so nervous I was almost hyperventilating behind my now-soggy mask. Whenever a baby got "hung-up" in the delivery process, I started sweating about lost time, hypoxia, injury, brain damage. Dr. Markham's composure under pressure was impressive, but I was having a mini-coronary waiting for this baby's delivery!

To my delighted amazement, that dignified, diminutive physician now dropped to his knees, scrunching his head and shoulders down under the baby's towel-wrapped body. Swiftly and adroitly, he slid a pair of forceps in and around the head, and without a single adjustment in their position, gently closed them. "Now lift," he said quietly, but urgently, to the resident. The baby's body rose at an angle as both physicians performed their manipulations, Dr. Markham on his knees, the resident on his toes as his arms pulled up on the bundle of baby. And *voilà!* It was done! Finally out, forceps off, the baby, blue and still, was rushed to the warmer and the impatient pediatricians. I hurried to offer my assistance, but two nurses and two physicians had already surrounded the newborn. Superfluous for a moment, I allowed myself to slump against the wall, holding my breath as I waited to hear a sound, any sound, from the baby. Drying, stimulating, suctioning, giving oxygen, listening to and counting the heart rate through a stethoscope, listening for breath sounds, watching the skin color—everything happened simultaneously. Eight expert hands moved with speed and proficiency, urging this body to respond—breathe! Cry! Move! Live! Live! After only a couple of minutes, time that seemed endless, a thin watery wail drifted up from the warmer, followed by sounds of laughter and parental sobs of relief. A roomful of people relaxed, rejoicing over that wail, each subsequent cry acting as a tonic to our nerves.

"He's pinking up! Looking good! Heart rate normal. Lung sounds clear and strong! Hot dog! You little devil! Had us on pins and needles there for a minute, didn't you? Yeah, go ahead and cry, scream and holler, it's music to our ears! Didn't pick a very considerate way to come into this world now, did you?" The pediatricians joshed the baby, all the tension in the room evaporating with every movement and sound from that kid. What a high!

I learned an important lesson that day about passing judgment on a physician before I'd seen him work. Dr. Markham's poise and expertise averted a potential catastrophe. He delivered that baby with such casual effortlessness that even on his knees, smeared with birth secretions, he commanded my respect.

Fortunately for my nervous system, most births are not so complicated or demanding. As I became proficient in attending to all my duties during a delivery, I was able to watch and enjoy the emergence of a new baby, even if only briefly. All my senses become engaged in the event. The grunts and groans of the mother's pushing efforts, the encouraging voices of the nurses and physicians, the laughter and excited exclamations of the family members, the mewling or caterwauling of the infant, the clink of instruments, the hiss of oxygen and suction tubes, the throb of the fetal monitor, the hum of the lights, all assail my ears. Distinctive odors fill my nostrils: the sharp metallic tang of blood, the stinging ammonia of urine, the stench of fecal matter, the briny sea scent of amniotic fluid. I can almost taste these smells sometimes through my paper mask, the filtered air I breathe in through my mouth still redolent with their richness.

My hands accept the warmth of the child, its smeary, wet, cheesy limbs soft and pliant under my fingers. I wrap it in warm blankets. I bathe the mother's genitals with cold antiseptic fluid and warm water. Enclosed in thin, clinging plastic, my fingers lift ice chips to her lips. My hands manipulate the cool glass of a medicine vial, the rigid cold of steel stirrups and instruments, the sweaty roundness of a gravid (pregnant) belly, the stickiness of monitor gel, the deadly sharp slenderness of needles.

Over my mask, my eyes take in the colors: bright red of blood and scalpel-exposed muscle, deep plum of placenta, pale gray-blue of umbilical vessels, salmon pink of infant skin, white glare of lights and flashing cameras, black of suture threads, rose flush of exertion and gladness on the mother's cheeks. Each birth, in however sterile a room, is so lush with vividness, it is almost always a sensuous experience for me, however strange that may seem. Like most obstetrical workers, I have grown somewhat inured to all this stimuli, but on some primeval level, I am ever touched, viscerally, within.

The enjoyable part of a delivery, the actual birth of the infant, is also the most frightening. There is no way to predict how a baby will look or act when he leaves his mother's body. The uncertainty in those last few minutes is what keeps an L&D unit sharp. No one can be absolutely certain that the baby will do what he's supposed to do. Every obstetrical team member must be on the alert, at the ready, if a baby comes out and doesn't breathe. After the head and shoulders are delivered, the rest of the body slips out without trouble. This is when I watch with intense concentration, assessing the newborn's first responses to extrauterine life. Is the baby limp and blue? Is it waving its arms, kicking its feet, grabbing at all this sudden new space around it? If it is, it's going to be a "good baby." The limp, blue ones may take a little stimulation, oxygen, and time to get going, to breathe and respond to their new world. The kicking, grabbing babies have already begun. Their muscle tone, respiratory effort, color, heart rate, and grimaces all indicate a healthy response to the world. All I have to do to ensure their safety is dry them off, keep them warm, and get them to a food source within the next few hours.

I also have to legally identify each baby, with identify bracelets and/or footprints. The bracelets have an I.D. number and are attached to a wrist and an ankle. A matching bracelet with the same I.D. number is placed on the mother's wrist; she must wear it until her discharge. The baby's number is checked against the mother's each time the baby is returned to the mother from the nursery. Some hospitals also tie a matching bracelet on the father's wrist so he can collect the baby from the nursery himself. If I print the baby, I also print his mother's right thumb on the print document which remains in his legal medical record.

The Apgar rating is a system of scoring the newborn's physical status immediately after birth. At one minute and at five minutes after delivery, five characteristics are assessed: heart rate, color, respiration, muscle tone, and reflex. Each characteristic may be assigned a score of zero, one, or two, so a total perfect score would be a ten. If the heart rate is absent, the baby gets a zero. If it is slow—below 100 beats per minute—he gets a one. If it is over 100 beats, he gets a two. Likewise, with respiratory effort, the breakdown is as follows: absent breathing—zero; slow or irregular—one; good crying— two. If the baby is completely limp, zero points; if there is some flexion of extremities, one point; if there is active motion, two points. With color, we give zero for blue or pale skin, one for a pink body and blue hands and feet, and two for a completely pink baby. Reflex response is scored by watching what the baby does when suctioned. If there is no response to a bulb or catheter in his nostrils, he gets a zero. If he grimaces, he gets a point, and if he coughs or sneezes he gets two points.

Good Apgars are eight to ten; most healthy babies lose points for color, since the extremities are often blue. A score of four to seven indicates a baby who has some problems right after delivery and may require treatment but probably will do fine, while a score of zero to three indicates a "bad" baby. All of us hate zero-to-three scores. Doing Apgars sounds complicated, but with practice, it becomes routine.

The main problem with the system is that different people see different things. What a nurse may see as "irregular respirations" may be viewed by the doctor as "a lusty cry." This has lead to innumerable arguments, because the doctor has a vested interest in delivering a baby with good Apgars. Low scores mandate additional close observation of the baby, at the very least, and probable additional lab tests and treatment. In my experience, the nurse receiving the baby from the obstetrician had the final say over the scores, unless a pediatrician is present.

I had been working only a couple of months when I had my first experience with a blue baby. This baby had delivered precipitously, which meant that the pushing stage of labor had been quite rapid. The baby had descended through the birth canal like a cannonball, with no effort on the mother's part to expel him. I was alone in the delivery room with the first-year resident who had guided the ignorant hands of a new intern through this, his first delivery. I received the baby on the warmer, dried him and did his Apgars and identity bracelets, as I simultaneously prepared the Pitocin injection for the mother's IV fluid after the placenta was delivered. The baby looked fine for the first ten minutes, pink and breathing well, with occasional full-bodied wails to register his complaints about the lights and cold air.

The resident departed for "a few minutes," leaving the intern to wait for the placenta. As I worked on my documentation, I watched the baby. Suddenly, he began to lose color, turning first pale and then a dusky blue, lying still with no evidence of respiratory effort. Immediately alarmed, I tried to stimulate him by rubbing him with towels, but received little response. I flew to the door, yelled loudly "I need Peds stat!" and flew back to the warmer. I didn't know what to do. The intern knew even less than I: he stood between the mother's legs staring aghast at me, as I rubbed the baby and slapped its heels hard. Within a minute, thank God, a pediatrician was there, applying oxygen, listening to the heartbeat, then bagging the baby briefly, forcing oxygen into his lungs. The color returned, respirations improved, and the baby began to holler again. I sagged against the wall, unbelievably frightened by how rapidly this baby had faltered and livid with anger at the resident who had left me alone.

I cornered him in the hallway later. For the first time, I let a doctor know how angry I was. "Don't you *ever* leave me alone in the DR again! You know I'm new and inexperienced. How could you be so irresponsible? I had absolutely no idea how to resuscitate that baby. He could have died while you were out of the room. You're just damned lucky the peds are so close by. Don't you ever do that to me again!"

"Oh, Susie, you handled it just fine," he said with a laugh. "The baby's okay and you did fine. Have more faith in yourself."

I couldn't convey to him how terrified I felt watching that baby slip away from me, from life. I couldn't sleep that night. I kept seeing that baby turn blue. I kept realizing how little I knew about keeping a faltering baby alive. After a tortured night of tears, I made it my business to learn about applying oxygen, practicing with the mask and bag, begging experienced people to walk me through neonatal resuscitation efforts. I also learned to be wary of precipitous deliveries. Babies who arrived rapidly merited more than initial alertness. I learned the hard way that even though the baby might appear perfectly normal for the first five to ten minutes, if he came out fast and if he had a bruised blue look to his face, he needed to be more closely observed for the first hour. If the transition from intrauterine to extrauterine life is rapid, the neonate appears to have more difficulty in establishing and maintaining homeostasis. The respiratory system starts up okay, but then slips gears, as if the brain hasn't quite realized that breathing is now an obligatory function and not just the practicing of breathing that can be seen in utero through ultrasound. Maybe, I thought, the process of slowly being squeezed and pushed through the tight vaginal tube sends neurological signals to the baby's brain that extrauterine life is about to begin, so get ready. When the baby squirts out in a hurry, the brain hasn't had time to process the demands.

The next time I had a blue baby, again a precipitous birth, another nurse was present. We reacted without thinking, stimulating the baby, applying oxygen, and calling the pediatricians to the room. I was pleased afterward by my own calmness and my unerring efforts to sustain the baby's oxygen supply, but still frustrated by my basic ignorance in neonatal resuscitation. As I moved from one job to another, I was horrified to learn how few L&D nurses really know how to resuscitate a newborn. In the tertiary care (high risk) hospitals, pediatric residents are in-house, available around the clock, and are required to be present at any at-risk delivery. But during normal deliveries, when nothing untoward is expected, the nurse is responsible for baby care. Assessing a newborn is a relatively simple task with a normal baby, but every nurse will eventually be confronted with a nonresponsive infant. To rely on the availability of pediatricians is, to my mind, unsafe practice. I carried on a continuing argument about this with a succession of head nurses, who failed to understand my terror of being alone in a delivery room with a baby in need of help. Their assurances that the peds were right down the hall did little to assuage my fears, since I learned the peds were *not* always there. Sometimes they were on another floor or, commonly at night when I was working, they were asleep. The time lost while they were being paged was unacceptable to me.

At one hospital where I worked, most high-risk mothers were transferred to other facilities, so the majority of births were normal and uncomplicated. Nonetheless, I watched with incredulity as nurses gathered up blue, non-responsive babies and ran down the hall to the neonatal intensive care unit (NICU). Most of these nurses did not have any training in neonatal resuscitation. Even though all the necessary resuscitative equipment was on hand and religiously checked each shift, the nurses did not know how to use it and preferred to rely on the NICU if a baby went bad.

After I completed a neonatal resuscitation course I was even more distressed by this situation. The first four minutes of extrauterine life are the most critical: the baby *must* be adequately oxygenated or permanent, lifelong injuries may occur. Too many times I watched nurses spend two or three or even five minutes rubbing, slapping, and suctioning a baby to little avail, while yelling for Peds, and then rushing the baby to the NICU for resuscitation. I would fume at these nurses that the baby must be stabilized before being transferred and argued for mandatory classes in neonatal resuscitation.

Every hospital I worked in relied completely on the pediatric staff, but to my dismay, many of the residents and pediatricians did not have formal training in neonatal resuscitation. Each physician had his own routine: some followed procedure fairly closely, but many that I observed just did their own thing. Some never listened to the heartbeat, some spent two or three minutes stimulating a baby, some didn't know how to suction an infant properly. It scared me. After my course, I became more agressive about baby care. I made it my business to push right in there if the baby looked anything but normal, and I didn't hesitate to direct traffic: "Listen to his heart rate, give me the suction tube, let's bag this baby, dry him off," and so on, if the personnel present were dawdling with the resuscitation.

Because I never know what might occur at delivery, I get a real kick out of the babies who surprise us, like the posterior or "sunny-side-up" babies. That little mashed face and the usual surprise of the obstetrician just tickles me. It is also amusing to see a baby's body deliver more rapidly than anticipated. Once I watched two physicians grabbing frantically at a baby boy who shot out of his mother like a bullet. The doctors scrambled and grasped at that wriggling, slippery little body like two football players madly going after a fumbled ball. Some babies baptize their obstetricians with an arc of urine or a smear of meconium—baby shit—before the cord has been cut. One young physician almost fainted because of what a baby did to him. He had delivered a baby girl and was reaching inside the mother to check for suspected retained placental fragments when a second, unanticipated twin reached out and grabbed his forefinger! He fell off his stool with surprise.

Frequently, a baby will catch hold of the umbilical cord as it waves its arms and grabs with its hands. Several times I have watched with amusement as an obstetrician struggles to pry loose a tiny hand that has locked onto the cord or the doctor's gown. A newborn's grip can be astoundingly strong, capable of holding its own body weight if lifted by the hands. Some babies are quiet, crying only if really irritated by the hands that dry them or by the suction bulb or tube thrust into their mouths and noses. Others cry so lustily it hurts the ears. Many babies try to open their eyes immediately, if the light isn't too strong. Occasionally, I get a baby who is so alert, so obviously aware that it just knocks me over. Frequently such a baby is post-dates, or late. The extra time in utero has given it that much more time to mature, so its neurological system is farther advanced and its responses to extrauterine life more obvious.

One such baby was a girl named Amy. Her mother was two weeks overdue when this baby finally arrived. The birth had been natural—meaning no narcotics or other medications had been given to the mother. When Amy was born, her eyes opened as soon as her head emerged. She looked around and yelped, as though startled by what she saw. On the warmer she responded immediately to my caressing hands and voice. Her eyes looked focused, unlike many babies whose crossed eyes give them a drunken look, and she followed my face and voice with her eyes and her body, turning toward me with her whole torso as I spoke to her. I held her upright and brought my face close to hers.

"Oh my goodness, little girl! You are really here with me, aren't you? Look at you watching me. Wow! Happy birthday! Hey, Mommy, Daddy, look at this little girl! She is so alert. Look how she watches me and listens. Don't anybody tell me this kid doesn't know where she is. She is all here, for sure!" She watched me, her little face moving in mimicry with mine, eyebrows lifting, mouth opening and closing in little moues, smiles struggling to break across her tiny face. I could *sense* her personality. This wasn't just an unfeeling little blob of protoplasm I was holding. This was a real person, brand-new and without experience, but still very much a person, taking everything in, absorbing everything as rapidly as her brain could process it.

I wrapped Amy in warm blankets and laid her on her mother's breast. Her father and I leaned in close and watched her study her mother's face. As her mother talked to Amy, I could see her body grow still and turn toward her mother's voice. She was looking at her mother and attending with every bit of her little self to this face and voice. It was delightful!

The next day, I stopped by to see her on the postpartum ward. Her mom was changing her diaper. Amy was kicking and making little baby noises, waving her arms, looking for all the world like she was engaging in conversation with her mother. When I leaned down and spoke to her, both her mother and I were amazed at her response. She stopped moving her arms and legs and turned toward me, her eyes searching my face.

"Wow! She knows you, Susie! She recognizes your voice!" her mother exclaimed. By God, that one-day-old baby looked at me, listened to me and then smiled at me, one of the most lovely little smiles I've ever received! Before Amy left the hospital with her parents, they searched me out to say good-bye. I sat holding Amy, talking to her. Again she responded to me, just as an older child or an adult would. "Amy, you are a special little girl. You are beautiful and so cheerful. I'll miss you. You be a good kid and learn all about the world from your parents and have lots of fun growing up. Someday, maybe I'll pass you on the street. I bet you we'll just know each other right off, just like we do now. You're one special little baby." She watched me solemnly and then gave me one last smile. Her parents and I were all in tears as we hugged each other good-bye.

Amy was the first baby I'd seen be so responsive and alert, but as time went by, there were many others. I was never surprised to read research findings about the neurological sophistication of newborns; I knew from experience how responsive newborns really are. I felt sorry for parents and hospital personnel who were under the impression that these babies weren't really aware of their surroundings. I encouraged mothers and fathers to talk immediately to their babies, to hold them close so the babies could focus on their faces. I explained that the babies could see, hear, and recognize them, and that they also would know their parents' unique smell within a few hours.

One night I was taking vital signs on a mother who was two days postcesarean. Her baby, a funny-looking, elfin-faced, bald-headed little girl, was awake, lying in her mother's arms, looking up at her mother's face. I admired the baby and watched with pleasure as the mother began to talk to her daughter.

"Yes, hello, my little girl. You are such a good little baby! You nursed so well this time from me, didn't you?" She crooned to her baby, her voice high and soft, her face close to the baby's. She was completely in love with her daughter, smiling broadly at the baby's expression of concentration. The baby's face mirrored her mother's expressions. As we watched, this tiny girl worked with her mouth until it shaped the same broad smile on her mother's. We laughed, and she did it again! I crowed with elation:

"Look at that! She's smiling back at you! Fantastic! Don't let anyone tell you that's just gas! That is an honest-to-god smile! She is responding to your face! Hot dog!"

Later that night I heard the mother talking with another nurse. "I just finished writing in my journal," she explained. "I'm trying to keep notes on each of these days with the baby. I just wrote: 'First smile. *Not* gas!' "

Every time I receive a baby at the warmer, I am deeply moved by the significance of my work. Except for the obstetrician or midwife, the first contact this fresh new human being has with its species is me, an anonymous nurse. My hands are the first to stroke its small body, my words the first its mind will hear and begin to process. This is a great honor for me; it is somehow imperative that I acknowledge this beginning. I know this baby is absorbing all the myriad sensory stimuli around it: light, space, air, color, temperature, sound, texture. My interactions with the baby provide many of those first impressions. I try to convey to it a warm, welcoming gentleness, so that somewhere in its unconscious memory the trauma of birth and the physical separation from its mother's womb are ameliorated by my touch, my voice, my tenderness.

It is a privilege to watch a child's beginning, to shape with my touch and care a baby's initial experience as a living, breathing human being. Because I firmly believe that my presence is imprinted on each baby's memory, regardless of whether he or she is ever able to recall it, I want my presence to be a positive one. At least the beginning of each child's life should be a joyous one, so I try hard to make it that way. I'll never see these babies again once they leave the hospital. Their futures are unknown and filled with every possibility. But I want the first hands that touch them, the first voice that reaches them to be loving. So I greet them with as much enthusiasm as I can muster, while I wonder how they will be cared for, who they will grow up to be, what they will accomplish, how much love they will know in their lives.

"Hello, little one. Welcome to the world. Aren't you a beautiful little girl? Come over here, Daddy, and greet your daughter. Go ahead, touch her. Put your hands on her, let her know you're here. This is your daddy, little girl. Open your eyes and see your father. Oh, Mommy, you have made such a lovely baby. Look at how beautiful she is, how alert. Happy birthday!"

Twice I have been allowed to officially deliver babies myself as opposed to those babies I "caught" before the doctor arrived. The first time occurred one night in my third year of work, after a long sprawling conversation with the resident on call, Dr. Martin. He listened to me rambling on about how exciting I thought it was to participate in a birth. I asked him if he would let me do it sometime. As it happened, that very night we had an excellent candidate for just such a teaching session. Our only patient was a two-time mother for whom we anticipated a normal, unmedicated, uncomplicated delivery.

As the other nurse wheeled this mother into the delivery room, Dr. Martin was reviewing each step of the delivery with me as we scrubbed, gowned, and gloved. I was so excited I barely listened to him. As I stood between the woman's legs, I was conscious of how very different the perspective is for the doctor in the delivery room. All of the nursing tasks that I routinely attended to were only of peripheral importance. What held my absolute attention was the vaginal orifice before me. Countless times I had watched a perineum bulge and thin with the crown of an infant's head, but never before had I been the one responsible for the actual delivery.

I knew what to do without being told. All the times I had watched med students fumble with instruments, towels, and ultimately the baby had imprinted on my subconscious so that now I knew to provide support to the perineum by gently pressing against it. I knew how to place my hands just so on the baby's head as it emerged. I knew how to apply downward and then upward pressure for the delivery of the shoulders. It felt absolutely routine as if I had done it many times already. I was a little clumsy with the baby's body; I hadn't paid a great deal of attention to holding the infant without tangling it in the cord, while keeping its head down; usually, at that point, I was waiting anxiously to receive the baby at the warmer.

What I didn't know was how it would feel physically and emotionally to lift a child from his mother's body. The first thing that amazed me was the sound I heard from the baby before his head was even fully delivered. I've never heard this before or since: with only his forehead and eyes released, his face from the nose down still gripped by the vaginal walls, this little one was making crying sounds: *"MMMMMMmmmnnn! MMMMMmmnnnn!"* It sounded like he was trying to yell at me through a mouth-gag: "Get me out of here!"

Then, as he slipped into my arms, I brought him up close to my body, clasping his slithery wet little self securely against my belly, fearful of dropping him. He was hot! Fresh and hot with his mother's internal body heat! It startled me: when I received the babies on the warmer, even within a few seconds of birth, they had already begun to cool.

What a rush I had just then, cradling this heated little being in my arms! Deep inside me was a longing to hold him close always, to maintain the warmth of him with my own heat. In that instant, I felt again the shape and feel and warmth of each of my own two babies. It was a marvelous, merry-go-sorry experience for me, thrilling and new and old and nostalgic all together. With that delivery, and in times that followed when I birthed a baby because the doctor wasn't available, I had the opportunity to actually be the first human to touch these new little creatures. I hope they felt my excitement, my awe, my sense of being gifted by them.

Not all babies respond to me, of course. Each one is unique, with a personality just waiting to be discovered. Some babies look so angry they make everyone laugh at the unrelenting fury of their crying: bodies beet red, faces grimacing, fists pounding the air, feet kicking furiously at my hands. Some are cozy snugglers from the get-go, curling toward the warmth of my hands, tucking themselves into the fetal position, cradling their cheeks with their hands, apparently at ease with this new environment. Others look bewildered, eyes roaming around vacantly, sometimes crossing, sniffing and whimpering, tentatively reaching out little fingers as if to test the air. Occasionally a baby just won't stop crying until he gets his mother's nipple in his mouth or hears his mother's voice and feels her arms around him. But oh those alert ones, those post-dates babies, like Amy!

Joseph junior was one of them. This kid made my day! He was big, almost ten pounds, and he was noisy, hollering and jabbing his fists at me. I laughed at him as I dried him, talking to him the whole time. "Man, are you a big boy! You have a big voice, too, don't you?"

At my command, his enormous, heavily muscled father came over to the warmer, grinning with delight as he looked at his firstborn. He bent over the squalling baby and touched him tentatively.

"Hey Joseph junior, how you doing, big guy? What're you crying so loud for? It's okay, baby. Your daddy's right here now."

To our mutual surprise, the kid shut up instantly. He rolled toward his father's voice, his body assuming that intense look, almost rigid with concentration.

"Go on, keep talking, Dad. He knows your voice."

"Of course you know my voice. I talked to you all the time, didn't I? I just put my head on your mommy's tummy and talked to you and sang to you, huh, Joseph junior?" The father looked at his wife on the delivery table. "Honey, look at this. He knows my voice!"

I reached over to put his identity bracelet on his leg. When I picked up his ankle, he started yelling again. "Good lord, kid, I'm sorry. He doesn't want me bothering him, does he?"

His father started stroking his belly and talking to him; again he gentled and quieted immediately. It was obvious this baby knew his father, who was now touching him all over.

"Man, look at you! You are a big baby, huh? Look at these hands. Look at these feet! Honey, this baby has some big feet, I can tell you!" The father was gleeful, so thrilled with this baby. I couldn't resist teasing him. I tapped his hand to get his attention and then lightly touched the baby's penis, which was actually much larger than a typical newborn's. "It isn't just his feet that are big, Dad. Check this out!"

When I touched the baby, he kicked at me and started yelling again. His daddy and I convulsed with laughter. "Gracious, I'm sorry, Joseph junior. I disturbed you, huh? I'll keep my hands to myself. You sure don't want anyone but Dad to touch you, do you?"

"Okay, now, Joseph junior, it's okay. You don't want this nurse to be messing with your stuff, do you?" his father soothed him as we laughed together. His wife asked what was so funny. "Well, Ms. Diamond here says it isn't only his feet that's big. He takes after me, honey, and not only with big feet!" Everyone in the room laughed, enjoying this man's joy and pride in his son.

Writing about Joseph junior reminded me of a baby that I'm sure would have broken any record in *The Guinness Book of World Records*. I was assigned to mother-baby (that is, postpartum) care one shift and was told by the outgoing nurse during report to be sure to take off one baby's diaper when I did his assessment. She would say nothing more, just insisted that I be sure to change this baby sometime during the night. Because I was very busy, another experienced nurse, with at least twenty years of working with babies, did the required assessment on this particular infant. She returned from the nursery, grinning: "Well, Susie, nothing much surprises me anymore, but the other nurses are right. You have to change that baby's diaper sometime tonight! And do it in the nursery, not at the bedside!" She wouldn't say any more, either.

Later that night, I took the baby to the nursery at his mother's request and dutifully stripped him down to weigh him and change his diaper. Oh my God, what a shock! Even with a good idea of what to expect from all the giggling, I was astounded when I saw this newborn's penis! Most boys' penises, naturally, are quite small in accordance with the size of the rest of the body. I've never measured any newborn penises but estimate most to be around an inch long, tops. This baby's penis was easily two and a half inches long, in the flaccid state. It touched his belly-button! Simply unbelievable . . . if I hadn't seen it with my own eyes. Needless to say, there was a lot of very discreet snickering at the nurses' station that night.

It was surprising to me when I first began working as an obstetrical nurse to find that I had no desire to work with the babies in the nursery. In my first jobs, the nurseries were separate units, physically removed from the labor and delivery units and, more significantly, from the intensive-care nurseries where the pediatricians spent the bulk of their time. The two or three times I was asked to fill in because of short staffing, I was vehement in my refusal. It was one thing to be responsible for the babies immediately following birth: I knew how to assess a newborn immediately and how to resuscitate it if necessary, plus there was always a doctor present in the delivery room to back me up. But being thrust into a room of babies, a good distance away from the physicians, filled me with fear.

I didn't know enough, I insisted. The only neonatal training I had was an extremely brief rotation in pediatrics during nursing school. I couldn't just walk into a nursery and be legally and morally responsible for a bunch of babies without at least an orientation to the nursery. If I were given such an orientation, I would have a minimal basis for providing care, but without it I was practicing irresponsibly. I didn't know how to do routine tests such as PKUs and glucose checks, how to do required physical assessments, how to calculate and administer medications, or what to look for in the babies' behavior that might indicate how well they were adjusting to extrauterine life. In addition, I didn't know how to chart what I didn't know how to look for, which meant that everything I charted, and everything I didn't know to chart would leave the hospital, the doctors, and me open for future legal action. I didn't want the babies, or my license, put on the line because of short staffing. For the most part, I was successful in avoiding the responsibility.

Staffing problems like this were and remain significantly controversial for nurses. Most people believe that a nurse is a nurse is a nurse. Worse yet, hospital administrators and harried ward managers, knowing full well the fallacy of that belief, still act on it when staffing needs demand a warm body to fill a slot on the ward or unit. The difficulty is that a nurse today simply cannot provide appropriate care for any given patient in a hospital. Medicine, and therefore nursing care, has become so specialized, so technically complex, and so legally dangerous to the caregiver, that it is madness to send a labor and delivery nurse into a cardiac care unit, a neuro nurse into an gynecology clinic, a psychiatric nurse into a medical-surgical unit. All nurses have the same basic training: they can take and assess vital signs, they can provide general nursing care, and most of them can tell if a patient is doing well or having problems. But they don't know the medications used in each specialty. They don't know the machines and monitors and devices particular to a unit. They don't have the knowledge about the disease or condition that is essential in providing safe care. Because of what they don't know, anything they do for the patient is risky, both medically and legally.

For instance, as a new nursing graduate with no work experience, it took me a full three months to learn enough on labor and delivery to be trusted to work without my preceptor, and another three months before I was left on the unit without another nurse. Every specialty and every unit require lengthy orientations for their staff: this is hospital policy and is demanded by the hospital accreditation boards. After such an orientation, further training via inservices and specialized courses are required for most specialties.

And yet, everywhere I've ever worked, there have been times when too many nurses call in sick, or are on vacation, or the schedule of staffing has been inadequate to cover the demands of a unit. Every time this happens, a nurse has to be scrounged up from another, less needy unit to cover the staffing gap. Very few nurses want to go to another ward on short notice: it's jarring to come to work anticipating a normal routine, only to be told to go to another unfamiliar unit and spend the shift trying to take care of patients you don't know, with routines, medications, paperwork all equally unknown. Of course, the fact that the short-handed unit is desperate for another nurse usually means the unit is having an unusually busy time, which means there will be little advice, assistance, or guidance for the visiting nurse. It's not at all unusual, either, for the harried nurses on the unit to dump the worst patients on the visitor, just to give themselves a break.

So most nurses hate like hell to be pulled to another unit, myself included. Sending me to the nursery was bad enough, even though an argument could be made that as a maternal-child nurse, I should be able to wing it with the babies without an adequate orientation. But I have been sent to gynecology wards, the operating room, outpatient surgery units, and even a surgical intensive-care unit, simply because the patient census was low on labor and delivery and a nurse was legally required on another, understaffed unit. Even when I tried to make myself see the reassignment as a challenge and an opportunity for a change of scene and people, I still couldn't avoid the very real fact that I was putting the patient, the hospital, and myself in jeopardy. It scared the hell out of me! I became very assertive about refusing to be pulled because of my legitimate concerns about these risks.

To utilize nursing personnel more efficiently, every hospital I have worked in eventually initiated cross-training programs for the labor and delivery, postpartum, and nursery nurses, lumping us all under the designation maternal-child nurses. It didn't matter that each of us had been hired in a specific area of expertise. Nurses who had been working only in the nursery or in labor and delivery for decades were forced to learn another specialty if they wanted to keep their jobs. With the guidance of experienced nurses in each specialty, we were obligated to work in each area for a specific period of time, to attend inservices specific to each specialty, and to complete clinical and written tests.

Upon completion of this cross-training, every nurse in the maternal-child department could work in any of these areas, to meet staffing needs, regardless of the nurse's preferred specialty. I escaped cross-training until my last job at the birthing center. During my orientation there to mother-baby care, I realized that while I knew how to do postpartum nursing, newborn nursing was a weakness, so I screwed up my courage and requested several additional twelve-hour shifts in the nursery, working with a seasoned, highly proficient nurse. Under her expert guidance, I gained confidence in my ability to work competently with new babies and my abhorrence of the nursery disappeared rapidly.

I found myself enthralled with these little people. Many of my intuitive conclusions about the individuality of newborns were reinforced by the behaviors I observed. Ironically, I also found myself irritated with my previous reluctance to venture away from my area of expertise, labor and delivery, to expand my own nursing knowledge and skills. I had limited myself unnecessarily because of my bad experiences in nursing school with pediatrics and because of my own lack of confidence in my ability to be a nursery nurse. In doing so, I had restricted my marketability. More important, I had missed the chance to appreciate the marvel of newborn babies.

Some babies are so physically beautiful that they take my breath away. Most people think newborns all look alike and are pretty ugly, to be honest. But I have seen some *gorgeous* babies. A Mexican girl, all of eighteen years old, gave birth to one of the most exquisite baby girls I've ever seen. She had thick curly black hair, long enough for a ribbon, almond-colored, satiny-soft skin without a mark or scratch on it, black eyes with the longest curling eyelashes, and a tiny Cupid's bow of a mouth. Lord, she was beautiful!

A little blond-haired baby boy seduced me with his skin: I couldn't get over how unblemished and satiny it was. Most fair babies will mottle at birth, when they're wet and cold. Many babies are daubed with vernix, a protective cheesy substance, and may have peeling skin and lots of wrinkles. This little boy was velvety smooth, fair as fresh cream, and begging to be touched. The softness and beauty of his skin invited caresses. Another little boy looked so finished, so polished it was hard to believe he was newly born. His hair, his features, his mannerisms all gave the impression of a Little Lord Fauntleroy. He looked like he had just been prepped for a magazine photo session. I could easily see him modeling clothes in *GQ* in twenty years!

In spite of the commonly held belief that newborns are unthinking blobs of protoplasm, I have always felt, even from when I was a child, that newborns are thinking, feeling, aware human beings. Scientific studies have begun to detail the myriad ways in which newborns experience and respond to the world around them. Even the long-held belief that neonates were neurologically immature and therefore unlikely to experience pain to the same degree as mature humans is no longer routinely assumed, although surgery on newborns, from circumcisions to cardiac operations, is often still performed without benefit of anesthesia.

Working long hours with brand-new babies made it quite obvious to me that babies are just as sensitive to painful stimuli as anyone. Whenever I had to do a heel-stick on a newborn to obtain a drop of blood for a glucose level, I felt like a wicked witch! Every baby did precisely what you'd expect a person to do when stuck with a sharp object: the foot jerked in my hand, a look of dismay, shock and/or pain flashed over the baby's face, and objections to the affront were voiced in loud, furious howls.

When a sleeping baby suddenly started crying, the very first thing nursery nurses did was to check its diaper. The majority of the babies in the nursery did not enjoy having wet or poopy diapers; quite often a clean bottom was all that was necessary to restore the baby to its sleeping state. Any kind of physical manipulation of the baby's body was likely to be received by the baby with distress. Upon arrival in the nursery after birth, each baby was subjected to a complete physical assessment. After taking vital signs—rectal temperature, blood pressure, pulse, and respirations, the body and head were measured. The skull was examined, feeling for the fontanels, or "soft spots," and the soft separations, called sutures, between the bones of the skull. Eyes were assessed for movement, color, secretions, or bruises. Mouths were opened, looked into for any abnormalities in the palate, tongue, or gums, then a finger was inserted to check the sucking reflex. Skin was evaluated for bruises, swelling, lacerations, rashes, color. Nipples were felt, along with a gentle grasping of each testicle within the scrotum to rule out abnormalities. The spinal column was felt and visually examined for any irregularities in its shape or position. Hands were grasped to check the baby's grasp reflex and then abruptly released to see if the baby jerked its arms and hands in the startle reflex. The baby's legs were flexed at the knee and rotated outward from the body to check for problems with the hip joints.

All these activities, and others not mentioned, involved handling the baby: turning it over, lifting it up, moving its limbs around, probing with thermometers, Q-tips, fingers, and hands. Rarely would a baby respond quietly to all this stimulation; crying, and sometimes downright outraged, beet-red fury, was the norm. And even this response was evaluated, along with the baby's ability to be comforted once the physical assessment was completed.

Doing the assessments was a challenge for me initially. I was so clumsy and slow and the babies' discomfort was so upsetting that the babies and I suffered together. As I became more adept in my manipulations, the babies were tormented less and I began to take pleasure in interacting with them.

Invariably, baths were not enjoyed by the babies—or me. Cold air on wet skin, being lifted and turned over and scrubbed, having water on the face, just wasn't a newborn's idea of fun. However, I was amused to discover that washing the hair was different. After the trauma of the bath, which was given in the isolette, I would swaddle the baby in a warm blanket and tuck its tightly wrapped, cocooned body against my side, under my arm. Standing at the sink, I would gently lave warm water over the baby's head. Almost without exception the response was the same: each baby would startle at the first touch of water, begin to screw its face to cry, and then as I continued to bathe the head, I could feel the body relax, the head actually push back against my hand, neck extended and face bearing a look of fierce concentration on this new sensation. I actually laughed out loud when I went for a haircut myself, reclined in the chair at the washing sink, and felt that luxurious pleasure of having one's hair washed and scalp massaged. I believed that pleasure was one the newborn babies recognized instantly: "Ah, now this feels good!"

On several occasions, I found myself getting emotionally involved with some of these infants, in spite of my resistance to working in the nursery. When I received a newborn from the labor and delivery nurse, I was responsible for the next two to four hours of that baby's life. In between taking its vital signs every fifteen minutes, in the first hour, I did the physical assessment. Sitting on a stool beside the warmer in which the baby lay, I listened with a stethoscope to the baby's heart and lungs. Listening to the sound of air rushing in and out of these newly functioning lungs, counting the rapid heartbeat demands total, focused attention. Everything around me had to be completely shut out for me to hear any abnormal breath sounds or a heart murmur. I always felt a sense of protectiveness toward the baby. The strangeness of it touched me. There I was, totally unknown to this person, listening to its body's interior workings, my actions safeguarding its helpless, vulnerable little self. It seemed so personal, so intimate, even though I performed my tasks with the requisite detachment of a professional.

As I did my work with each baby, this sense of being privileged permeated my feelings about the baby. After these few hours, I would have no further contact with this child. I wouldn't know its family or anything about the life it was just beginning. But I was permitted to touch it, examine it, bathe it, feed it, dress it in the first clothes it would ever wear, listen to its body's sounds. Inexplicably, that felt like an unanticipated gift to me; I tried to convey my gratitude in the way I cared for the baby. I talked and crooned to it, stroked it gently, tried to hold it with respect and delicacy. After several hours of such concentration on a little person, I felt I knew each of them in some indefinably special way, if only for those few hours. I felt proprietary about them, and shared every little action and reaction of theirs with their families, who lined the windows around my work station, watching me attend their babies. Some of the other nursery nurses thought I was nuts to spend so much time out in the hall with the families, crowing over how remarkable their baby was, but I couldn't help myself. I wasn't doing it just for the families, I was doing it because the babies had captured my enthusiasm and I wanted to share it.

Probably the most enjoyable little mental game I played in the nursery was trying to figure out what kind of people these babies would be, based on their behavior the first two or three days of life. It is remarkable how patently obvious the distinct personalities of each baby are, even given the normal developmental phases newborns exhibit during their first few days. All babies sleep, eat, cry, mess their diapers, and respond to stimulation, but the manner in which they do so is uniquely their own. There were two or three babies that I just knew were going to have a hard time with life. These kids simply couldn't handle all the things that were happening to them and all the bodily functions that were expected of them. They cried inconsolably when awake; spit up after every feed, gagging and choking with distress as their formula soiled their beds; had diarrhea or couldn't poop at all; had sticky gunk seeping from the corners of their eyes and scratches on their faces from their own fingernails; startled and screamed at the slightest noise or touch—and were just generally unhappy little people. I laughingly called them my neonatal neurotics as I tried without much success to keep them clean and comforted.

Other babies were zonked out completely, except when it was time to eat or have a diaper change. They lay in their beds, snoozing away without any apparent awareness of all the noise and dither, the bright lights and activity of the nursery around them. They cried only when really stimulated by an overlong bath or a heel-stick. These babies I fancied would be laid-back, easygoing characters, incipient couch potatoes, who could handle whatever life dished out as long as they got a nap now and again. The ones I really got a kick out of were the eager beavers, the kids that didn't want to sleep or lie in their cribs because they wanted to see what was going on around them.

Some of these hyper-alert babies I found truly fascinating. I would receive such a baby from the delivery nurse and begin the several-hour period of close observation of this child. No matter what I did with or to the baby, it was obviously paying strict attention. The baby—eyes open and tracking my movements, responding immediately to my touch, and easily comforted by caresses and a soothing voice—was taking everything in and processing each sensation with a look of total absorption. One baby in particular just tickled the hell out of me.

She was a big girl, eleven-plus pounds, and I spent one whole twelve-hour shift facilitating her avid curiosity about the world. A fat, firmly fleshed body, sturdy neck, and chipmunk cheeks were topped by fine, black, straight hair about an inch and a half long that stuck straight up, punk fashion. This little girl did not want to sleep or suck on a pacifier and be quiet in her bed. She took her formula well, messed her diapers appropriately, and dozed only for a few minutes after every feed. The rest of the time she cried until I picked her up, put her high on my shoulder, and let her look at the world. She held her head up straight and studied everything around her, the whole night. She reminded me for some reason—maybe her hair—of the cartoon character Lulu, so most of the night, as I carried her around, talking to her, grinning with pleasure at all the families and visitors watching her alert little face through the windows of the nursery, I introduced her to all the other babies as Lulu. The next night I was off. I couldn't stop thinking about Lulu and how much fun I'd had with her. I missed her! When I returned to the nursery two nights later, the nurses told me she had slept soundly the entire previous night, exhausted, I surmised, by her first explorations of this world!

When it is slow on L&D, I like to go to the nursery and check out the babies. One hospital where I worked had upwards of sixty babies at a time. I walk down the line of basinettes and peruse the little faces. So individual, so different, each one of them. Some with long hair, some with tight thick curls, some bald or with only a bit of peach fuzz. Some crying, some sleeping, some sucking their pacifiers, some flailing their arms and legs. Their newness, their potential, their purity touches me. It is almost voyeuristic to stand there watching them sleep, cry, suck. They have no privacy. Strangers guard them, providing them with warmth and nourishment. They are completely vulnerable.

I grow pensive watching them and finally leave them with good wishes for long, productive lives and good parents who will treasure them. Looking at them renews my sense of purpose. It is for these little beings that we work: to bring them safely into the world and guard them until their parents can assume their care. It isn't just a job, it's about new humans, the little people for whom I am responsible, and I try to feel delight each time I take one of these babies in my arms.

Chapter Three

🌿 PREPARED CHILDBIRTH

Before I became a mother, I used to smile indulgently when female conversation at parties would invariably move to the topic of childbirth. Why did women always gravitate to that subject? I wondered. Are their lives so boring that they have nothing else to talk about? Are they so wary of other subjects, or of each other, that they avoid discussions of politics, religion, the arts, whatever? I believed—and still do to some extent—that many women were socialized to leave the so-called significant issues to the men. To talk with passion about politics or philosophy or science wasn't acceptably feminine. Thus, I assumed, they were reduced to discussions of childbirth and childcare. Years later, it was easier to recognize that these women were just discussing the primary concerns of their daily lives. In their early twenties and thirties, they were in their prime parenting years. Naturally they talked about birth and kids.

But women I knew socially through my husband's work, professors and attorneys who were older than I, also frequently gravitated to the topic of birth. During my two pregnancies, I was in fact the catalyst for many of these dinner-party conversations. My gravid belly drew forth memories of their own pregnancies and birth experiences. I began to realize that for most women in our culture, labor and childbirth are the closest analogous experiences a woman has to that of combat. It is an experience of physical and psychic travail, a time during which one's body takes over and engages in a monumental endeavor—to thrust a new being out of itself. This ineluctable process startles many Western women in a profound way. We privileged women have become so separated from the physicality of our bodies: we don't work in the fields, we don't do hard labor every day, we don't have a constant, abiding sense of the muscles, the bones, the tissues that make up our selves. Our culture and our civilized manner of living have removed us from the physical. We take our bodies for granted. When they malfunction, we seek medical aid. We grow up believing that pain is an unacceptable concept: Take an aspirin, swallow an antacid, take a laxative, smooth on a soothing ointment, apply a local anesthetic.

When we get pregnant, our bodies demand attention. All sorts of untoward events occur. We gain weight. Our hearts pump a lot more, a lot harder. Our breasts tingle painfully and swell, along with our hands and feet. We can't breathe as easily and eventually can't eat as much. Clothes don't fit. Food won't stay down. Bowel movements become irritatingly difficult and hemorrhoids may blossom. Our skin often striates with permanent stretch marks—"maternal combat ribbons." Some of us lose our hair. Some of us grow a dark line down our bellies, others a butterfly of blush across our cheeks. We are afflicted with episodes of near narcolepsy, our bodies nagging us to sleep, *sleep!* We become experts at locating toilet facilities, no matter where we may be, as the need to urinate becomes frequent and relentless. Our minds boggle with visions of bizarre foods, the pickles and ice cream syndrome, and we gorge our bellies with strange sustenance: lead paint curls from the wood-work, orange sherbet by the quart, chalk, Big Macs, dirt, you name it. Our sleep is perfused with weird, often nightmarish, dreams. Our attentiveness and our ability to concentrate diminish with each passing month. We grow absentminded and emotionally labile, weeping at inconsequential things that not being pregnant, we wouldn't have even noticed.

We become exquisitely sensitive to the slightest stimuli: smells, tastes, textures, and music all are experienced with intense clarity. An uncooked piece of meat or a slightly soured glass of milk may send us rushing for the toilet, our stomachs churning in protest. A broken fingernail may result in a flash of temper. A Brahms lullaby may provoke a cascade of memories of our own childhoods. A child's cry in the grocery store may wrench our hearts with the desire to comfort and soothe. Small children and babies fascinate us and we notice them everywhere. When pregnant, we are more . . . everything! More susceptible, responsive, compassionate, gentle, tempermental, grouchy, excitable, irascible, intuitive, delicate, more robust. We are on a roller-coaster ride of emotions and perceptions unlike any other time in our lives.

The nesting instinct emerges as we prowl the malls, search the cata-logues, discuss the best buys in baby furniture and equipment. We give serious thought to paper versus cloth diapers, bottle versus breast, and begin to spend many hours thinking about our own mothers. For many of us, as it surely was for me, the physical facts of pregnancy are beguiling: every minute change in our bodies captivates us, absorbing all our attention. There is often a feeling of such overwhelming gratification over our fertility that we are rendered buoyant with gladness. Some of us are more animated and light-hearted than ever before. Others float through the days of gestation with a serenity, a tranquility that lends an elegance and charm to the rooms we inhabit and the people we live with. Pregnancy is, for many women, a time of intense spiritual and emotional centeredness. Our bodies are performing their primal female function, to our ceaseless, fascinated self-satisfaction. The pure joy of harboring new life within our bodies, the feel of each kick or hiccup within, is sometimes almost too extravagant to contain.

Our bellies grow, inexorably. Initially, a small hard lump is felt in the center below the navel when we lie on our stomachs. When we feel the first flutters of the fetus moving within, known as *quickening,* it seizes our attention completely, and a lump lodges in the throat when we realize that no, it isn't gas, it's the baby. We pass through the months of gestation, growing familiar with the lurches and kicks and tumbles of that person within. A person, a human body is in there—kicking, swallowing, turning, sucking, peeing, heart beating, blood coursing, fingers waving, elbows and knees tapping out indecipherable messages. All of it in there, intact, growing, and subsisting on our blood, cradled in our bony pelvises, awash in our amniotic waters, tethered to our muscle by placenta and umbilical cord, living off of us, a human parasite hosted by its mother.

When labor begins, the inescapable nature of it is intimidating to most of us. Classes attended, books read, stories recounted, due dates longed for—none of it matters when we face the reality of labor. This is going to happen whether we like it or not, whether we cooperate with it or not, whether we are awake or unconscious, whether we smile or scream. Trapped in our pregnant bodies, we cannot escape this process. It is the great challenge of womanhood, yet it is a task performed by millions of women throughout the millennia, a universal female experience and yet uniquely, individually, our own. The body *demands* the fulfillment of this task: the fetus must be expelled. If the body can't do it by itself, other people must see to it that the infant is delivered. However blindly we began this adventure, a single act of vast consequence, regardless of motive or intent, has resulted in this final event: birth. Is it any wonder that we discuss it endlessly, that we are filled with curiosity about the myriad permutations of the process, of how completely different each labor and delivery can be, of how life-changing the experience will be?

Most Western women have never been physically tested until we go through labor and birth. Most of us are fortunate enough to never have gone eighteen or twenty-four hours without food or sleep. Few of us allow ourselves to go a day and night or two days and nights without a bath or shower, without brushing our teeth and doing our hair and makeup. Even fewer of us would allow anyone else to see, smell, or touch us, unwashed, sweat-soaked, naked, oozing mucus, blood, and feces from our nether regions. When faced with the forces of labor, we can't hide the fear, the anxiety, the responses to pain. We are laid open in a hospital bed, vulnerable and trapped in the physical process. All the inhibitions and trappings of our social selves are peeled away as our bodies thrust and heave, vomit and grunt, cry and leak. The animal is there for everyone to see. The civilized, social self is just a veneer, easily lost when the contractions overwhelm our modesty, our control, our dignity. To add insult to injury, there are strangers present, people with expectations of us, observing and passing judgment on our behavior. Afterward, our perceptions of how we endured the process profoundly affects our sense of self, our very identity.

It's a very simple process, actually. The uterus, a large bag of muscle, opens its mouth, the cervix, so that it can then push its contents, the baby, down the vaginal pathway out of the body. It's also an amazingly complex, mysterious biochemical and physiological process; a wondrously elegant fusion of hormones, muscles, and nerves into a stately dance, beginning with a closed cervix, climaxing with a delivered infant. The medical masters have analyzed and studied the process, dividing it into distinct stages and phases.

In the first stage, the cervix dilates or opens from zero to ten centimeters and effaces—or thins out—from zero to 100 percent. To do this, the uterus contracts and relaxes repeatedly, much as the muscles of your mouth and cheeks contract to open your mouth into a smile or a grimace. As it contracts, the uterus squeezes the fetus inside, pushing its head against the cervix, using this pressure as additional force to get the cervix open.

In the second stage, the open uterus continues to contract, pushing against that little body and moving it down, past the bones of the pelvis, making the baby stretch the vaginal folds and squeeze out into the light. The third stage is after the baby is delivered: attention may be focused on this new child, but the uterus still contracts to slough off the now unnecessary placenta. When the placenta is expelled, labor is over, according to the textbooks, but the uterus still has a few weeks of recovery ahead. It takes time for the organ to squeeze itself back down to the tidy little mass of muscle it was before pregnancy.

Of course, all this effort does not pass unnoticed. The uterus resides inside a thinking, feeling female whose response to this physical process is what becomes so fascinating to most women:

"How was your labor?"
I was in labor for 36 hours . . .
I couldn't stand the pain . . .
I was so hungry and tired . . .
We had a great time, my husband and I. He helped me so much and I handled the labor just fine!
I pushed for three hours . . .
It was much easier than I expected . . .
It was so fast; I was lucky . . .
It felt so good to push that baby out . . .
I tore badly . . .
My husband was wonderful . . .
Thank God for epidurals . . .
They had to put me to sleep . . .

I had to have a cesarean . . .
We held that baby together and cried and laughed and felt so glad.

Talking about childbirth aids the understanding of it and ties us to one another. It is the women's shared experience, like that of men in combat, or any group of people who undergo the same physical and psychological crisis.

The women of the childbirth organization I joined after Michael's birth took their interest a little bit further. They were enamored of birth, as I was, found it endlessly fascinating in all its variety. Some of them were fanatics, some radical feminists: these women breast-fed their babies past age three, shopped at the organic food store, attended home births, and were adamantly and vociferously anti-establishment, anti-hospitals, and anti-doctors. Others were just mainstream, middle-class mothers who needed something extra to occupy their minds and time, who wanted to assist others in the process of labor and delivery, who enjoyed the vicarious thrills of others' birth experiences.

Wives and mothers, very few of the women in the volunteer organization for childbirth education had jobs. They managed their homes, husbands, and children while yearning to be involved with the process of giving birth. They attended monthly meetings, shared countless telephone calls, typed minutes and teaching notes, read books about birth, organized classes for expectant parents, opened their homes for the meetings and classes, and thought and talked endlessly about their birth experiences, which were the common denominator for these women. They wanted to prolong their involvement with the process of bringing new life to the earth, despite physical and financial limits that held them to a finite number of children of their own.

My involvement with this volunteer group was an effort to fill the aching emptiness I felt after Michael's birth, knowing I wouldn't be having any more children of my own. I also wanted to try to prevent, through education and support, the kind of emotional abuse I was subjected to by my own obstetrician. I was afire with indignation over the way he treated me. I couldn't change the character of that experience, but I could try to positively shape other women's labors.

Over the next three years I learned how difficult it would be to realize that goal. I was in training for seven months before I was allowed to stand alone in front of a class of expectant parents. I read and wrote reports on dozens of books: books about the physiology and psychology of childbirth; books about natural childbirth; Grantley Dick-Read, Bradley, Kitzinger (all pioneers in prepared childbirth techniques); books about the management of pain, the fear-tension-pain syndrome, fetal development, the first year of life, breast-feeding, nutrition in pregnancy, and so forth. I attended classes with my cotrainees, memorized the right way to describe the events of labor, practiced the relaxation and breathing exercises. I constructed visual aids, cutting up pieces of colored felt to slap on my visual-aid board. I ordered supplies: a fetal doll complete with umbilical cord and placenta, a red knitted uterus to stuff the doll in, a flip chart, and posters and graphs of every aspect of pregnancy and birth.

After a seventy-page take-home exam and a closed-book exam in my last training class, I was judged ready to begin coteaching. A class was selected and an experienced instructor chosen as my preceptor, or tutor. During several phone calls, she outlined precisely what I would be responsible for in the first class.

I practiced the lessons, saying the words out loud into a tape recorder, trying to memorize them and spit them out smoothly and graciously. I was as nervous as a cat; two days before the class I prevailed upon my best friend to let me rehearse with her. We stuffed cookies into the hands of our toddlers and got down on the floor, she patiently pretending to be pregnant and ignorant of the exercises I was to teach her. She giggled on occasion but I was deadly serious; I was going to do this right, dammit! I was terrified. For five years I had been at home with my children, my social contacts limited to dinner parties with my husband's colleagues and long lunches with a couple of female friends and their small children. I was appalled at the presumption that I could present myself to a room of total strangers as an expert on childbirth.

First-night jitters were almost incapacitating. As I drove three times around the block of the instructor's house, I cursed myself for ever getting into this. *Oh, it was going to be so bad. I wouldn't be able to remember anything I had learned. I would get the exercises mixed up. I would forget critical steps in each exercise; What would I do if someone asked me a question? Oh God, I can't do this!* I chain-smoked four cigarettes before popping a stick of gum in my mouth, then hauled my books and charts to the front door, literally trembling with anxiety.

What a ninny I'd been! My preceptor was turned out to be a mellow, easygoing mother of three, a nurse on a part-time basis, whose relaxed demeanor began to calm my fears. When the couples arrived, I realized that I had a wealth of knowledge in my head from all the weeks of studying and reading; all I had to do, for chrissakes, was teach them a few relaxation exercises. How hard could that be, anyway? I had also completely forgotten how much I loved an audience. The little girl of three who would dance and show off for anyone in sight still resided in this housewife. When I started my spiel, after a casual introduction that informed the couples of my in-training status, I was onstage. It was a piece of cake! The words flowed smoothly, humorous ad libs about body shapes and unwieldy bellies were offered; I remembered everything and had a great time!

The couples who came to my classes intrigued me. It was the beginning of my awareness of the undeniable individuality of each couple, an awareness that would grow into a sensitivity to the aura of each patient I would eventually care for. My limited, personal mental construct of pregnancy and of marriage was shattered and then expanded as I observed, talked with, and helped each of these people step toward the reality of a baby. That everyone is unique seems so ridiculously obvious, but to a sheltered homebody this was an absorbing realization. Not every woman enjoyed pregnancy as I had, and many of them downright hated it, felt crippled by it, resented the changes in their bodies, or felt ugly, even though they were eager for their babies. I watched them, listened, and learned. I became adept at reading body language and figuring out which couples had marital problems or ambiguous feelings about childbirth. Often I could predict who would cope well with the demands of labor and who would respond to it with horror. After so many years of being a housewife, I was invigorated by my exposure to these couples. I wasn't interested in knowing the details of their lives; what they did for a living, how well-off they were, where they lived. I only wanted to know how they felt about having a kid. What did they fear? What did they expect? How could I help them realize their fantasies about their child's birth?

Over time, and through many classes of six to ten couples each, I worked and learned about childbirth and about teaching. I moved from quoting directly out of my instructor's manual to an easy, conversational mode of teaching. I laughed and joked and kidded my couples about everything. Nothing was sacred in my classes; we talked about the primitive aspects of giving birth. I described how messy it could be and told them about shitting on Dr. Mauller's shoes as my son came forth. When a mother would accidentally pass gas while practicing the pushing technique, I got her and everyone else to laugh about it, smoothing over her embarrassment by reassuring her that "after all, there's not much room in there for extra air!" I had them all stretch out on the floor with their pillows, then moved among them, touching and stroking limbs as we practiced the relaxation and breathing exercises. I tried to get them used to being touched by a stranger in intimate places, their inner thighs, their pubic bones, their necks. I made them close their eyes and do mental imaging while they concentrated on specific muscle groups and controlled breathing. I made the husbands "be the wives," insisting that they know and demonstrate all the techniques their wives were using. I tried to shake their concentration by fussing at them or asking them to change position during a "contraction." We played with different scenarios, to bring the lessons to life, to practice the techniques in "real" situations.

Childbirth classes offer a variety of breathing techniques and relaxation exercises. There are a number of different approaches offered to the expectant couple: the Lamaze method, the Bradley method, the Kitzinger method, and so forth. But for all intents and purposes, the main objective in all of these classes is to prepare the couple for the experience of labor and birth. Through lectures, exercises, role-playing, imagery, movies, books, and charts, the instructor strives to educate the couple about the physiological and psychological process of labor and birth; the obstetrical practices, routines, and procedures that occur; and methods that can be used to exert control and maintain the couple's dignity and autonomy during the experience. The theory behind this education is that ignorance leads to fear, fear leads to tension, tension leads to increased pain, increased pain leads to greater fear, and so on. By breaking the fear-tension-pain cycle with knowledge, specific breathing patterns, and relaxation techniques, the birth process can be enhanced and can become a positive event for the couple.

In my classes, I placed emphasis on achieving that positive goal. I explained the theory that the brain can only focus well on one stimulus at a time, so that if the mind actively concentrates on a breathing pattern, the pain messages being sent from the uterus will be blocked, or at least diminished. I also argued that it was almost impossible to panic and lose control, in any situation, if the woman forced herself to concentrate on controlling her breathing. That old adage, "Take a deep breath and count to ten," when you are about to lose your temper, like most folk remedies, has a solid base of truth to it.

The theory of conditioned, learned response is incorporated in these classes. By repeatedly practicing the breathing and relaxation techniques the mother is supposedly conditioning herself to respond automatically to uterine contractions with controlled breathing and relaxed muscles. Having her coach practice with her is believed to be an important adjunct to the conditioning: his touch, the words he uses, and his tone of voice are supposed to contribute to her automatic learned response to labor.

Three types of controlled breathing were taught, each to be used at specific times as the labor progressed. The first, slow deep-chest breathing, was simply that: the mother was to slow down her respirations so that she breathed no more than six to nine times in sixty seconds (normal respiration rates are fourteen to twenty per minute). She was to inhale deeply into her chest, feeling her ribcage expand, and then exhale just as slowly. This breathing pattern was to be initiated when she could no longer walk or talk through her contractions, and employed for the duration of the contraction.

When or if the contractions became so uncomfortable that the mother found it difficult to maintain slow, deep-chest breathing, she was then to utilize the second breathing technique, a shallow pant, one every second. If she reached a point where panting didn't allow her to maintain control, the third technique was to be used.

This breathing pattern was a series of pants and blows. Picking whatever number of pants the woman desired, she was supposed to pant that number of times and then follow the pant with a short, sharp blow or puff, such as she might use to blow out a candle. For example, she might pant twice and then blow, or she might pant five times before blowing. I demonstrated each pattern and then had the men and women perform for me while I watched and critiqued their methods. "Pant up in your throat, so it feels like your breath doesn't go down into your chest. Pant just like a puppy, mouth open, tongue relaxed. You can say 'hee-hee-hee' or 'heh-heh-heh,' whatever works."

We practiced these techniques at every session, along with forceful blowing efforts used to counter the premature urge to push, if that became necessary. The couples also stretched out on the carpet while I taught relaxation techniques. "Okay, now tighten all the muscles in your right arm. Real tight. Make a fist. Hold it. Hold it. Now let it relax, let all the tightness go. Dad, check your wife's arm. Lift it gently and see if it's completely relaxed. Now tighten your legs, flex your feet, curl your toes . . . etcetara." Through these exercises, I was trying to condition the mothers to relax tense muscles on command. The idea was that complete relaxation of the body would enhance blood flow to the uterus, making for more efficient, effective contractions. In addition it provided another way for the mother to concentrate: if she was focused on maintaining relaxed limbs, she would be less aware of the contractions.

The techniques, both breathing and relaxation, weren't so important in themselves. Practice of them, however, made the mothers more conscious of their physical bodies. Most women in our society, unless they are athletically inclined, don't pay much attention to how their bodies feel. The focus is more on how their bodies look. Awareness of individual muscle groups, of muscular tension, of joint flexibility is not common, at least as far as I've observed. I wanted my students to get in touch with their bodies, to feel centered in this physical form. If nothing else, I wanted them to have some exposure to the positions they'd be assuming during labor and to being touched by strangers. I walked among them, putting my hands on their legs, their feet, their shoulders. I stroked their legs from the crotch to the ankle. I kneaded their buttocks and tapped their inner thighs. And I made their husbands do all this over and over again. The initial shyness they felt, lying on the floor with a bunch of strangers, evaporated swiftly as they grew accustomed to performing in front of one another.

I spent a full class talking about analgesia and anesthesia. Analgesics such as aspirin, Tylenol, Percocet, relieve pain, while anesthetics, like Novocaine or Lidocaine, eliminate the sensation of pain entirely. I emphasized that there was no right or wrong about using medication; that it was there if they needed it, and there shouldn't be any sense of failure if they did. We spent a class talking about cesareans, how and why they happen and what to expect, right down to details about having the pubic hair shaved and a catheter inserted into the bladder. We talked about what "informed consent" really meant. We talked about breast-feeding and newborn care. I always tried to convey the personal joy I had felt with my own babies, openly expressing my sentiments about the magic of giving birth, the awesome beauty of new life, the privilege of bearing a child. My classes invariably ran three hours, but no one was ever in a hurry to leave. The final class always amused me, because I couldn't get those couples out of my house. They would tarry at the table, finishing up the snacks and drinks, jabbering away, until I would have to laugh and physically push them out the door with reassurances that they would know what to do when the time came.

There is an inherent bias in prepared childbirth classes. In order to be effective, the instructor has to focus on the couple's belief that childbirth will be something they can control. Ideally, as I have said, the intention of the classes is to arm the couple with enough knowledge and information so they will be able to deal with the events of their labor in a controlled, dignified manner. Presumably, the more they know about the physiological, psychological, and emotional aspects of giving birth, the better equipped they will be to handle the stress of this event. Additionally, the more they know about how labor and delivery are managed in a hospital setting, the easier it will be to respond to the routines and procedures that are commonplace there. The objective is to make the couple partners with the doctor and nurses. These ideals are hard to realize. For one thing, the instructor inevitably brings her hidden agendas to the class. Why is she teaching? Is it because she had a negative experience herself with childbirth, or is it because she just wants to supplement her income? Does she have an axe to grind against doctors or hospitals? Is she antimedication or anticesarean or anti-anything? Does she present the material in a nonjudgmental, informative manner, or is she shaping the way in which these parents will perceive their experience, through her word choices, her descriptions of procedures and routines, what she elects or forgets to mention? How well informed is she? Does she know what happens in the specific hospitals where these couples will be admitted? Does she understand why many of the routines are used or does she jump to conclusions based on word-of-mouth horror stories and assume the medical professionals are out to torture her couples?

Then the couple's biases enter the picture. What brings them to these classes? Is it simply the thing done in their peer group, or is it because they're frightened of the big event and want whatever help they can get? Are they the type of people who always read *Consumer Reports* before making a purchase or do they just want a general idea of what to expect? Is the woman hoping to gain techniques that will help her with pain or is she just interested in having an informed partner to guard over her? So many motivations, so many agendas.

Hospital personnel have their own biases. Many a time I've listened to L&D nurses and obstetricians voice their objections, frequently in obscene terms, to natural childbirth classes.

Those damned instructors, they tell these people they don't have to agree to an IV.
We need an IV, dammit.
They think they can make it without an epidural. Hah!
She's refusing to be monitored.
She's refusing to stay in bed.
She says she is going to eat because her instructor told her she could.
She insists on being able to walk around.
She's refusing to be catheterized.

The problems are complex. The parents attend six to eight two-hour classes. They are told all about the stages and phases of labor and delivery. They are taught breathing and relaxation techniques. They are instructed about analgesia and anesthesia, monitoring, IVs, and cesareans. They often have a hospital tour to familiarize them with the physical setup of the unit.

Then they go into labor. They come to the hospital without their instructor and are met by total strangers who will be managing their childbirth experience. Their expectations are shaped by the content of their classes, every labor story they've heard in the past nine months, and their own needs and personalities. The hospital staff doesn't know what they've been taught or what their hopes are. The staff is focused on getting them delivered safely and expeditiously, so the room will be free for the next patient. The routines and procedures of the L&D unit may be more or less flexible, depending on the philosophy of the nursing management and the physicians who utilize the unit. In many cases, individual nurses and doctors make an attempt to meet some of the demands of the couples, to try to individualize their care, but policies and procedures are nearly written in stone. Bending the rules takes courage on the part of the nurse and requires assertiveness and interest in the patient's expectations.

Most nurses find it easier to simply say, "IVs are the rule. . . . No food is the rule. . . . Continuous monitoring is the rule. . . . Two visitors only is the rule. . . ." While one of the objectives of prepared childbirth classes is to produce informed consumers, it is not in the interest of a smoothly running, usually understaffed L&D unit to encourage patients to be actively involved in their own treatment decisions. It is less complicated to care for a woman by the Policy and Procedures manual than to explain each procedure, to ask her opinion, to ask her permission, to keep her informed. It is easier to send her coach out of the room, to ban other visitors, to prohibit cameras and tape recorders, than it is to approach the event as a team, working toward the goal of maximal comfort and safety for the mother and baby, with a little celebration of new life thrown in. So it is not surprising to hear the negative comments and belligerence that are voiced by staff members about prepared childbirth couples. They are resented because they require more effort and more time.

They are also resented because they are seen not as informed consumers but as obstructionists, as people who make the work more difficult. When a mother "succumbs" to her pain and fear and begs for relief, the staff quite often relishes her "failure," just as Dr. Mauller sneered at me when the contractions hit me like a sledge hammer. The antagonistic glee some doctors exhibit is appalling: *I knew she would be hollering for an epidural. These people think they know everything from their classes and then the real world hits them!* Perfectly reasonable human beings who go to great lengths to guard their own loved ones from abusive treatment in hospitals sometimes become almost sadistic in their vindictiveness. They want to see the patient's plans fail so they can say "I told you so." They want to swoop into the room with an epidural cart and play the savior, self-righteous about their years of experience with laboring mothers.

The mother is in no position to defend herself. She can't calmly discuss the pros and cons of 100 mg of Demerol, or of continuous fetal monitoring, when she is locked into the rhythm of hard contractions, without sleep or food, cut off for hours from all that's familiar to her. Even if she or her coach have questions about the necessity of certain procedures, the staff routinely uses language that in effect blackmails her into acquiescence:

We need to be sure of your baby's heartbeat.
We're worried that your baby may be stressed too much by these contractions.
We are afraid you might have an infection.
We have to get blood from the baby's scalp so we can know for sure if he's in trouble.
If something goes wrong, we need an IV line to get emergency medication into you.

How can she argue with this? She wants her baby to be safe; that's why she's in the hospital. Additionally, many times these statements are honest and necessary: the mother's and the baby's safety are the paramount concern of any labor and delivery unit.

The medical approach to childbirth sees it as a pathological event in which the goal is to prevent injury and/or death to the mother and baby, and to micromanage the event so that it happens as quickly and safely as possible. Concerns about the mother's emotional needs, about a warm, loving, positive birth are always secondary to concerns about the pathological characteristics of the birth process. In other words, obstetrical teams are trained to treat childbirth as an illness, an abnormal event, rife with danger to the mother and baby, rather than as a healthy act in the normal reproductive life of the mother. The fact that medical teams identity the mother as a patient, underscores the philosophical bias of the caregivers.

A "bad" baby is simply to be avoided at all costs, even if that means using procedures and routines that may cause embarrassment or pain to the mother. The fear of malpractice lawsuits colors the entire environment of a L&D unit. It shapes the very words that are written in the charts and spoken to the couple. Most staff members become adept at screening their words and facial expressions and at guarding against any behavior that might be construed as ammunition for a potential lawsuit.

After several years as an L&D nurse, I realized that most L&D staff members, nurses and doctors alike, have no idea of what actually occurs in prepared childbirth classes. They don't realize or remember that a bond is created among the class members; that for these couples, the hospital experience is just the culmination of a long process of learning and understanding. The staff interacts with the couple during a discrete period of time, the actual labor and delivery, without any awareness of how the parents have prepared themselves for that particular period. The couple is on a continuum that carries them from prepregnancy to parenthood, while the staff interacts with them during only one part of that continuum. There is no advance exposure to each other, there is no time beforehand to incorporate any understanding of the couple's expectations or fears.

The only advantage that the medical personnel see in childbirth classes is that the couples receive prior explanations about routines and possible occurences during delivery, which saves the staff some explaining. It is not surprising that often the most effective, most supportive L&D nurses also teach prepared childbirth classes. Those who don't, or who haven't attended classes, or who haven't given birth themselves, just don't really comprehend what the parents have incorporated into their mental construct about childbirth. This explains some of the hostility exhibited by L&D nurses toward prepared couples: they feel threatened by what they don't understand, yet feel empowered by their experience with innumerable births and their clinical perception of the process, which of course the expectant parents don't share.

After four years as a childbirth instructor and eight years as an L&D nurse, I was able to see more than one side of the issue. Even though everyone involved in a birth has the same underlying goal of a "good outcome," a healthy baby and mother, the conflicts inherent in achieving that outcome often seem insurmountable. As an instructor, I moved from preaching about maintaining control over your own birth experience to attempting to support the doctor-patient relationship by providing my couples with explanations of hospital routines. Very quickly I realized that I could affect the childbirth experience in either a negative or a positive way. If I chose to present the hospital personnel as bad guys, as people didn't care about their patients' hopes and plans, as people who only wanted to get the patient delivered, I would be guilty of introducing an element of conflict between the patient and her caretakers. I didn't want to do that; labor is stressful enough without anger and hostility curdling the atmosphere. Eight weeks before a due date is too late to have an impact on a couple's choice of doctor or hospital. I spent two years trying to create a hospital consumer guide that would provide couples with detailed information about what was and wasn't allowed in each of my city's hospitals, only to realize that such information was not of interest to the couples until they neared their delivery date. At that point, it was too late to switch doctors or hospitals.

After much thought and many conversations with couples, other instructors, and hospital staff members, I chose to define myself as a facilitator. I stressed objective information: this is why IVs are used, this is why monitoring is done, this is why a cesarean may be required, this is why you won't be allowed to walk or eat, this is why you cannot have narcotics or you can have an epidural. I told my couples that, above all, the dreams or fantasies or plans they had about the approaching event must be flexible: no one can predict what may happen in the course of labor and they must always keep in mind that the safety of the mother and infant is the primary concern.

Bring your written birth plans to the hospital, review them frequently with your OB in your weekly visits, go into the experience with all your hopes and dreams, but always be ready to go with the flow and cooperate if there is any untoward event that challenges your plans. In this way, you establish yourselves as informed consumers who can participate in the team effort at the hospital, while allowing yourselves the necessary flexibility to deal with unexpected events, without wrecking your self-esteem and your dreams about this birth.

I insisted that couples be active participants in their own childbirth. We acted out various scenarios, to give them some practice with gentle self-assertion. I'd play the mean or indifferent nurse or the abrupt doctor and make them ask me questions. I tried to ensure that they recognized their right to question *and* the rights of the medical personnel to perform the procedures they might be required to initiate.

In each class, I reiterated that I was not an expert. I could only give them what knowledge I had and try to steer them toward more information. I reminded them that I wouldn't be with them to run interference, that they were responsible for their own experiences and that they could be as actively involved as they chose. If they wanted to lie back and be cared for according to hospital protocols, fine. If they wanted to participate in decision-making, they had to speak up, and they could speak up without being hostile or beligerent. Quiet questions and a courteous manner would get them far, so I told them.

The most gratifying aspect of my four years as an instructor were my reunion classes. For six weeks before their deliveries these people came to my house for class. I watched the women's bodies change as they neared their due dates. At the end of the course, I sent them home with my best wishes and my phone number. Thanking them for sharing this special time with me, I gave them my own gentle wish for a wonderful birth and a healthy baby. We were close by the end of the series of classes. When they called with the news about their deliveries, we celebrated over the phone.

After their deliveries, the couples would return for one last night, babies in arms, loaded down with diaper bags and blankets, to relate their experiences. These were always joyous evenings, crowned by the feeling that attending my classes had helped, in whatever small way. The best part of it all was the fathers. To hear these men talking animatedly about how "it was just like you told us it would be," to have them praise their wives' stamina and courage, to listen to them speak with awe over their wives' bravery in the face of such arduous labor, to see their faces as they described greeting and touching their newborns were gifts to me of immeasurable value.

One father told me, with tears in his eyes, that he had never dreamed of what it would be like to become a father: "It was as though a door opened to a room in my mind, in my heart, that I never knew existed, and I felt emotions of such sweetness and strength that I was overwhelmed. I have been ecstatic, absolutely joy-filled, since the moment I laid eyes on that little baby." Another father, a young brawny steelworker, very macho in his dress and manner, paced around my living room, crowing loudly with pride in his wife and volunteering to be anyone's coach: "Man, she was so brave! I never knew how strong my wife is, you know? I just always thought of her as being delicate and beautiful, and man, she was so strong, and so beautiful, it made me dizzy to watch her. I loved being a part of it! I want to do it again and again! Man, Susie, I'm serious, if you have anyone who needs a coach, I wanna do it! What a high!"

Chapter Four

LABOR PAIN

The pain of childbirth is a much belabored subject—pun intended! Cultural, familial, and personal expectations affect the woman's experience of labor and birth and, as prepared childbirth advocates have been preaching for years, fear contributes greatly to the amount of pain a woman feels, and her ability to cope with it. While influenced by the theories I've studied, my observations about childbirth pain are largely personal ones. It fascinates me to watch a woman go through labor.

Each labor is distinctly unique, as each individual brings to it her own singular responses. Yet there are similarities, regardless of age or background. After eight years of experience, I can usually tell what stage of labor a woman is in by observing her behavior. During early labor, as the cervix dilates to about five centimeters, most women are able to converse between contractions, and sometimes during them, although at those times they may only be verbalizing how much they hurt. As labor intensifies, women tend to withdraw, concentrating on getting through the contraction or else yelling for help. As the cervix nears eight to ten centimeters, women may be near panic, if not already hysterical. The contractions come close together and are excruciatingly intense. On palpation, the belly feels like a rock.

The body language of labor pain intrigues me. My own experience with pain, mercifully, is limited. I vaguely remember struggling with an inexplicable bellyache one long night, years ago, that resulted in an appendectomy. I distinctly recall the surgeon's hands as he palpated my abdomen. I reached out with my own hands to press his against the pain; they felt so warm and comforting. There was a real sensation that these hands would heal me, free me from the grip of pain. That experience taught me, in a visceral way, the true meaning of "hands-on care." At twenty years old, I was blissfully healthy and ignorant of my body's limitations. I found myself surprised by the postoperative pain: I was embarrassed to tell the doctor that I hurt. Real pain was simply not something I had ever been forced to confront.

My experiences with the birth process have already been described. I was fortunate, I suppose, in comparison with many of the women I have cared for during labor, to have had such easy labors, so the pain I felt left no lingering psychic scars. However, a herniated disc in my lower back at age thirty-nine made pain a familiar adversary. After months of more conservative attempts to alleviate this pain, I finally opted for surgery. When I regained consciousness in the recovery room, I remember seeing my surgeon's face and telling him with several expletives how badly I hurt. I vividly remember that this pain was so overwhelming that I wanted desperately to get out of my body. My being felt trapped inside an envelope of agony. Fortunately I lost consciousness and all memory of the next few hours.

Two weeks later a cerebrospinal fluid leak complicated my recovery, requiring treatment that consisted of placing a catheter drain into my spinal canal. This procedure, often painless, was not in my case. As the catheter was inserted, it touched nerve endings. Without warning, I was introduced abruptly to all the nerves in my legs: sharp needles of fire all over the surface of my legs, radiating in little branches; deep, dull, heart-clanging pain in the bones; and red-hot waves in the muscles—all terrifying, as my legs jerked and shivered involuntarily. These sensations lasted only a few minutes, but this was long enough to cause my legs to spasm, my breath to leave my chest, and cold sweat to pop out all over. The resultant seven-day "spinal headache," as fluid drained out of my spinal canal, was a nightmare of pain. Unable to move my head or to eat, I passed the time waiting and asking for the next injection of Demerol. When the catheter was removed, the nerves were brushed again: for the first and only time in my life, I lost all control and screamed in agony. The only thing that kept me anchored to reality was a nurse's hand that I bruised with my grip.

I recount these personal experiences only to explain how my consciousness was raised about laboring mothers' pain. There is no way anyone can truly understand another person's pain. We health-care professionals are more exposed to human suffering than any other people. We deal with complaints of pain daily, and we spend a great deal of time and energy trying to alleviate it. Unfortunately, we also inflict a great deal of pain.

In labor and delivery, we draw blood, start IVs, do vaginal and rectal exams, give enemas, administer medications that cause nasty side effects, give injections, cut episiotomies, tear off tape and all the body hair under it, vigorously massage cramping postpartal uteri, force a post-op cesarean-section patient to move from a litter to a bed, or shift her from a bed to a chair when her body is screaming at her to lie still, *lie still!* We pour hydrogen peroxide into a separated C-section incision and pack it with gauze; we poke and prod at edematous and newly sutured perineal tissue. We even do crash, or emergency, cesarean sections without adequate anesthesia.

We must attend each woman in the throes of a labor that may last from twelve to thirty-six hours. We make her change positions frequently. We ask her to urinate on a bedpan. We strap her belly with monitors, her arm with a blood pressure cuff. We puncture her other arm with an IV. We place a catheter inside her uterus to measure her contractions and we screw an electrode to her baby's scalp to monitor it. We invade her back with a long epidural needle and a catheter for anesthesia. We pile all of these invasive, inhibiting devices and procedures on her and give her only IV fluids and ice for sustenance. She must cope with all of this in addition to the awesome internal forces of labor.

In my experience, the younger the parturient, the less tolerance she has for pain. In most cases, teenage girls have little factual knowledge about their bodies and even less about the process of childbirth. They are blithely unaware of the inevitable process in which their bodies are engaged. A frequent reaction to labor contractions is absolute astonishment. They want to be told, as do almost all women, how long it will take. They demand relief and stare at me with horror if I cannot immediately remove the pain. I have had fourteen-and fifteen-year-old girls go through labor clutching a teddy bear or a blanket from their own infancy, or sucking their thumbs as they regress to the little girls that they are, despite their gravid bellies. Their surprise and shocked disbelief reminds me of my bewildered reaction to an inflamed appendix. "No one told me it would be like this! You can't expect me to put up with this. Stop this pain, now!"

Once I had a thirteen-year-old girl in labor. She was mammoth, weighing nearly three hundred pounds: physically she looked like a fully mature female. But her emotional level was that of a preschooler: she whimpered and sobbed with the contractions, pleading for relief, tossing and turning in the bed, fighting off the hands that tried to examine her or adjust the monitor belts. *How awful*, I thought, *this huge young child struggling with this pain, having to endure strange hands and needles, wires and tubes on and in her body. She's not mature enough to deal with all of these invasions, much less the wracking pain of labor.*

She was, however, mature enough to conceive and carry a child, mature enough to be the victim of several sexually transmitted diseases. When she was delivered of a daughter, she looked up at her mother with fatigue and bewilderment, silently asking with her eyes, "Is it finally over, Mama?" I left the delivery room fighting tears of anger and sadness, the image of my thirteen-year-old son in my mind.

Another thirteen-year-old was so undeveloped that her pelvis wasn't mature enough to accommodate her six-pound infant. As we prepped her firm little belly for surgery, I cursed inwardly at the necessity of a cesarean; to cut into this immature little body seemed so wrong. Yet there was a child within, unable to get out without our help. So another girl was thrust suddenly into the reality of surgery—an incision, post-op pain, and so forth. As the surgical team prepared instruments and drapes, she kept asking me, "But where's the medicine? When do I get the medicine?" She hadn't understood that an epidural would be used for anesthesia and that she would be awake during the operation. I explained several times. Finally she stopped asking where the medicine was and looked at me pitifully as she whispered, "Well, then, will you hold my hand?"

"Yes, honey, I'll hold your hand. I'll do better than that; I'm going to get your mama in here, to sit here beside you and hold your hand and talk to you through the whole thing, okay?" I felt such anger at her mother; I wanted to slap her and yell, "How could you let this happen to your little girl?" As the mother of two teenagers I understood rationally how these things happen, but my emotions couldn't be denied.

I distinctly remember a seventeen-year-old black girl, still pudgy with adolescent fat, with a baby-girl face, who lay stiffly on her back, going rigid with each contraction, holding her breath except for strangled gasps. Her mother sat in the room, her presence the only support she seemed able to give, her loving concern obvious in her face.

I talked with the girl briefly, explaining what the contractions were doing, and showed her how to breathe, talking her through a couple of contractions. Then I involved her mother.

"You want to help, Mama? Okay, good. C'mon up close to the bed, just pull up the chair. There, that's good, no, you're not in my way there. I'm used to working around these chairs. Good, now hold her hand. Watch your mom, honey, she'll tell you where you are with the contraction."

I taught her mother how to watch the contractions unfolding on the monitor tracing so she could talk her daughter through the pain. I waited quietly through two contractions, making suggestions in between and praising their efforts. Then I left, saying, "Holler out if you need me." What a joy to watch that girl dig in, her apparent determination and inherent strength reinforced by her mother's presence and active support. Whenever I returned to her room for vital signs, she almost looked peaceful, greeting each contraction with a calm, silent fortitude and slow, deep-chest breathing that awed me. This young girl had never been to a Lamaze class. She just listened intently to my instructions and then put them to work. She went through labor, including the pushing, with a stamina and quiet dignity that made me love her. Her proud, shy joy as she held her baby in her arms is a treasure I carry with me still.

As a former Lamaze instructor, I was surprised, very early in my nursing career, to see some of the theories I had so blithely espoused get blown to the wind. One of the tenets of the natural childbirth philosophy is that the woman conditions herself to respond to contractions in a specific way; practice was considered essential to this method, for without practice the response wouldn't be a conditioned one. Imagine my delight in discovering that many women could pick up the breathing techniques immediately, maintaining control, and their dignity throughout labor. I learned that this ability depended on their personalities, their self-esteem, and the way in which they had been socialized to deal with pain.

Many black women use their hands and arms quite expressively. They raise their arms in the air and wave or vigorously shake their hands, fingers outspread as if reaching for help, often calling for God or their mother. "Oh Lord, help me, Jesus, help me! Give me strength! Mama, help me, save me! I'm dying!" Some will grab my hand and cling to my forearm or upper arm with their other hand, pulling at me as if to climb into my arms or yank strength from me. Sometimes one hand squeezes mine so tightly I'm bruised, while the other grasps my hip or my ribs, literally hanging onto me for dear life.

One night we had a woman whose expressiveness was downright entertaining. Her skin was dark chocolate in color and she wore her hair in an elaborate cornrow style. A statuesque, somewhat heavy woman, her limbs were well muscled and almost too long for the hospital bed. Her physical presence was so commanding that she overwhelmed the tiny, equipment-filled labor room. With huffing and puffing and loud prayers, she made it through the first stage of labor, but as the baby descended in the second stage, the urgency of its descent and the fullness in her pelvis inspired her. She began to holler:

"The baby! The baby! Get the baby!"

The resident and I rushed into the room. She was almost crowning and she didn't need to push; the baby was coming out on its own. She lay on her side, her upper arm extended, forefinger jabbing at the ceiling as she cried:

"The baby! Get it! Get the baby!"

We moved her quickly to the delivery room after unplugging and un-tangling all the tubes and wires and lines. All the while she urged us on, pointing to the sky and then jabbing her finger down at her perineum as she shrieked:

"Get it! Get the baby!"

The resident answered her every cry:

"I'll get it. I'll get it. I'm getting it. I'm getting it."

Their duet continued until the entire L&D unit and everyone on the postpartum ward heard the resident's triumphant *"I've got it!"*

The patient was a wonderfully good sport about the teasing she received for the next three days from patients and staff alike. Strolling down the hall, she'd hear "Get it!" and would raise her arm in a power salute and cry, "He got it, honey, oh boy, did he ever!"

As labor progresses, a telltale sign of increasing pain in the more controlled woman is the movement of her legs. At first it may show only in her feet, which flex as a contraction builds, but eventually many women will begin to draw their legs up and then stretch them out, pushing them into the bed, almost as though they were riding a bicycle in slow motion. It looks like an attempt to walk away from the pain while lying down.

Many women will assume the most awkward-appearing positions: body catercornered across the bed, head hanging down between the pillow edge and the side rail, forehead pressed hard against the rail, upper arm thrown over the railing, hanging limp between contractions, and clenched stiff during them. One beautiful young girl, no more than eighteen years old, simply could not be still during contractions. Petite, almost elfin, she crawled, writhed, and hopped around in bed, moving on her knees to one end and then the other, sobbing and grabbing at me and her mother. As she scrambled around, she became entangled in the sheets and IV and monitor lines, almost strangling herself in the process. She looked like a crazed, caged, wounded animal, desperately attempting to move out of the pain. I remembered how I had wanted to leave my body in the recovery room after spinal surgery and found it painful to watch her futile efforts to crawl away from herself.

We had problems with a laboring woman who insisted on sitting up or kneeling in her bed. Because her baby had been showing ominous signs of stress on the monitor, we tried repeatedly and unsuccessfully to keep her in a sidelying position to improve bloodflow to and oxygenation of the baby. Eventually, when I left the room briefly, she tried to climb out over the side rail. I found her straddling the rail, rigid with indignation and pain. Spitting with fury, she demanded that we let her go home if we weren't going to give her anything for the pain. Her labor was progressing so rapidly we didn't dare medicate her; there was no anesthesiologist available for an epidural; and we didn't dare further stress the baby with narcotics. Incensed, she refuted our explanations, saying that she didn't care about the baby, her body would take care of the baby, but we by God better take care of her or she was going home! Only the intensity and frequency of her contractions prevented her departure. Thank goodness, her labor was completed rapidly.

One night I walked into a room to investigate a drop in a fetal heart rate I'd seen on the monitor screens at the nurses' station. I found a young woman on her feet by the bed, literally jumping up and down, holding her belly with both hands. She immediately yelled at me, "This hurts, it hurts, it hurts!"

Some women cry throughout their labors. It may be silent tears or wracking, wailing sobs. One woman, a schoolteacher, said my name with every panting breath: "Susan. Susan. Susan." Never before have I ever heard so many feelings expressed in my name. There was accusation: "You can't let me go on like this!" There was pleading: "Please, please give me something, take away this pain." There was anger: "You aren't helping me, why aren't you helping me? How can you stand there and let me suffer?" There was helplessness and despair: "I just can't, I just can't." There was fear and panic: "I'm out of control, it's going to kill me!" An articulate, talkative woman earlier in her labor, she had voiced most of this to me between contractions and now telescoped all these emotions into my name. Needless to say, it was almost unbearable to hear. I was finally able to get her an epidural, which relieved both of us greatly.

One girl cried little sobbing hiccups in between contractions, her green eyes swimming, then brimming over with tears as she tried to convince me: "I'm tired. I'm hungry. I want to go home. You don't understand. This is just too much. I just want to go home. I want my mother." During the contractions, she yelled and cursed like a sailor, flinging her outrage at her husband and me: "I *can't* do it! I can't breathe. It doesn't fucking work! Jesus Christ, don't tell me to try! Shit! I *can't*!"

Another woman came to the unit before her labor got real active. She was very thin, a heavy smoker, and she looked like an inordinately tense person: scraggly dirty brown hair, nails chewed to the quick, hunched shoulders, with an acne-scarred, thin, ferretlike face. As labor progressed, she started to get mean. She was pleasant to me, but began to verbally abuse her cowed husband. If he touched her, she swatted his hands away, cursing him: "Don't touch me, you son of a bitch. This is your goddamned fault!" When he tried to talk to her, she snarled at him to shut up. Still relatively inexperienced, I was distressed by her anger and seemed to be unable to work with her successfully because she was resisting me and her husband with an incredible fury. Finally I decided to go along with her, to use her anger to keep her from totally losing control.

"Man, Edna, are you angry!"

"Yes, I am!" she panted at me.

"Well, use it, come on, be angry at these pains. Wow, they really hurt, huh? Piss you off, right? Well, curse them away, use your breath to curse them away." Surprisingly, it worked, except that in the delivery room, she reached up in the middle of a final push and scratched bloody hunks of skin from her husband's cheek and neck, as though determined to make him suffer along with her.

Another tenet offered by natural childbirth advocates is that labor doesn't have to be painful; that it is our socialization that creates the perception of labor as painful. This may be so, and may be a useful theory for people who have the inclination to educate themselves about childbirth before they experience it. But in most cases, the L&D nurse has to deal with women in full-blown labor, who aren't capable of listening to and understanding the theory. The contractions hurt something awful, and the nurse is expected to take the pain away. I can't count the number of times I've talked to women who have pleaded with me: "Help me, oh help me, I can't do this, I'll never make it, I can't stand it." Their bodies lean toward me, yearning for comfort, their hands reaching for mine: "Don't let go. Don't let go. Don't leave me.

Give me your hand, don't let go." Their eyes lock on mine, searching for the truth: "Do you really mean what you're saying? Are you sure? Do you care?" Many of them only believe me after they ask me, almost accusingly, "Have *you* ever had any kids? Have *you* been through this?"

I have learned that my hands are my most valuable aid in my work. My physical presence is somehow reassuring; when I enter the labor room I can see the relief on the woman's face. But when I hold a laboring woman's hand, I am giving her an anchor. My touch, my grip, grounds her to reality. Caught in a maelstrom of phenomenal physical forces, her body has taken over. The uterus will not be denied. It surges into a contraction, tightens and squeezes until the force alters the woman's perception of everything around her. Measured time has no meaning; a contraction seems to last forever and the moments in between are oh too brief. But I offer a hand that she can cling to, grasp tighter and tighter. Through this contact she can convey the force and share the pain with the woman whose hand she grips. My hand keeps her in the real world, lets her know she's not going mad. It even sweats with her.

My voice is my other asset. I talk to her, usually very quietly, although sometimes I have to speak loudly, with force and authority, to break through the ocean of pain in which she is immersed. In between contractions I ask her to think of the hardest physical thing she has ever done.

"Have you ever chopped wood, scrubbed floors, run a race? Well, that's what this is, hard work, probably the hardest work you'll ever do. But you can do it. Your body's designed to do this. It's a really tough act but you can help your body do its job. Work with it now. Breathe with it. Watch me, look at me, and breathe with me. I'll get you through. Don't hold your breath. Breathe, that's right. Just like this. Okay, keep going." I use the monitor as an adjunct to my voice, telling her where she is with the contraction, helping her pace herself through it.

"You're at the top now, it's not going to get any worse. Now it's coming down, just a little more, good, you're doing great, it's almost gone, slow down your breathing, that's right. Good, now rest." My voice gets hypnotic: I go for a rhythm and try to get her to keep it with me. I make her open her eyes: "Keep them open so you're not turned inward. Look at my eyes, keep looking at my eyes, lock on me." She does: my hands, my eyes, and my voice are her lifelines.

Sometimes the looks we exchange during a contraction are almost palpable. It is as though there is a steel-strong crystal filament between our eyes, binding us together and keeping her afloat during the contraction. This is an extraordinary experience. It is quite unusual in everyday life to maintain eye contact for a full minute with anyone, much less a total stranger. If she looks at me in this way, if she allows herself to use my eyes, I let her in as far and as deep as I can. I shut out everything around me and give her my eyes. I put all the support, encouragement, and strength I can into my eyes. I smile at her and show her I can see her pain, her effort, and her strength. I have absolutely no idea what she sees, but I expose my face, my eyes, and my expressions to her scrutiny, giving myself to her, trying to be as honest as I can. I don't know or care what she thinks about me later because it works. When the contraction ends, the barriers come down again. I turn my eyes from her and am the professional again, allowing her to regain her privacy momentarily. I can see the change just in her eyes, from wide open fear, need, trust, agony, and vulnerability, to a slow lowering of her eyelids: then the guarded self is there again, taking stock of what has just occurred and how she feels. We hold each other off until the next contraction, the need builds up and her eyes search for the anchor of mine.

In many cases, I can successfully transfer this visual strength to the woman's labor companion, usually her spouse. Sometimes I don't need to, because the connection is there between them; she knows she can draw on his strength without question.

One night, a couple who epitomized this synergy of man and wife came to the hospital. The woman was in hard labor, seven centimeters dilated and oblivious to everything around her except her husband. She rested on her side, holding one of his hands and rubbing his side with the other as he stood at the bedside. She never took her eyes away from his. He stroked her hair and cheeks with his free hand, smiled at her and talked her through each contraction. When a contraction ended, he would lean down and kiss her delicately and sweetly, while she wrapped her arm around his neck and held his face close to hers. So intimate was their interaction, I had to leave the room. I felt like a voyeur. I stood at the nurses' station crying because I envied them so.

Such intimacy and trust are magnificent to behold, but often it is somehow safer for the woman to expose herself to and take from me, a stranger, rather than her husband. I come to her without all the complexities of a relationship. I won't be going home with her after this time of exposure and vulnerability. I know nothing about who she really is. But I am someone who's seen it all before, who will not be threatened by her need, and I am female.

Not shy about physically engaging with my patients, sometimes I feel like I've been through labor myself by shift's end. If a woman needs more than my hands, it doesn't bother me to have my arm, waist, shoulders, or neck clutched. I've had one arm around my neck, another around my waist, and a head scrunched against my breast as a woman pushed with all her might. When I support a woman in a sitting, curled-up position for an epidural, I often find myself locked in an embrace with a stranger. She leans into me, head on my breast, arms around my waist, inhaling my scent. My face brushes hers as I lean close to whisper instructions and encouragement.

The intimacy and the physicality of it is not at all disagreeable to me. It makes me feel involved, truly engaged in this woman's work, sharing it with her in a tangible manner.

Of course, not all nurses allow or participate in such physical interactions. One incident can graphically illustrate differences in nursing styles. I was assisting another nurse in the transfer of a patient from her labor bed to the delivery table. I wasn't her nurse, hadn't even met her, didn't know her from Adam. As we were pulling the bed into the delivery room, a contraction surged over the woman. The baby was crowning and this mother had no control over the explosive forces of her body. Screeching, "It's coming! It's coming! I can't stop it!" she reached out and caught me around the neck with one arm. Her other hand gripped my arm like a vise.

"Let go! Let go, so I can get you on the table!" I pleaded in her ear. She had me in a wrestler's headlock. There I was, trapped between the bed and the delivery table, bent over almost double, being strangled by a screaming, flailing woman!

"Oh, it's coming! Help me! It's coming!"

"Let go of me so I can help you! Just let go, honey, please!"

The other nurse was hollering at her. The doctor was staring, open-mouthed, at the woman's bottom as I tried to break her grip on me, with my face buried in her neck, unable to move or see anything! Suddenly, her arm tightened even more, almost cutting off my air.

"Arghh!" We both cried out as the baby's head literally popped out of her vagina. Only then did she let me go. I laughed without restraint as I righted myself and helped with the rest of the delivery.

After everything was over, the other nurse couldn't stop talking about how unmanageable the woman had been.

"Jesus, she was awful! She wouldn't listen to us. She wouldn't do anything we told her to do. I can't stand it when a woman behaves so badly. And you, Susie! God! I thought she was going to strangle you. Why did you let her get you like that? That was horrible! I can't stand it when a patient grabs at me. How can you take that? How can you allow it? I don't want them to touch me or grab at me. I don't see how you can tolerate that."

I hooted with laughter. "Jeez, Ann, I didn't have any choice about it! I just made the mistake of being close enough for her to catch. She needed something to hold on to and I was there. It didn't bother me, except that I couldn't help you. I thought it was hysterical!"

For a couple of days, my neck hurt, my back hurt, and I had blood blisters and bruises on the arm the woman had wrung in her frenzy. I teased the mother about my wounds. At first she was embarrassed and apologetic, but as we talked about the urgency of her labor, I kept emphasizing how funny I must have looked, locked in her embrace! She relaxed and laughingly introduced me to her family as the nurse she almost strangled! For me, the bruises, the aching hands and arms, and the sore back I sometimes take home are my combat ribbons. I wear them with pride; they are physical evidence of the help I give and of the bond between me and my patients.

After four years of working as a staff L&D nurse at a military hospital, this close physical interaction with laboring women, so gratifying for me, changed when I assumed a management position at a different hospital. The L&D unit in this hospital was large: twenty labor beds compared with the five I was used to, fifteen to twenty babies delivered in a twenty-four-hour period instead of one to three.

As the night manager, I was responsible for running the unit during my twelve-hour shifts. I made assignments for the nurses, directed the flow of traffic, coordinated personnel and equipment for cesareans and vaginal deliveries, and made sure stocking of equipment and supplies was accomplished, leaving me precious little time for direct patient care. Although nights were quieter than days on this unit, it remained a busy place. I adjusted fairly well to the demands of the job. I never cried on the unit, something I'd done in the past after particularly stressful shifts. I was frequently angry and frustrated, but for the most part managed to maintain my composure. The worst part of the job, which I failed to recognize for several months, was not being able to use my skills with laboring mothers.

At first I enjoyed the diversity and the high-volume environment. But after a while I began to realize that the sheer number of patients and deliveries made it difficult at best to provide truly supportive care. While the nurses rarely had more than two patients at a time, they didn't have time to give one-on-one care. As a result, it was customary to encourage the use of epidurals for labor pain. The nurses were so pressed for time and so stressed by staff insufficiencies and the volume of patients that most of them opted for the easy way out. It takes an enormous amount of physical and emotional energy to stay with a woman in labor, to breathe with her, to encourage her, to hold her hands, to rub her back, to soothe her fears. Working twelve-hour shifts meant that some nights a nurse might have up to six patients to admit and care for, or three or four deliveries to attend. Under conditions like these, it is nearly impossible to give of oneself to so many people night after night.

Initially, this situation offended me. *What was wrong with some of these nurses? Why wouldn't they spend a little time with the patient, instead of calling for an epidural at the first sign of trouble? A little hands-on care would go a long way,* I thought self-righteously. Eventually I recognized the nurses were doing what they had to just to get through their shifts. They were exhausted by the ceaseless flow of patients, the never-ending pain, the endless paperwork. They didn't have any reserves left to hold a hand or rub a back.

As a result, the worst thing about this place were the sounds on the unit. Many a night I listened to quadrophonic screaming. Four or five or eight women in hard labor or pushing or delivering—all screaming, wailing, sobbing, grunting, cursing, retching. It was unbearable. One Asian woman keened, a shrill, high-pitched ululation that was worse than chalk screeching on a blackboard. Over and over, with every contraction, she pierced the atmosphere, until I realized I was grinding my teeth in rhythm with her sound.

Another woman let out the most blood-curdling screams I have ever heard, worse than any horror movie scream you can imagine. Two other patients on the unit at the time were so frightened by these screams they tried to walk off the ward. *For God's sake, get her an epidural* was all I could think as I worked to calm the other patients. A woman who had borne three other children arrived one night, fully dilated. She was educated, articulate, well dressed, athletic, in excellent health: all attributes one might expect to predispose her for a certain measure of control. Nothing doing. She shrieked at the top of her lungs, completely hysterical, totally unable to respond to our instructions and attempts to get her back into control. Another woman cooperatively followed my instructions about pushing, but was unable to contain the savage, throat-rending grunts that tore from her as she pushed. They reverberated through the unit like the growls and roars of a caged tiger.

I need to emphasize here that under most circumstances, I never minded if a woman was noisy during labor. I believed then, and still do, that whatever a woman needs to do to get through labor and birth is legitimate and acceptable. Locked into the inexorable activity of their bodies, many women aren't even aware of the sounds they are making or of how they are moving their bodies. The movements and noises are either unconscious, or are simply part and parcel with the tremendous effort in which their bodies are engaged. Many patients have apologized to me for their behavior, chagrined by their perceived loss of control. I insist repeatedly that whatever they are doing is acceptable and appropriate, given what they are feeling. "I don't mind your noises. Every woman has to do whatever helps get her through this. If you need to cry or grunt or moan, that's okay with me, as long as you can still hear me and respond to my instructions. If you're screaming so loud you can't hear me, then we have a problem."

If a mother is shrieking so loudly that she can't hear me, or if she's flailing around so violently that she's in danger of hurting herself, it's extremely difficult for the nurses and doctors to protect and deliver her baby. I try to explain these difficulties to her during lulls between contractions. Usually, I'll put my mouth right on her ear and whisper to her, "Shh, quiet down, listen to me, listen to me. Don't scream, just hold your breath and push. Shh, shh." Quite often this approach is effective, but sometimes I can't get through to her with a soft voice. I have to speak to her loudly and firmly like a drill instructor or football coach, to break through the wall of incomprehension and noise. Then I'm the one who's apologizing afterward, trying to explain why I was yelling at her.

I don't ever want a woman to feel ashamed if she isn't quiet or in control.

There is no right way or wrong way to give birth. I've never subscribed to the belief that a birth that isn't silent isn't dignified. For instance, it didn't occur to me to think, as Ann did, that the woman who nearly strangled me was behaving badly. But over time I've recognized the judgmental bias that develops in nurses and physicians. None of us enjoy trying to do our work in the middle of chaos. We are focused on accomplishing the tasks our jobs demand—inserting IVs, strapping on monitors, manipulating forceps or oxygen masks, trying to position legs into stirrups, or even just holding legs open so a baby can get out. Without the mother's cooperation, we can't do any of this efficiently or well. It becomes a battle between the caregivers who must do their work, and the woman, whose frenzy eliminates any possibility of control.

Over time, all nurses become judgmental, often without even realizing it. We describe quiet deliveries or peaceful labors with positive words—"she was so calm"; "that was such a quiet, peaceful birth"; "she never complained"—reflecting our biased evaluations of these births. A noisy, restless, or volatile patient is "a wimp," "awful," "a pain in the neck." Even if we acknowledge the intensity of what she is experiencing, we say she is out of control. It is almost impossible to avoid these judgmental traps, however unfair it may be to the mother. After years of experience with hundreds of laboring women, most nurses' tolerance for unruly patients has worn thin or disappeared completely, particularly if the nurses work on an understaffed, busy unit.

On busy nights at this new hospital, I found myself fully commiserating with the nurses as they called for anesthesia. The cries and wails, groans and screams made me feel like I was trapped in a lunatic asylum. I'd drive home with the noises echoing in my ears, interfering with my sleep, putting my nerves on edge. It was an unendurable cacophony. For a while I coped through humor, as did we all. A woman who had a remarkably deep, masculine voice spent an entire night dry heaving, making the most godawful retching sounds that a closed door did little to soften. In my report, I warned the day shift to put in their earplugs after they heard a sample of her basso profundo heaves. I thought seriously of making a tape of all this pandemonium so I could play it for Halloween trick-or-treaters. Voicing my idea brought gales of laughter from the nursing staff. Eventually I recognized that all these sounds, these cries for help, however verbally inarticulate, were ripping me up inside. I simply could not bear it any longer and resigned.

Thankfully, for me, many women give birth without such attendant sounds. I doubt I will ever lose my admiration for these women. There is no way to predict who will labor silently and who will scream. The emotional, cultural, physical, and psychological factors that shape a woman's response to pain are so complex that I've given up trying to predict how a woman will behave. Again, I don't condemn those who have their babies in a clamorous uproar, but oh, the joy of a patient who goes through labor with composure, quietly maintaining her sense of self.

A young woman in labor with her third baby astounded me. Unless I palpated her abdomen or looked at the monitor, there was absolutely no indication that she was having contractions except that her face would flush a bright rosy red during each contraction. Her breathing didn't change, her body didn't tighten up, her facial expression remained calm and composed. When I expressed my admiration to her and her husband, he blithely commented, "Oh that's the way she does it, nary a sign, eh?"

I cared for a pediatrician once. She maintained perfect control during her labor, breathing carefully and with full concentration during each contraction. Her husband was a masterful assistant: he counted, coached, and supported her with great effectiveness. After several hours, her cervix was only about five centimeters dilated. Apologetically, she asked for an epidural: "I just can't make it any longer without help."

"Hey, that's okay. That's why we have epidurals. This isn't an endurance test, you know," I told her. The epidural didn't work too well and had to be repeated. Through it all, she was quiet and controlled. I complimented her. "You should be in the Lamaze movies! You are doing a terrific job." She disagreed, as do most women when I praise their efforts.

It's very difficult to accurately assess one's own behavior in such a stressful situation. Most women think they're not living up to society's expectations. I admonish them: "Look. I'm an expert on labor behavior. I've watched hundreds of women go through this. If I say you're doing a good job, trust me, you are!" This pediatrician was beautiful to watch. She labored and pushed and delivered her baby with an equanimity that moved me. I felt privileged to be a part of her birth experience. Somehow her efforts, her husband's devotion, and their intense focus on keeping it together made the process feel holy. Every action, every response was directed toward the end result: their baby. I had a sense that I was participating in a ceremony or ritual of some sort, so that when I placed the baby in the mother's arms, it felt like the final blessing of a spiritual act. This aura of holiness clung to me for several days. I walked around feeling as though I had been included in something incredibly profound, even though in outward appearance it was only another birth. But this is the way I wish all new beings could come into the world. Her parents labored together for her, endured the hours of pain, thirst, hunger, and exhaustion knowing she would be worth the effort. They were commited to making her arrival one to be remembered with pride and with joy.

Another woman I took care of touched me in a similar way. Margie had been in latent labor for thirty hours before she finally began to contract effectively enough to cause cervical dilation. When I came on duty, she was exhausted. An epidural had been inserted but wasn't working. We went through the application of a second one. All the while she was contracting every two minutes. Her belly was like a rock; these were intense contractions. She panted through each one, clinging to her husband's hand, focusing on his eyes, never crying out or losing her concentration. She was lanky and muscular, with the firmness of an athlete. Cropped black hair framed her square face. She was sweaty and rumpled, but very much in control.

Finally, she began to get a little pain relief. We chatted. I got her some ice chips, washed her face, and replaced her wrinkled, sweat-dampened sheets with cool fresh linen. At my direction, Margie rested, her body sagging, her features haggard with the effects of coping with her labor. After a couple of hours, she was completely dilated and ready to push.

We pushed. Her husband and I helped support her, giving her our hands to pull against, counting and encouraging. She sat up in the bed, gripping behind her knees, chin down against her chest, face frowning and red with strain. Her husband hovered at her side, supporting her shoulders with his arm, leaning his weight into the bed. I sat on the bed facing her, watching her vulva, lifting her feet into my hands, holding them up and wide apart, using all my strength as I pushed against her feet. I'm telling you, we *pushed*!

After two hours, Margie was really hurting again. The epidural had completely worn off and been redosed, but her contractions hurt, even with pushing, and she was truly exhausted. Her back was killing her. In between each contraction she would move tentatively around in the bed, trying to alleviate the fierce pain she felt in her back. We shifted her to lying on her side, but she felt less effective in that position. She didn't cry. She didn't moan or scream or curse. She just matter-of-factly described how much she hurt, looking at me for relief. I felt so helpless. My inability to help was painfully frustrating. There wasn't anything I could do except stay in the room and endure it with her.

I kept encouraging her, praising her, stroking her legs and arms between contractions, rubbing her back, smoothing her hair, trying to convey how impressed I was with her stamina, her dignity, her will to continue, despite her obvious pain. After three hours, the doctors began to talk to her about the probability of a cesarean. They explained that they would give her another half hour because they thought the epidural had interfered with her ability to push and they wanted to give her at least a two-hour trial of effective pushing. Just as they finished talking, a contraction came. Her husband and I began our routine, holding her hands and legs, me talking quietly:

"That's it, Margie, just like that, keep it coming, you're doing great, now breathe and once more," while her husband counted smoothly, "One, two, three. . . ." He stopped counting. I looked up at him. His tired face was contorted, eyes squeezed shut, mouth unsuccessfully trying to clamp back his sobs. He cried unashamedly as I continued the count. Margie didn't stop for a second, even after she realized he was crying. She kept on pushing, with a determination that awed me.

After the contraction ended, she sank back against her pillows, silent, chest heaving. I reached across her bed and stroked her husband's shoulders as he wept, unable to comfort him. Another contraction came. She began to push as he blew his nose and picked up the count from me. We kept on trying. The doctor came in and donned sterile gloves. With both hands, she pulled and stretched down on the vaginal walls, urging Margie to push just a little harder. We worked together, the four of us, the doctor trying to manually open the last few centimeters of vaginal muscle and tissue. It worked. Suddenly I could see the head move down into the space the doctor was creating. The baby crowned after six or so more contractions and we went to the delivery room for the birth, after three hours and forty-five minutes of pushing.

I hadn't left this couple all night except to get ice and once to go to the bathroom. When I got Margie settled in her room after the delivery, I went to the nurses' station. The other nurses grinned at me: "Boy, you must be wrecked, Susie!"

"Oh, man, I am flying! I am so proud of her. God, did she work! She just impressed the living daylights out of me! What strength! What dignity! What endurance! Man, am I glad she didn't get cut!" Even though I was a physical mess, sweaty and rumpled, I was exuberant. I was so glad Margie had managed to avoid a cesarean: she earned her vaginal delivery with every fiber of her being. After so many long hours of pain and effort, it wouldn't have been any kind of failure to have the baby via surgery. But the determination and effort, the stamina she displayed, impressed me so. I found myself skipping and jumping down the hall and back, dancing with delight, relief, and pride in this woman.

After taking the baby to the nursery, I went into the room and stood at the end of the bed. Margie's exhaustion was still evident in her face, but she had brushed her hair, her eyes were sparkling, and there was a rosy flush to her face. Her husband's previous fatigue and dismay had disappeared. He was bustling with a second wind brought on by the successful completion of their arduous task and the reality of an exquisite baby son. I grinned at them and then stuttered self-consciously: "I have a little speech I want to make now. I hope you'll forgive me, but I need to tell you something." Margie and her husband looked at me expectantly.

"I just want you to know how incredible I think you are, Margie. Your courage, your endurance, your willingness to keep on trying just impressed the hell out of me. I want you to take this thought home with you, to remember always that you passed one of the greatest tests a woman ever has. No matter what life hands you in the future, I want you to always be filled with pride in yourself for the way you went through this labor, and to know that you can handle anything. You were magnificent. Both of you were. You were a terrific coach, Daddy, and I'll never forget the love you demonstrated for your wife when you cried tonight. I consider myself truly privileged to have been a part of your baby's birth."

All that I had shared with these two people—the intense exertion, the increasing disquiet we felt as the possibility of a cesarean loomed ever greater, the gentle consideration and concern they demonstrated toward each other, and finally the triumph of a healthy, squalling baby—swirled together in my thoughts. My emotions got the best of me, bubbling up as I spoke. Trying unsuccessfully to control myself made my words sound stilted and stiff. Before I was finished, I was crying through my smile.

Margie held out her arms to me, eyes shining. We embraced, a good long hug of gratitude and appreciation. Then her husband and I hugged, as they both thanked me for my help. But it wasn't my help that was important. It was the manner in which they endured, their love for each other, their concern for each other and the baby, that enriched their struggle and honored me.

I've made similar speeches a number of times over the years, always straight from the heart. Each time it follows a similar set of circumstances: a painfully long labor, a mother and/or a couple whose courage and fortitude shine brightly, somehow demanding a formal acknowledgment from me. It is almost impossible to convey how I felt after these births. In the grand scheme of things, these were just acts of reproduction. However unmarked by the larger world, to me these were times of great drama, when all the most admired human attributes were displayed before my awed eyes. I won't ever forget how they performed or how I felt working with them.

Each time is a triumph, a victory over difficult odds, and I can't ignore my conviction that such achievement deserves to be marked. If I could I would give them a gold medal, crown them with laurel wreaths, clothe them in flowers. So my awkward little orations are my fanfares for these humble heroes! Sharing such an experience with them, doing what I can to help is why I do this work. The emotional high afterward is the icing on the cake.

Probably the most difficult aspect of working with women laboring in pain is maintaining a sense of compassion for them and an appreciation of their pain. As I have described, it takes a great deal of energy to truly assist a woman in labor. Many factors enter into the task of supporting the patient. The first is staffing. In many hospitals the nurse-patient ratio is rarely an ideal one-to-one. Most L&D nurses struggle to balance the various needs of two or more patients. There have been times when I was assigned the care of four laboring patients, and times when, as a nurse manager, I attempted to care for five women while simultaneously orchestrating the entire unit. Needless to say, at such times the care given is the bare minimum. Dealing with the patient's pain at such times means calling for an epidural or pushing narcotics as rapidly as possible, the goal being to simply shut the woman up, as cruel as that seems, so that another patient can be attended.

The second factor that inhibits supportive nursing is burnout. It's almost inevitable that nurses working on an understaffed L&D unit will reach a point of exhaustion. It becomes nearly impossible for them to respond appropriately to a woman in pain. In order to survive the shift, the job itself, L&D nurses become hardened to the suffering of their patients. As I've noted, many of them will make snap judgments about a patient's behavior, ignoring her pleas for help on the grounds that she is a wimp. Most nurses will call for an epidural as soon as it is practical rather than encourage and support the mother with comfort measures, breathing assistance, and their presence. If the patient doesn't cooperate with whatever assistance is offered, the nurse may react with coldness, hostility, and indifference. The first time I saw two experienced nurses lolling in chairs at the nurses' station, eating pizza and laughing together, while screams of agony emanated from a labor room, I was speechless with disbelief. Years later I was able to understand, to a point, their apparent indifference.

When a loud noise is made near him, a newborn will react initially with the startle reflex, followed by crying. If the sound continues, eventually the neonate will habituate to the sound, accept it as part of his surroundings, and shut it out. The same phenomenon occurs with L&D nurses. As their time on a unit extends through years and hundreds of patients, they become habituated to the sounds of labor. Their compassion, their ability to relate to each woman as a unique individual and relieve her suffering wane, until they perform their nursing tasks with a humdrum routineness, inured to their patients' pain and fear. In fact, I'm amazed when I see nurses who can still appreciate an individual patient, who can still be attentive to that patient in a caring way. Such attention and compassion is extremely difficult to sustain if the nurse is overloaded with patients.

Another serious factor is the attitude of many physicians, particularly overworked residents and HMO doctors who are expected to care for too many patients at one time. An attitude develops. The doctor will actually say—how many times have I heard this?—"It's not *my* fault if she's in pain. This is labor." Another doctor might snort. "What did she think when she got pregnant? That it would just slip out of her without any pain? Too bad. She's just got to take it. I didn't get her pregnant." And so on. Doctors will refuse pain relief if labor is just beginning, because they don't want to stop it or impede its progress. Doctors will refuse pain relief if the mother is too close to delivery. Doctors will also refuse pain relief because they just don't believe the patient is really in pain.

I have watched young, inexperienced doctors refuse pain relief because the patient's labor isn't following the "labor curve"—the textbook pattern of labor progression. Never having experienced any serious pain themselves, many young doctors simply have no concept of what the patient may be feeling. No one can ever truly know what another person is feeling, as I've said, so if the patient isn't in active labor, the physician assumes she's a wimp. The underlying, usually unspoken attitude is that she deserves what's happening to her. Sometimes that attitude is even voiced: she should've known better, she shouldn't have gotten pregnant in the first place, she has no courage, she hasn't been cooperative, or simply because she is female.

Yes, unfortunately, there are obstetricians out there who don't like their patients because they're women. I have watched physicians do cervical exams with a viciousness that resembles rape, totally impervious to the woman's discomfort. If she fights the doctor off, the response is quick and brutal. How disturbingly odd it is to watch a man get furious with a woman who attempts to shake off his hand, to forcibly withdraw his fingers from her vagina. The indignation the doctor will express—"Don't touch me! Keep your hands away from here, from me!"—is astonishing. I wonder how many doctors would permit another person to invade their bodies with such abrupt, assaultive actions and not try to fight them off.

If a woman is out of control, it isn't unusual to see a male physician shrug his shoulders with disdain or hear him make disparaging, sexist remarks about the patient—"What do you expect? She's a typical female!" I think back on the way I was treated during my labor with my son and believe my obstetrician exhibited the same distaste for me. Sometimes doctors will punish the woman by withholding pain medication or performing an episiotomy or a forceps delivery without adequate anesthesia. This misogyny is so subtle that it is difficult to confirm, and most nurses, myself included, are very hesitant about confronting the offender.

One resident was completely unaware of how painful his cervical exams were. I believe he assumed that exams were supposed to hurt, never considering in his blithe ignorance that his technique was the cause of the pain. Most women simply endured his exams, writhing under his hands, weeping soundlessly as he dug around inside them. One woman in hard, active labor was so incensed at his insensitivity that she vehemently threatened him with bodily harm if he didn't get his hand out of her. "If you don't stop, if you don't get out of there, I'm going to slug you in the face!"

Another obstetrical resident was blatant in his misogyny. He hated his OB patients, hated the rotations on the labor deck, and made no bones about it. A number of patients refused to be examined by him; several actually left the hospital rather than submit to his hands. One husband assured me that he would "beat the shit out of that bastard if he comes anywhere near my wife!" Curiously, while being inundated with complaints about his insensitivity and brutality from obstetrical patients, I heard several gynecology patients sing his praises to the skies!

I have held the hands of women during cesareans while they screamed, moaned, and sobbed with pain. "I can feel that! I can feel what you're doing! Oh God, you're killing me!" The anesthesiologists standing at the head of the operating table would actually tell the woman she wasn't feeling what she was feeling. "It's just pressure you're feeling. It's just a pulling sensation!" These residents believed their monitors, their dosages, their medications, and simply refused to acknowledge the patient when she didn't behave according to their expectations. One woman told me after her cesarean that she actually believed she was going to die and that we didn't care.

On many occasions I have watched an exhausted, irritable doctor repair an episiotomy while the woman literally screamed, ignoring her pain or commanding her to be still. The doctor simply didn't want to take the time to give pain medications and allow them to work before doing a repair. I've witnessed similar torture scenes during the manual removal of a placenta. A doctor who wouldn't consider doing a D&C—dilatation and curettage, a widening of the cervix and scraping of the uterine lining—without anesthesia will casually reach his or her whole arm up inside a woman to pull out a placenta or explore for placental fragments, while the patient goes crazy with pain.

If I challenge the doctor, asking her to let me give the patient some medication, frequently the response is hostile: "This will only take a minute if she'll just be still. I'm almost finished." It is as though the physician has forgotten that the tissues she is stitching, the uterus she has her fist in, the cervix she is pulling at are actually connected to a thinking, feeling being. The doctor's priority is to finish the task, complete the surgery, find the source of the bleeding. The patient is a faceless, anonymous thing that is keeping the doctor from attending to other tasks, like getting a meal or sleeping. When the patient or the nurse voice objections, however justified, the doctor becomes perplexed and irritable, surprised that his actions are perceived as unreasonable. Sometimes the doctor will order heavy-duty narcotics with the aim of "snowing" the patient, putting her to sleep so the doctor doesn't have to listen to her complaints. Occasionally this is appropriate, but often the end result is a mother who can't function and can't interact with her newborn for several hours after delivery because of the opiates in her system.

A final factor that contributes to the difficulty of sustaining compassion for laboring women is, on occasion, the patient herself. Every once in a while, a woman will use her contractions as devices to manipulate those attending her. I have had quite a number of patients who acted out to an extraordinary degree while their significant other was in the room. A woman may be hollering throughout her contractions, weeping and cursing in between them, while her support person hovers anxiously over her, remonstrating with the staff over our apparent indifference to her distress. When this person leaves, for whatever reason, the patient suddenly becomes cooperative and quiet.

These patients usually appear to have some sort of dysfunctional relationship with their support persons. They have an underlying psychological need to perform for their relatives or spouses, and derive some secondary gain from such performances. No amount of placating, no comfort measures, no encouragement seems to help. In many cases, the support person causes, or at least contributes to, the behavior by his or her actions and words. He or she may be aggressive with the staff, questioning everything belligerently, or becoming extravagantly effusive with concern over "the poor thing's terrible pain."

One example of this behavior stands out in my memory. This young woman was absolutely infuriated when her husband was ordered to a distant military unit. Throughout her pregnancy, she expended much effort with everyone in a position of authority in her attempts to have her husband recalled to her area. Finding her extremely difficult to deal with, the obstetricians called for a psych consult. The psychologists got her involved with a support group for wives of deployed soldiers. She was advised by members of the support group to "act crazy and then they'll have to bring him home."

What a challenge! This girl was something else! She was stick-thin and heavily made up. She simpered onto the unit, clutching the arm of her companion, bending over and grasping at her belly, swearing she would die from the pain. When we examined her, with much difficulty as she wriggled around on the exam table, she was only one centimeter dilated. A monitor tracing of her contractions helped confirm the diagnosis of early labor. We tried to get her to walk around. She refused. We tried to send her home. She refused. Finally, we threw up our hands and admitted her; I was assigned to be her nurse. She refused everything I was supposed to do for her, while excoriating me for allowing her to suffer. She was completely uncooperative. She cried loudly for her husband, calling his name over and over. She refused to get into bed. She refused to change positions. She refused the monitors. She refused the IV. She was abominable. I explained, cajoled, argued, and pleaded with her. I'd finally convince her to get into bed only to have her leap up with a contraction, whining and whimpering. She would insist that she had to go to the bathroom and then wouldn't get up and go, urinating in the bed. I tried to start her IV four times. Every time I brought the needle anywhere near her arm, she would yell and pull away from me. I could feel my blood pressure going up. My face got hot and red, my hands trembled, and I was perspiring heavily. Irritation and then downright anger clogged the back of my throat as I attempted to do what needed to be done.

I rarely lost my patience with any laboring woman, but this time I was so aggravated by her obnoxious intransigence, I had to physically remove myself from her presence. I walked out of the room, near tears and shaking with anger, to ask the charge nurse for assistance. Only by speaking to this woman in harsh tones, treating her as a misbehaving child, and threatening her with expulsion from the hospital, were we able to manage her during labor. Her histrionics made working with her an unmitigated ordeal. When her support person left for a break, she was more reasonable, but still blatantly attempted to manipulate the residents and nurses. In the end, she was successfully delivered and discharged from the hospital with enormous sighs of relief by all who had interacted with her.

Much to my dismay, two of the worst patients I ever worked with were nurses. I really think the first woman was psychotic. During a contraction, she would scream at the top of her lungs, lunge around on her bed, slamming her legs and arms against the side rails, lifting her body up and smashing it down again against the mattress, hurling curses at everyone. As soon as the contraction was over, she would lie back against her pillows and casually pick at the polish on her fingernails, calmly speaking about how terrible the pain was and what bastards we were to punish her in this way. She accused us of torturing her, keeping her prisoner, wanting her to suffer and die. No manner of consolation was accepted. She didn't want us to help her; she just wanted to abuse us. After she attempted to kick me in the face, missing by bare inches, it became necessary for me to take turns with another nurse in giving her care. Neither one of us could tolerate being in the room with her for more than fifteen minutes. The entire staff was shaken by her viciousness. I felt like I had truly been through the wringer by the time we finally got an epidural into her, even though she had only been on the unit for three hours.

The other nurse was the first nurse I'd ever had as a patient. She tried to manage her own labor, questioning every activity and every decision, arguing about techniques, criticizing every effort. We weren't doing anything right, according to her, and she knew because she'd "been in this business for a long time." When her labor intensified, she grew abusive, calling us names and accusing us of denying her appropriate care. She slapped one doctor and spit in my face as she screamed at me to take away her pain. I was horrified and deeply embarrassed by her behavior. I had to struggle hard to contain my anger at her. I wanted to slap her and yell at her about her unprofessional behavior. It was a surprise when I realized that I expected her to "behave better" than other laboring women precisely because she was a nurse. This was, of course, an unfair expectation and I fought against it, but her actions made it very difficult to suppress my underlying feelings.

Sometimes the patient is her own worst enemy in the opposite way. There are women who think they have to suffer to have their babies, that it is expected of them, and that they must do it silently and efficiently. While these women can be a pleasure to work with since they are so undemanding, it is easy to overlook the severity of their pain because of their silence. They will apologize when they make noises or cry. They will try to maintain good manners in the midst of hard labor, croaking out their pleases and thank-yous, when getting through the contraction is all that matters. Not only is it possible for the nurse to miss the patient's real, justifiable need for relief, but such behavior conditions the nurse to judge even more harshly the women who aren't as stoic in their need.

Any combination of the above factors can make caring for a patient in labor an onerous task. Balancing the patient's needs, the safety of the mother and the baby, with all the other agendas held by the doctors, the anesthesiologists, the nurses, the support persons, plus the layers of cultural and social expectations that each of these people bring to this birthing experience, can be challenging at best and harrowing at worst. If the nurse perceives herself as the patient's advocate, as I do, then on occasion she will undoubtedly be in conflict with her colleagues. Usually, it is easier to acquiesce to her co-workers than to stand up for the patient.

This is a continuing battle for me. After a lifetime of avoiding conflict and confrontation, I must make the effort on a daily basis to accurately determine the real priorities; to force myself to question, prod, and plead with physicians and other health-care workers to obtain the best care for my patients, even though those patients won't ever see me again, while I must get along with my co-workers in order to survive on my unit. Many times I have failed my patients by neglecting to fight for them because it's easier not to. The fact remains that giving birth is a painful process. The body is stretched, literally and figuratively, to its limit. It is imperative that I maintain my awareness of this fundamental fact and dedicate myself, patient by patient, to rendering the most supportive care possible, to alleviating whatever pain I can, so that the mother's experience can be a positive one. If I am unable to do so consistently, then I shouldn't be a labor and delivery nurse.

Chapter Five

🌿 NURSING SCHOOL

For more than two years I taught prepared childbirth classes in my home. Six weeks for each group of parents, sometimes two classes running simultaneously—which could be quite confusing: What had I told each class? In the beginning my organizational skills were nonexistent, but of necessity I learned to keep notes, arrange topics, set priorities. I struggled with two small children, an active social life of dinner parties and long afternoons with friends who were also the mothers of small children, the increasing demands and meetings of the childbirth organization, and my marriage. I was making the transition from being solely a wife and mother to being a working woman, even though the work I did was for the most part unpaid and volunteer.

My husband wanted my attention. My children needed my attention. The parents in my classes paid for my expertise. The childbirth organization desperately needed my time. I spent hours and hours on the phone in my kitchen, talking about the problems of childbirth in my city, of how to address the pertinent issues and provide consumer advocacy for our couples. I wiped runny noses, drove carpools, made breakfasts and lunches and dinners, arbitrated two small children's squabbles, and worried about the menus for the elaborate dinners my husband and I hosted. I have vivid memories of stirring Hollandaise sauce while discussing cesarean rates, of searching behind the kitchen cabinets for a treasured Lego doll while arguing about the necessity for a hospital consumer guide, of nuzzling my baby's neck while listening to a mother describe her baby's birth. All of this was simply my personal experience of the feminine issues of the seventies, the struggle to define for myself what my role as a woman should be: Housewife? Mother? Prepared childbirth instructor? Consumer advocate? All of it? Some of it?

Priorities, setting priorities. If I wanted to pursue my interest in the birth process, I had to discover ways to do that while meeting my obligations to my family. Nothing new. Many women face the same conflict. My husband supported my interests, but grew increasingly frustrated with my activities, because they interfered with a smoothly run household, and worse, because I wasn't being paid for my efforts. It was hard to handle the conflict I felt on class nights, as I devoted myself to strangers' needs while my children were tucked into bed by their father. The core of my identity, my sense of self, was *mother*. Before anything else, I was Rebecca's and Michael's mother. I had never yearned for a career; I had no desire or need to work, to earn a living. In the implicit contract of my marriage, my job was to be housewife and mother, my husband's to bring home the bacon, which he did, and well. He had always assured me that if I wanted to work, we could afford to hire help. But he grew accustomed to my being at home, and never seriously considered my going to work, knowing how vehement I was about raising the kids myself.

But now, something had shifted in me, catching both my husband and myself by surprise. My need to be involved with childbirth, my hunger to be active in this sphere fired me up while leaving my husband cold with indifference. Slowly my interests and activities began to coalesce into a definable goal. My fascination with pregnancy and childbirth intensified as I began to realize that teaching my couples wasn't enough. It was frustrating to be off-stage during the critical event. I met with these people for six weeks before their deliveries and once afterward. Our classes focused on a life-changing event and the preparations and expectations for that event. But I wasn't there for the birth. I missed the fireworks. I laid the groundwork but didn't get to be a part of the actual experience. I knew my contribution was valuable, as evidenced in the feedback I received from my couples after their babies were born. But I wanted more. I wanted to see if the content of my classes really was pertinent. I wanted to know firsthand which techniques were effective, and why. I wanted to be there!

I was asked to be the labor coach for a woman whose husband wasn't available for her delivery. After meeting privately with her, teaching her the breathing and relaxation techniques and getting to know what her expectations and concerns were, I was finally called one night to meet her at the hospital. Her labor was brief and uneventful: a lovely second son was delivered safely and satisfyingly to the happy mother. But for me, it was a pivotal experience. The sights, sounds, and smells of the labor and birth, the effectiveness of my coaching, the significance of my presence all combined to push me exuberantly into another world. Watching that baby emerge from his mother, standing right there at her leg, so close I didn't need to stretch to touch his wet little head, was such a high! Everything was so vivid! I was completely involved, yet detached enough to observe even as I participated, and I loved it. I wanted to do it again, to be more involved, to know more, do more, affect more of what happened to the mother. I didn't like being an outsider, having to defer to the nurses. I wanted to put my hands on the baby as it emerged. I wanted the credentials and the right to be there, to be part of the team of people who orchestrated the entrance of a new being into our world.

Thus I decided to go to nursing school and get a nursing degree as the first step toward a long-term goal of becoming a nurse-midwife. I didn't want to be a doctor: I was too old and too devoted to my kids to give up the years it would demand. I didn't even want to be a nurse, but recognized that I wasn't radical enough to be a lay midwife at home deliveries and that a bachelor of science in nursing was one of the necessary credentials for becoming a hospital midwife. Books about nursing, midwifery, and childbirth cluttered my kitchen and my bedside table. Course descriptions and requirements and college applications arrived in the mail. The master's degree in English literature, which I had been pursuing desultorily for several years, was left unfinished as I investigated the different nursing programs in my area. I took night classes in sociology, introductory psych, and education at a community college as I negotiated with my chosen nursing school to accept credits from my first degree, completed nine years earlier.

By this time Michael was three years old and in nursery school half a day, and Rebecca was seven, in second grade. As my interests and activities outside the home expanded, my marriage grew increasingly troubled. As I struggled with everything—kids, husband, school, childbirth classes—I was also fighting serious depression as I confronted the break-up of my first long-term relationship. Overwhelmed by responsibilities and painful emotions, I went through the last year of my marriage in a fog of anguish. The only saving grace during that time of upheaval was the classes I attended. They offered me a few hours a week in which to slough off my wretchedness through intellectual challenge.

The dissolution of my twelve-year marriage coincided with the first real courses of my nursing education. As I waded through microbiology, developmental psychology, chemistry (the bane of my existence), and anatomy and physiology, I struggled to maintain my children's home and well-being. Drastic changes in my financial status accompanied whopping tuition bills. Cold sweats at the checkout counter in the grocery store were not uncommon: did I have enough money to pay for this food? I juggled my schedule so I could meet my course requirements without taking too much time away from my kids, whose father now lived in another house.

Housekeeping became a lost cause. Autumn leaves and spring growths threatened to overwhelm the yard. The third floor was rented out to a succession of college students, the basement closed off in the winter to save on fuel costs. I learned how to fix the plumbing, how to rewire an electric light, how to put up storm windows. I bought a car, negotiating alone with sleazy, sharklike salesmen, and learned to drive a manual transmission on the hills of my city, bucking the car up and down the streets, laughing and crying hysterically with the kids in my carpool as we lurched and stopped and groaned through all five gears. And I spent more nights than I like to remember, crying alone in my bed after spending hours trying to comfort two forlorn little children who couldn't understand what had happened to their family.

Through it all I went to school. Tests, quizzes, labs, classes. Teachers of vastly disparate ability: the incompetent ones were subjected to my complaints, criticisms, and written letters of protest to the administration. I had no time to waste. I wasn't nineteen, living in a dorm, having my bills paid by my parents. I was thirty-four, a single mother of two, in need of a livelihood, scraping by on the pittance that was child support. And I knew what I wanted to do: I wanted to earn a living through work with women in labor. Give me the knowledge, the technical skills, the credentials; make me an expert, a professional. Don't waste my time!

The good teachers enthralled me. I never missed my anatomy and physiology class: the instructor was the best college professor I'd ever had, through four undergraduate years and uncounted postgraduate courses. He made the human body sing for me. The exquisite elegance of this mass of bone and muscle, tissue and fluid revealed under his humorous, knowledgeable tutelage enraptured me. I spent hours marveling at the musculature of my hands, thrilled to be privy to the underlying structure of this appendage so long taken for granted. As I slipped into exhausted sleep at the end of impossibly long days, the thump-bump of my heart, the whisper of my respirations, the relaxation of my skeletal muscles coalesced into an intimate lullaby: It all works right and I know how it works.

Finally the time arrived for actual clinical experience. Two months of twenty-hour days during my sophomore summer were devoted to learning patient care. A white uniform and nurse's cap, white stockings, a stethoscope, scissors, blood pressure cuff, and the all-important comfortable nursing shoes were purchased. Photographs were taken of Mommy in her nurse's uniform, grinning like a idiot out on the sidewalk by the house. Aid was enlisted: my youngest brother came for the summer to help me with the kids and the house, to free me for the rigorous hours and efforts of clinical work. Friends and family pitched in with money for tuition, time for the kids' care, and oceans of emotional support as I ventured out, into the world of hospitals and sick people, doctors and nurses and lab techs, machines and medicines, monitors and operating rooms, bedpans and emesis trays. I was terrified, elated, anxious, angry, and eager. I was changing, growing into a new role, a professional identity—a nurse.

The nursing school I attended was part of a small women's college in the heart of the midwestern city that was my home. Most of my classmates were eighteen to twenty-two years old. There were only five or six women who were returning to college after years spent out in the world. We were the continuing education students, occupying a rather ambiguous place in the class. One woman was in her fifties, a postmenopausal biology teacher who wanted a new challenge in her life. Another was a beautiful woman in her late twenties who'd been married and a mother early in her teens. With her daughters now teenagers themselves, she was pursuing the education she'd missed. Another, the daughter of a minister—one college degree under her belt already, a year of missionary work in India behind her, nearing thirty and getting married for the first time during our nursing-school days together—became my closest friend.

The rest of the students didn't know quite what to make of us older women. Our life experiences, our emotional and physical maturity, and our avid pursuit of education set us apart. We were irritants in class. We always sat in the front row. We asked questions and demanded satisfactory answers, whereas the girls just wanted to take notes and get out of there. After a few weeks of lectures, every time I spoke up I could hear rustlings and mutterings behind me. Students back there were thinking, and sometimes saying loud enough for me to hear, "Oh, please, here she goes again!" But even as we irritated, we enlightened. When we studied adult development and sexuality, the classes rocked with arguments and hilarity as two of us older, "experienced" women related the changes in our sexual appetites and activities. The girls sat, mouths agape, as we assured them graphically and passionately that sex in middle age was something to look forward to; that they couldn't begin to know how fantastic a sexual future awaited them in their mature years. At one point I exclaimed, "I'm in my *prime!*" and my cohort stated, "I wouldn't go back to the fumblings and insecurities of my twenties for anything in the world!"

The girls began to seek us out for advice about assignments and reassurance when they felt uncertain about their performance. I hadn't thought of myself as an adult until then, even though I was married with two kids. It was seeing myself reflected in the eyes of these young women that made me recognize how far ahead of them I was. I really didn't feel any different, physically or emotionally, than I had felt when I was in college nine years earlier. I was still intimidated by professors, worried about reading lists and tests, scared of sounding foolish in class. But as I watched the girls in class and in the hospital, I realized that, by God, I was a grown-up! After one particularly hilarious sexual development class, one young student stopped me in the hall.

"I just wanted to thank you for what you've contributed in this class. I've been having problems with my mom. She and my dad divorced just a year ago and she's dating now. It's caused me all kind of confusion. But listening to you, realizing that my mother is just a couple of years older than you, all of a sudden I was able to see my mother as a woman, not just as my mother. I feel like I'm seeing her as a person for the first time in my life, and I can see that she has needs and desires similar to my own."

As I thanked her, I swallowed my shock over being old enough to be her mother, which I was, and felt glad about the consciousness-raising we "old ladies" were accomplishing in our classes. Another day, as we struggled into scrubs for a clinical rotation, all of us anxious, I said something about how jittery I felt before each of these forays onto the wards. One of the girls, a thoughtful academic achiever stopped dressing and looked at me with amazement. *"You're* nervous?" she asked dubiously.

"You better believe it. My stomach is in an uproar!"

"But Susie, how can you be nervous?" she asked.

"Huh?" Now I was puzzled. "What do you mean, how can I be nervous? God, I worry about whether I'll remember the drug info, whether I'll remember to wash my hands, or what happens if I get a patient and don't know a thing about his illness? Jesus, Martha, I have the same fears you have, you know, performance anxiety, I guess. Why does that surprise you?"

"Well, I never would have thought it, Susie. I mean, you come across as the most confident, competent, self-assured person I know."

I whooped with laughter, thanked her for the compliment, and couldn't stop thinking about the exchange. Was this how other people saw me? It sure wasn't the way I thought of myself. But I realized that I must be growing into this new identity if I was already projecting such an image. This was the first of what were to be many instances over the next ten years when I was able to step aside from myself and actually recognize personal growth. Until then I hadn't had time to reflect on my life since becoming a wife and a mother, and I was not consciously aware of how those roles had changed me. Thrust back into the sanctuary of a college campus, side by side with just-emerging young women, I came face to face with my adulthood.

Some of the nursing instructors weren't quite sure how to deal with us older women, either. It took some time for me to surmise that a couple of my professors were actually threatened by my presence and active participation in their classes. One teacher described, in class, a dream she'd had about trying to teach the class while all the students turned into crying wild babies over which she was unable to exert any control, until I stepped in and helped her. She thought it was funny; I thought it was revealing. Another instructor was unremittingly aloof and hostile to me in our individual conferences. She went out of her way to reprimand me for my manner of interacting with patients, which she felt was too informal. After she assigned a lower-than-expected grade to my research paper, coauthored with my best friend, I was forced to admit that no matter how hard I tried, or how good I was at my work, she simply had to assert her dominance over me. Upon careful examination by people other than just myself, it seemed obvious to me that her objections to our research paper and to my clinical skills were groundless and in direct contrast with the top grades and excellent evaluations my friend and I earned from other professors.

The first days in the hospital were a homecoming for me, an unanticipated recognition that all this was familiar from my days as a doctor's child. My fears and insecurities were countered by an unexpected realization that I belonged here; all I had to do was learn what I needed to know to do the job. The skills and knowledge were almost incidental to the discovery that I was where I belonged. Just let me at those patients!

The first patient I was assigned to care for was a tiny, white-haired, frail, seventy-six-year-old woman whose hip had been replaced. I charged in, all gung-ho to finally be doing patient care. Within an hour I was frantically searching for help, after trying by myself to change her bed linens while she was in the bed. She was half-hanging out of bed, breathless with exertion, close to a serious fall, while I left her unattended. How humbling, and how lovely she was in her patience with me, encouraging me, brushing off my effusive apologies for getting her all tied up in the sheets, denying the pain my efforts had caused. "You have to make mistakes to learn things, honey. I'll be okay, don't you worry about me," she assured me.

Each mistake, each endeavor was a learning experience. I was flushed with excitement over it all. I couldn't wait to start each day. Walking into a patient's room and introducing myself was exceedingly difficult the first few times. Why should these poor people have to endure my fumblings, my ineptness? But each one of them welcomed me, appeared to enjoy the one-to-one attention, having their own private nurse. Little did they realize how little I knew, until of course old blabbermouth Susie told them: "I'm a brand-new nursing student. I don't know what I'm doing. Will you teach me? Tell me how I should do this so it will be the most comfortable for you." Every one of them helped me. They were wonderful and I loved our interactions, even while I cursed the hours, the nurses' notes, the quizzes, the clinical conferences. I had little interaction with the doctors, to whom nursing students are invisible, or the nurses, who were just glad to have us doing patient care for them.

Not surprisingly, I flourished in my maternal-child health course. The years of Lamaze teaching had provided me with far more knowledge than I had realized. Curiously, the clinical rotation on the labor and delivery unit left me feeling dissatisfied. The hospital in which we trained was huge and the care given was impersonal. I hated the indifference the staff displayed toward providing family-centered care and watched with dismay as women were treated as though they were on an assembly line. *Get an epidural, roll her into the DR, expose her to the lights, slice up her perineum, throw on some forceps, and get that kid out.* That was the way it looked during my brief rotation, so it wasn't hard to decide that I wasn't going to work in that baby factory.

Nursing school was difficult, far more rigorous than my first college experience or even my graduate school courses. There was a calculated effort on the part of our instructors to make the program as stressful as possible, to weed out those who couldn't handle it. Implicit in all our assignments and clinical rotations was the philosophy that being a nurse was an extremely taxing job with enormous responsibility and little authority. If we couldn't tolerate the pressures, the hours, the burdens imposed in nursing school, we wouldn't make it on the job. Our work was attacked, our appearance maligned, our efforts belittled. We were inundated with useless information and trapped in boring classes that dealt with obscure, never-to-be-used data.

Great emphasis was placed on the importance of identifying ourselves as professionals, which necessitated the acquisition of a solid foundation of theoretical knowledge. Clinical skills were always secondary to our understanding of the theories behind the diagnosis and treatment of a multitude of diseases. Truly excited by the intellectual stimulation, I burned with frustration over the lack of time to absorb all the theory and we all argued with the instructors about how little we were being taught when it came to clinical skills. "Don't worry," they assured us, "you'll learn the techniques on the job. We want you to know why you're doing whatever it is you do for your patient. That's more important." None of us believed them. We were frightened about being on the spot and not knowing what to do.

The pressure to learn, to make the grade, to complete the assignments while performing without error was intense and stirred up a mini-revolt in my senior year. I didn't believe that anyone needed to be "broken" during their training to prove they could handle the stress. The woman who taught me psychiatric nursing and supervised my sophomore summer proved that excellence in nursing could be developed without undue harassment, without insulting or demeaning the student. She was strict and demanding, but she never humiliated a student. Working under her tutelage was stimulating and fun. Even as I participated in the student protests about the curriculum, hours, and unrealistic expectations of our teachers, I grew in confidence about my abilities to be an effective nurse. My professional identity was slowly and painfully being acquired.

Several experiences during my clinical rotations dramatically affected the development of that professional identity. With each rotation, most nursing students evaluated whether or not she or he wanted to continue in that particular field. Like medical school, nursing school emphasizes general, basic nursing skills. Courses and clinical practice are organized around specific areas of illness such as pediatric nursing, obstetrical nursing, and medical-surgical nursing, a catch-all term for patients hospitalized for an illness or surgery, but the education in those areas is, of necessity, a general overview of each field of study. After obtaining a nursing degree and passing state nursing board exams, the graduate now a registered nurse—can begin work in a specialty, such as neurosurgical nursing or psychiatric nursing, but must continue her training in that field. Seminars, workshops, specialized and mandatory training courses, conferences and daily exposure to the idiosyncrasies of the specialty are all part of this continuing education, which most states require for licensure.

Some students knew exactly what specialty they wanted, just as I had no doubts about being a labor and delivery nurse. Nonetheless, I approached each area with interest and curiosity: Would I find this specialty appealing? Med-surg, psych, community health? Curiously, I was surprised at how much I hated pediatrics. I'd always been good with kids and considered myself a good mother, but I despised every day of that rotation. The primary reason probably was because all my patients were hopeless. The horror of these lost children was just too close to home for me.

I took care of a three-month-old baby with cytomegalovirus, a virus that could cause brain damage and death; microcephaly, abnormal development of the head and brain; cleft palate, cleft face is more like it—she had a gaping hole instead of a mouth and nose, and a prognosis of only a few months of life. Her mother and father had completely rejected her. I tube-fed her and rocked her, writhing with revulsion and pity. Then there was the twelve-year-old microcephalic kid admitted for heart surgery: she was so severely brain damaged that she only responded to the world when she felt pain— and getting "pre-op'ed" for surgery was painful.

I observed a two-year-old diabetic child who had gone into a coma at her first birthday party. She had been in the intensive care unit ever since, carved up from the multiple surgeries necessitated by her malfunctioning little body, on a respirator, with a tracheotomy that had to be suctioned every hour; her brain a mush of old bleeds and crossed electrical impulses. I watched the intensive-care nurse bathe and dress her, manipulate her arms and legs through range-of-motion exercises while she jerked and spazzed in the large crib, her eyes sightlessly scanning the walls and ceiling, her mouth grimacing into tortured "smiles," her soundless crying accompanied by huge tears. When the nurse finished her morning care, she sat down in a rocker with the child on her lap and began to read Raggedy Ann to her, a book much loved by my babies. I completely lost it, stumbling out to the hall, leaning against the wall in the bathroom, crying hard at the hopelessness of it all. My instructor was irritated by my loss of control.

Two of the geriatric patients I cared for had similar impacts on me. The first was an eighty-year-old stroke victim in the hospital because she had fractured her ankle. When my instructor gave me the assignment, she told me the patient was aphasic—unable to speak.

"Great! Thanks a lot! How the hell do I do all the nursing process history and such if she can't talk? Why me?"

She laughed. "You can handle it, Susie."

This was only my second ever patient. I was scared. I had to spend three days with this woman and she couldn't talk! How would I communicate with her? How would I know what to do? When I walked into her room, I was terrified. She was big, probably weighing two hundred pounds, with a body grown flaccid and pendulous with old age and inactivity. If you looked hard enough you could see the shadow of what had once been an imposing, strong woman. Her shoulders were broad, her hands large and gnarled with arthritis and years of work on an assembly line in a textile factory. She had soft hazel eyes hooded by sagging skin and her wary distrust of strangers. A look of helplessness and defeat warred with flashes of anger and frustration over her helplessness. She couldn't talk, had minimal use of her right hand, and a broken ankle, swollen and wrapped in gauze.

Those three days were among the most rewarding and insightful days of my training. The woman was alert and aware of everything. She just couldn't talk. I made up for it: I talked and talked, loudly at first until I reminded myself that she wasn't deaf. I explained everything, working out an awkward system of communicating with my hands, facial expressions, and the process of elimination so she could tell me what felt good, what needed to be done, what hurt. Her verbal sounds were repetitions of the syllables "ba-duh-ba-duh," but her face and hands were remarkably expressive and I picked up on her body language rapidly. During a bedbath she grew frustrated with her inability to convey a thought to me. I felt her body stiffen under my hands. When I looked down into her face, I realized that she was near tears.

"It's okay. You can cry. This must be really difficult. I can't understand you and you're trying so hard to explain something to me. I'm so sorry." She wept. I stopped the bath, held her hands, leaned in close and tried to share her grief, her agony of being locked behind a wall of silence.

The next day I made up for my ineptitude in silent communication by washing her hair. She'd been in the hospital for eleven days; her hair was dirty! She moaned with pleasure, smiling broadly up at me, as I shampooed and lathered and rinsed. It was clearly ecstasy, a small sensual pleasure to lie in a bed and have someone wash your hair. As I finished the rinse, she raised both arms, took my face in her hands and pulled me down to her, embracing me tightly, murmuring her ba-duh-ba-duh's of gratitude. Briefly speechless, I hugged her back, both of us caught firmly in each other's arms, water sloshing all over the bed, as we two women acknowledged each other. It was a hug I'll never forget.

The last day together, we "talked." I asked her questions. With sign language and lots of guesses, she told me about her family, her work for forty years in a textile factory, her daily routine at home. I watched the way hospital personnel avoided contact with her and actually pleaded with the brusque, impatient intern who put a cast on her leg.

"She's in pain! You're hurting her. Can't we give her something first before you manipulate her ankle?" I realized my initial fear of this patient was no different from everyone else's: they were afraid of their inability to communicate with her, so they shielded themselves from her muteness by ignoring her. This is the way so many people have been socialized to deal with the handicapped: act like you can't see them or just ignore them. My instructor was correct: I handled it, but in truth, it was my patient's willingness to let me inside her barrier of silence that made the time so meaningful.

Another geriatric patient unknowingly had a profound impact on my sensibilities. He was an ancient, wizened black man, surely in the final weeks of his life. A foot had been amputated as a result of diabetes. The other foot was blackened, with skin like charred parchment, ready to pop and ooze at the slightest bump. He lay in his bed, lost to the world, hallucinating, crying out about his missing foot that hurt so much. Multiple problems, the results of his advanced age and the ravages of diabetes, were being treated during this hospitalization. I silently bathed him, changed the dressing on his stump, tried unsuccessfully to get some liquids into him and felt helpless in the face of his disintegration. At one point, he began grabbing violently at something in the air above his face, screaming incoherently at what only he could see.

"He's there! There! I got to get him! Oh Jesus, save me! He's come for me! I got to get him! Get away! Get away! Oh, my foot, how it do hurt!" He thrashed wildly, eyes bulging with apprehension, locked in a vicious struggle with a private reality. I held him down, fearing what would happen to his remaining foot if he were successful in his attempts to rise from the bed. His agony finally subsided and I watched him slip into unconsciousness, breathing stertorously.

Badly frightened, I called my instructor into a linen closet to describe his breathing and my fears. "He sounds like he's dying. I've counted forty-five seconds between breaths, and then he only inhales because I command him to '*breathe*'! What was he seeing? What are we doing for him? What if he dies on me? Why isn't he on an apnea monitor, or in an ICU?" Everything we were doing for him seemed so cold, so impersonal. We were treating his symptoms, but he was alone, disoriented, out of his mind, reduced to almost nothing. And slowly his disease was devouring his flesh. It wouldn't be long before the other foot had to go; it was already in the early stages of gangrene. I had an image of him being literally sliced and trimmed and nipped away, until there was no more flesh to support his ravaged soul. I felt sure he had hallucinated the devil, for surely what was happening to him seemed to my overwrought imagination to be evil. I don't know what happened to him after the three days during which I provided rudimentary care for him.

After working with many geriatric patients, I recognized that I truly loved being with elderly people for extended periods of time. With that time, one could learn so much. Long lives, with all their history and wisdom, foolhardiness and vanity, were there to explore. They could teach me so much and I was old enough to know how to listen, to glean the pearls of wisdom and reject the foolishness. I actually liked to study their bodies, to see how time and life had marked them, to search for the young adult and the long-lost child under the wrinkled folds of skin, the bowed legs, the fragile fingers, the clouded eyes. This intimate scrutiny, an effort to internalize and accept the aging process, was something I'd never done before, always taking for granted my own youth and health. Now, in my thirties, I was beginning to perceive hints of my own mortality in a way a twenty-something woman rarely does. To spend a day with an old human being, washing the aged body, dressing and soothing the hurts and wounds, afforded me an invaluable opportunity to appreciate the effects of long life, both the beautiful and the loathsome.

But how those geriatric patients could suffer, and how all our technology and science could extend their suffering. How diminished they became, how much we stole from them: their dignity, their autonomy, their privacy. I couldn't bear it. I didn't have a thick enough skin. I hated having to bathe and shave that tortured little old man, take his vital signs and change his linens. I wanted, in the worst way, to pick up his wasted old body, to cradle him in my arms and rock him in the rocker, crooning lullabies to him. I only wanted to soothe him, not cause him more pain. I was new and raw at this. I hadn't learned yet about inflicting pain, causing discomfort in order to accomplish a treatment and give the necessary care.

My experience on a locked psychiatric ward in a Veterans Administration hospital was another pivotal event in my training. During our orientation to the hospital, we were escorted to the psychiatric ward. At the door, the nurse educator brandished a huge black key, a key that surely locked the dungeons of a tyrant's castle.

"You will be given a key like this. You will keep it on your person at all times. You will not open the door for anyone unless they produce identification, verifying that they are staff and have a reason to go through these doors." She unlocked the door and we were ushered onto the ward. The door clanged shut behind me. I listened to the key being turned in the lock. I broke out in a cold sweat, my senses all working overtime. Oh, the smells, the drab gray walls, the drugged, expressionless faces of the patients shuffling down the halls, the dreary dayroom that reeked of cigarette smoke, stale bodies, and old magazines. I grew increasingly anxious. I couldn't focus on the orientation. I didn't care what anyone had to say. I wasn't afraid of the patients. I just wanted *out of there*! I almost fought my way through the crowd of students exiting the ward. Hyperventilating and fighting tears, I headed for my car, my best friend running to keep up with me as I tried vainly to explain my horror.

I talked to my adviser about this anxiety attack, voicing my fear of being locked in, the claustrophobia it produced within me. It was all so relative: What, I asked, really separated those locked in from those free to leave? There were times in my own life when I could have been one of those patients.

My adviser was understanding and supportive, cautioning me to take my time to recover while reassuring me. She felt my sensitivity was a quality that would enhance my interaction with the patients on the ward. I spent a month there and learned to control my anxiety about the locked doors, but I never could touch the key without horror. It was so blatantly malignant, that oversized, black-painted, old-fashioned key. It was a key of denial. It meant no freedom, no autonomy, no right to go about as one might wish. It kept the "crazies" and their keepers in, and fresh air and freedom out. Even though I was fascinated by the men locked in, particularly the Vietnam veterans, whose stories enthralled me, I despised that key.

The emotions I experienced in response to these various patients were understandably intense: I was an initiate in this arena of suffering, of diminishment, of lost hope, of the frailty of human existence. But those emotions, those reactions were also significant intimations of what would be problematic for me throughout my future as a nurse. My adviser addressed this issue in our last counseling session. She told me she knew I would make an excellent nurse, in part because of my sensitivity to and compassion for my patients.

"Your caring enhances all your interactions with your patients; it is what makes the difference between being a good clinical nurse and being an outstanding one. But I worry about you because you tend to be too idealistic, too judgmental; you see things too much as just black and white. There are very few situations in nursing that are strictly black and white, Susie. You need to be more accommodating. You'll never survive if you don't learn how to compromise. I think you will, you have great promise. And don't ever lose your compassion, your caring. If you find you don't care anymore, get out of nursing! Don't let yourself become jaded. Don't lose your ideals."

I listened. I agreed with her evaluation of me. I figured that with time I would get better at accommodating. I vowed silently to hang onto my caring, my compassion, swearing I would leave nursing if I couldn't care anymore. But I hadn't even graduated yet—my future patients were out there waiting for me. Ready and eager to be a real nurse, my adviser's words registered only superficially. I had to live the life before I could truly understand her message.

At the end of my senior year, exhausted from the sustained effort of four years, I seriously injured my back. Running in the street against all the rules, my dog was brushed by a passing car. I lifted her and held her as I assured the driver that she was okay. Then a disc popped in my spinal column and I spent the next month on the floor, nearly incapacitated by the pain. To be "floored" by the dog was just too ridiculous!

My final med-surg exam was taken lying on the floor of the classroom. A job-hunting trip was postponed. The week before graduation I wrote a speech for our pinning ceremony. Lying in my bed, reviewing the events of the past four years as I tried to integrate all those experiences into an understanding of my personal growth, I was overwhelmed by emotion. With tears streaming down my face, the words poured from me. They encapsulated four years of agony, of learning and doing and feeling, of training to be a nurse.

"Tonight we celebrate the end of our education and training as student nurses. With the receipt of these pins and our diplomas tomorrow, we achieve the status of graduate nurse. This achievement is the result of an arduous process through which we have suffered and matured.

"Remember how strange we felt the first clinic day of sophomore summer? How we all giggled about the dazzle of our new white uniforms and how we hated the caps? Remember how conspicuous and silly we felt? How scared we were to walk into that first patient's room, introduce ourselves and perform our first assessment? Or when we had to do our first morning care, our first dressing change, our first injection? Remember how uncertain we felt when a staff person or a client's family asked us questions? 'Who—me? I don't know anything. I'm just a student nurse!'

"We've moved from constant supervision, from being observers watching our instructors perform procedures, to being almost independent practitioners. From having every nurse's note, every med, every care plan checked, to caring for three or more patients simultaneously and doing our own charting and giving our own medications. We've moved from stumbling over our words and blushing with embarrassment when we had to make oral presentations in nutrition class to the completion of our research projects and those most professional research presentations of two weeks ago.

"We have absorbed an enormous amount of conceptual, theoretical, and factual information. We've been taught how to assess, plan, implement, and evaluate a multitude of nursing actions. We have agonized through exams, bellyached about grades and assignments and suffered many of the symptoms of stress and even burnout. We lost several classmates along the way, signed protest petitions, and burned with indignant rage at the workload, the woeful lack of time, and our own insecurity about really knowing what we were doing.

"We learned from our texts, our instructors, the clinical staffs we observed and with whom we worked, and especially from one another. But our most important resource in this learning process was, of course, our patients, our clients. They are the people I wish to acknowledge tonight.

"We've learned from class lectures and our texts that a person who is sick is vulnerable in many ways, unlike any other time in that person's life. Our patients revealed themselves to us, physically, emotionally, psychologically, and spiritually, in a manner that would rarely occur if they were not ill. They allowed us, total strangers, to touch, measure, probe, and stick them; to wash their bodies and assist them in the most intimate of physiological functions, because we were nurses—in white—authority figures. They told us details of their lives, their marriages, their families, their plans, their failures, their fears. Because we were there, with our charts, medications, and stethoscopes, we were privy to their anxiety, their pain, their humor, and their joy.

"I remember the ninety-eight-year-old man, chagrined because, in his words: '*Humpf!* Four women around my bed and I'm not worth a good goddamn!' I remember the ecstatic, glowing face of a young pregnant woman from Jordan with no English, as she watched on the sonogram the gently moving, ever-so-tiny arms and legs of her wee baby. I remember the awesome dignity and good spirits of the diabetic man who'd just lost his second leg to the disease and yet was thinking ahead about how he would drive with two prostheses. I remember the tears of pleasure of an aphasic, semi-paralyzed stroke victim, an eighty-year-old woman, who wept when I washed her hair for the first time in the eleven days she had been hospitalized. I remember the fifty-year-old cerebral palsied woman, who learned all of our names and thanked us every time we log-rolled her to change her bed, even though she hurt like crazy each time we did it. I remember the eighteen-month-old baby who didn't cry before or after eye surgery because I held him the entire time, until his daddy could take him from my arms and thank me with quiet relief and gratitude. I remember the mother of four who talked about what it meant to her to have a diagnosis of leukemia and to undergo chemotherapy. I remember the men on the psych wards at the V.A. hospital, sharing the pain of their experiences in the military and in Vietnam. And I remember one young man, a car accident victim, with multiple fractures and a massive hole in his leg from a bone infection, laughing and showing us the scrapbook of his accident and months-long hospitalization. These are but a few of my experiences: each nurse here could list her own similar memories.

"These people have no idea what they gave us. They thanked us for our help and encouraged us, patiently, as we fumbled and practiced and struggled with their linens, bedpans, emesis bowls, dressings, IVs. We owe them a large debt, for without them we wouldn't be here tonight. We must remember that we are not finished being students, because we will, of course, always be learning from our patients. And we haven't learned just nursing skills from them: we've learned life skills—compassion, generosity, courage in the face of pain and fear, dignity in the most undignified of circumstances, perseverance in the face of setbacks, tolerance of the indifference and even cruelty of others, and pleasure in the smallest of life's daily activities. *They* nurtured *us*, even as we tried to nurture them.

"This interaction assumes a significance in our professional lives and enhances our personal lives. In effect, we are entering into a covenant with all our future clients: a promise to look beyond the illness and the pain, into the eyes—the doorways of the personality or, if you prefer, the soul—of each of our patients. To *connect* with each other, to recognize and acknowledge each other, not only as caregivers and receivers, but also as unique individuals, exposed and vulnerable fellow human beings.

"If we hold this promised awareness clear in our minds as we work in the future, our patients' care will be more truly effective and supportive and we will be enriched beyond measure, by their gifts of gratitude and trust."

At the ceremony, I stood at the podium, my hard-earned nursing pin flashing gold from my uniformed breast, and read these words to my classmates, instructors, family, and friends. The people who had held my hand through my own passage were there to hear me, to accept my thanks, to share my pride in my achievement. It was a singular event in my life; now I was ready to find a job and really do this thing called nursing.

Chapter Six

DOCTORS

I've always been drawn to doctors: not surprising since my father has been a doctor for more than forty-five years. When I was a little girl, Daddy was the general practitioner for a small town in Texas, a big fish in a little pond. He radiated power: people were drawn to him, always, not just when they were sick or hurt. He was a big man, six feet-four, 230 pounds, blond haired and golden skinned. He looked like a Viking. He flew a little airplane, drove fast cars, went cave exploring, and drank with abandon. He worked eighteen to twenty hours a day in his enormous general medical practice, smoked heavily, and consumed gallons of coffee. Somewhere in all this activity he found time to keep my mother pregnant: nine pregnancies in thirteen years, seven living children.

My memories of my father when I was five, six, and seven years old were of a giant, a man with a loud voice, a huge body, and an aura of restless energy. He gave unstintingly to people, to his practice, day in and day out. He took his pleasures with ferocity and was rarely home to give directly to us. He provided for us, to be sure, listened to stories from my mother about our days and our adventures, and found interesting houses for us to live in, but when he was home he was exhausted. Our mother told us, "Daddy needs his sleep, we need to be quiet, we must be quiet so Daddy can sleep. He works so hard for us, he takes care of so many sick people." Sometimes his patients came to the house. I would spy furtively from around a corner, listen at the door, study them with a child's bald curiosity about illness. Careworn, in pain, anxious, bleeding, gasping for breath through asthmatic spasms, they would sit in the living room, waiting for my mother to fetch Daddy. They called at all hours. My mother always answered the phone, adept at screening calls, warning us children repeatedly to respect his patients' privacy.

I loved to go to Daddy's office, to watch him be a real doctor, and as the doc's daughter, I had the run of the place. I scoured all the desk drawers for interesting items, studied the medicines in the locked cabinet, handled the equipment and exam table. The most memorable times we had with Dad were going with him on nighttime house calls. After dinner, if he made it home in time to eat with us, he would pile several of us in the car and off we would go. In my memory it was always hot, but the night air coming in the car windows cooled us, evaporating our sweat. We would drive down long dusty roads to isolated houses in the Texas hills. I'd sprawl in the back, listening to the murmur of my mother's voice as she filled him in on the day's events at home and questioned him about his patients and the office activities. Sometimes he would tell us stories about his patients, or about some funny thing that happened at work, or he would describe who we were going to see and why they couldn't come in to the office.

These trips had a surreal quality: traveling down dark roads at night, keeping him company, helping him stay awake between houses and patients, participating however indirectly, in his caregiving. The isolation and the smells of the sandy cedar-scrub hills, the heat, the night air, and my dirty, tired siblings gave me the sense of being a family for brief bits of time. Then Dad would pull up in front of a stone house or a wooden shack, climb out of the car, reach in the back for his black medicine bag, and trudge to the front door; he was separated from us, burdened by his knowledge, his skills, the patients' needs, alone in his work. And we'd wait, sleepy, in the car.

Thirty years later, the first time I entered a hospital ward as a nursing student in my white uniform, sweaty with nerves, I experienced a sort of epiphany as I walked around to the inside of the nurses' station. I belonged here. This felt like home. Without knowing it, I had been waiting all those years to have the right to be exactly where I was. Finally I was allowed to pick up a chart and read its contents, to walk into a patient's room and talk directly to that patient. The ghost of my father followed me through the rooms, the routines, the banter, the work. The countless times he'd taken me on rounds; introduced me to patients, nurses, lab techs, doctors; all the illnesses he'd treated, the surgeries he'd performed, the bodies he'd touched, the care he'd given—somehow it was all with me. I understood him better on some level: now it was my turn.

So, doctors fascinate me. I've read innumerable books about, for, by doctors. My oldest brother, Dan, not coincidentally, is an astounding, dynamic physician in his own right, an ambitious, hard-driving doctor. Both my father and my brother influenced me vastly and powerfully. Much of what I do with patients and how I do it is a direct result of methods learned unconsciously from them. Sorting out what is me, my own, is a tricky business.

During my clinical rotations in nursing school, I was surprised to discover that the doctors routinely dismissed me as inconsequential. The student badge on my shoulder literally rendered me invisible. Not one doctor was interested in what I might think or say about a patient, even though I was spending an entire shift with that one patient. It was my first exposure to the pecking order in the medical world.

When I first started work after graduation, the doctors in the military hospital intimidated me. They were authority figures. They held sovereignty over everyone. No matter that I was fifteen years older than they; that as residents, they were still students, inexperienced in their work and their personal lives. No matter that they often hadn't the vaguest idea about what they were doing. I couldn't see that at first. I could only see "Doctor": Daddy, Dan, knowledge, medical school, effort, long hours, appalling responsibility, authority.

So I watched them and learned. I also loved them. Every time I did something for a doctor, I was doing it for my father and my brother. Most of the time I had no difficulty interacting with these physicians-in-training. My eagerness to learn must have been obvious to them. I respected their knowledge and truly desired to facilitate their work. I also clowned around a lot, was cheerful, encouraging, and supportive. In the past, I had watched my brother agonize through his years of training, while his family developed and grew without him. His devoted wife grew almost brittle with the effort of sustaining the family alone. I knew what some of the costs were to human beings who embraced medicine as their life's work.

It is, for interns and residents at least, all-consuming. It demands so much, takes so much time and physical and psychic energy, that they are permanently warped by it. A year after I started work I went to a third-year resident's farewell party and was scandalized by the adolescent behavior of the men and women with whom I had been working. They got drunk and wallowed in beer, wrestled and talked sports, sex, and medicine. They also assumed that any single woman wanted to get laid, and they tried, unsuccessfully, to ensure that one of them maneuvered me into bed. I was outraged by their presumptions, realizing that they didn't see me as a real person at all. Socially I found them at first pitiful, and then boring.

But at work I studied them. I wanted to see how each personality dealt with similar situations. I wanted to know them, understand them, learn from their strengths, and avoid their weaknesses. I watched them move through their residencies and grow into their role as obstetricians. Each year they did a three-month rotation on L&D, with increased responsibility each rotation. They were on call every third or fourth night throughout the three years, so we spent a lot of time together. On the professional level, I got to know them intimately.

Working nights, I was the one who roused them from exhausted, unconscious sprawls to assess a patient, to deliver a baby, to do an emergency cesarean. I saw them fresh in the morning in military uniforms, making rounds, and I saw them at night, wrinkled and stale with rumpled hair and bad breath after thirty hours hours on call. I watched them sweat through their scrubs and surgical gowns in the operating room, brought cold compresses for their necks while they sutured a uterus. I wiped beads of perspiration from their faces, smeared lubricant on their gloved fingers for internal exams, handed them speculums, swabs, and instruments. I massaged their necks while they wrote endless orders and notes, gave them backrubs in the quiet hours, made up beds for them, guarded their sleep, laughed and talked and argued with them.

And I was always, always asking them for something:

Mrs. A needs an order for Motrin.
Can Mrs. B have bathroom privileges?
Will you check the lady in room four?
Mrs. C has a fever.
Mrs. D is crying about her IV.
Mrs. E is pissed off and threatening to leave AMA.
Come now! The FHT's are in the 60s!
I need you now! The baby is crowning!
Mrs. F has bruises all over her hips, a rash, a cough, a fever, a distended abdomen . . .
She's bleeding, she's in pain, she's lost her baby . . .
I can't get this IV.
I can't find this baby's heartbeat.
I can't pick up these contractions.
I think she's ruptured.
There's meconium.
Why are we doing this?
Why aren't we doing that?
Will you . . . ?
Can you . . . ?
Would you . . . ?

I'm just one nurse, reasonably competent, reasonably adept at screening out unnecessary tasks and questions for the doctors. I'm also sensitive about abusing doctors. I'm aware of their exhaustion, their patient load, the demands on their time, knowledge, and abilities. I try to do what I can to spare them. But I am just one nurse. On that ward, in an average twenty-four-hour period, a single doctor interacted with a minimum of six nurses and nine nurses' aides and LPNs. The patient load would be at least six labor patients, twenty-four post-and antepartum patients, and, at night, twenty-five to forty patients on the gynecology ward.

The question then becomes: How do these young physicians survive at all? Knowing the stresses, all their little personality quirks, their irritability, lost tempers, physical complaints, and whining take on a new meaning. We ask too much of them. We expect them to be decent, polite, compassionate people while we flog them unmercifully with responsibility and need. What is amazing is how terrific most of them are.

Watching these residents develop was one of the benefits I derived from working in a teaching hospital. Early in my first job, before I understood the gradations of rank and year, I had a terrifying experience with a first-year resident. I hadn't been in the system long enough to even realize that he was first year and new to the role of managing the deck. He was responsible for what happened on L&D, backed by the in-house presence of the second-year resident (usually asleep), and the authority of the third-year resident (usually at home, with his beeper). Every decision he made was subject to question. He had to demonstrate just the right amount of independence and will to make decisions, but was strictly limited in what he could and could not do without consulting with his superior.

On this particular night, we had a patient whose amniotic membranes were ruptured prematurely, at thirty-six weeks. She had been a patient on the ward for two or three days. When she began to experience regular contractions, she was transferred to L&D. A cervical exam indicated that she was completely effaced and two centimeters dilated. The contractions were not causing her any discomfort; she appeared to be in the prodromal—the early, or latent—phase of labor. After a couple of hours, I was dismayed to see a variable deceleration, a decrease in the fetal heart rate, on the monitor. Until then, the fetal heart-rate pattern had been reassuring. I stood at the bedside watching the monitor. A couple of contractions later, the heartbeat fell precipitously into the eighties. (Normal rates for a fetus are 120 to 160 beats per minute.) I watched, hoping it would recover immediately, but when the slower rate continued for more than thirty seconds, I flew out of the room to get the resident.

"Roy, come quick! Mrs. Smith is having a decel!" I shook him awake in his chair at the nurses' station. Dressed in blue scrubs, wrinkled and smelly after fourteen hours of work, Roy was a dumpy little fellow. His body had gone soft in the years of medical school and internship. An incipient paunch hung over his pants and his arms were fleshy and pasty white. Unruly straw-like hair now stuck up all over his head, as he rubbed sleep from bloodshot eyes and ran his fingers through his hair.

Mumbling, Roy stumbled after me into the patient's room. The deceleration was now an episode of bradycardia—a heart rate below one hundred beats per minute; the heartbeat was staying in the seventies and eighties. Roy did a cervical exam: still two centimeters. I stood there, helpless, watching this baby's heartbeat putter along far more slowly than it was supposed to. This had never happened to me before; I didn't have the faintest idea what to do. To improve the blood flow to the uterus, I turned the woman to her left side, to no avail. I was waiting for the doctor to give me instructions. He stood there staring at the monitor, mumbling, "She's only two centimeters, she's only two centimeters."

"Roy, tell me what to do, what should we do?" I asked quietly. He didn't respond, just walked around in a circle. The patient watched us with growing fear in her eyes. I kept waiting for Roy to say something. Then, three minutes into the bradycardia, the LPN flew into the room. "Get up, get up, get on your hands and knees! Come! Quickly now! On your hands and knees, lean into the bed, yes! Get the doctor, we must do a C-section! Quickly now!" she commanded, as she put an oxygen mask on the woman, after positioning her on her knees to alter the fetal position, in case the heart rate was being affected by cord compression.

Galvanized by her presence and actions, I ran for the second-year resident. We had the woman back in the delivery room for a crash section in about four minutes, and delivered a stressed, meconium-covered baby, who rallied and recovered fully. I was terribly shaken by the whole event. My inexperience and total dependence on the doctor frightened me. His lack of knowledge, his inability to recognize the seriousness of the situation and call for help, also frightened me, and made me realize how much at risk that mother and baby were, alone on a labor unit with only an untried nurse and an inexperienced doctor to guard and protect them through the still hours of the night. Had it not been for the LPN, Roy and I might have stood there paralyzed with fright and incredulity forever. Needless to say, that was the one and only time I waited for a doctor to respond to what I perceived was an emergency. From that night on, I wasn't afraid to get a senior resident if I thought the first-year doctor was unduly hesitant about acting. I had learned in a frightening way about the inexperience and resultant indecisiveness of first-year residents.

With hindsight, I realize one of the most frightening aspects of caring for laboring patients is not knowing what you don't know. You can have all the theory in your head; you can read all the books and know lab values and labor curves and signs and symptoms and so on, but when you are responsible for the well-being of a woman and her unborn baby, you have to know how to recognize trouble and what to do when it occurs. That night I didn't know what to do. I'll never forget the feeling of terrified paralysis that overwhelmed me as I watched that monitor and waited for the person in charge, the doctor, to direct me. My idealism about doctors was challenged in a big way that night, when Roy seemed as frightened and uncertain as I.

Four years later I was caught off guard again by the doctor mystique. This time it was inexcusable, since I had watched four sets of first-year residents go through the agony of managing the labor deck. I had been off for a week, putting all thoughts of the hospital and my work aside, relaxing and recuperating after several months without any real vacation. I returned, refreshed and cheerful, to find a new obstetrics team on the unit. This was nothing new: every three months a new team arrived. But the doctor in charge that night was a new man, someone I hadn't met before. It was the first of

July, the traditional day when a new year of residency begins. It was also this doctor's first night on call as the first-year resident in charge of L&D. And dumb Susie, on vacation for a week, didn't make the connection.

A lovely young Asian-American woman showed up in the exam room, her husband holding her hand and looking concerned. I went through the routine with her, timing and palpating her contractions as I asked questions and took vital signs. She looked "active": the contractions were three to four minutes apart, moderate in intensity, and she was hurting. I taught her how to breathe with the contractions and calmed her down before I called the resident. He examined her and pronounced her to be one to two centimeters, which surprised me: she certainly looked farther along than that. I put her on the monitors and went to attend to another patient. It was a busy night; about an hour later I discovered that after reviewing her strip to make sure the baby was okay, the resident had sent her home. He had not rechecked her cervix.

The phone rang two hours later, for the umpteenth time. Hurriedly, I answered, "Labor and Delivery, Ms. Diamond, can I help you?"

"The baby's in the bed! The baby's in the bed!" A man's heavily accented voice yelled at me.

"Okay, slow down. Slow down. Tell me who you are and what's happening." I responded.

"This is Specialist Woo! I was just there with my wife. We came home like the doctor tells us, and the baby is now in the bed!"

Oh my god, it's the young woman we sent home, I thought. *I knew she was in active labor! Christ!* "It's okay. Now, is the baby breathing?" I asked.

"I don't know, I don't know!" he wailed.

"Well, is it moving at all? Is it moving its arms and . . . ?" I stopped. I could hear a baby crying loud and hard in the background.

"Okay, Specialist, it's okay. Just wait, I'll get someone who can tell you what to do now. Just hang on for a minute, don't hang up the phone, okay?" I ran to the residents' sleep room and roused the second-year resident, hurrying him to pick up the phone as I explained that the baby had arrived at home. I listened on the extension as the sleepy doctor instructed the man to call 911 for an ambulance to take his wife and baby to the nearest hospital. The father was so flustered he went to get a pencil to write down the number, thinking it was an extension of the hospital. The resident had to tell him three times, "just dial these numbers—9, 1, 1—and tell the operator who answers that you need an ambulance."

An hour later, I answered the phone again. This time it was an L&D nurse from another hospital. She was laughing as she asked me for prenatal information on Mrs. Woo.

"Is the baby all right?" I asked.

"Yes, he's fine, a little cold, but just fine. Who checked her over there anyway?'' she asked. I told her the first-year resident had sent the patient home; that I had been surprised because I thought she was in active labor and farther along than one to two centimeters. The nurse giggled, then blurted out, "The residents over here are having a good laugh about this; your first-year was an intern yesterday!"

Oh, good grief, I thought, *it's the first of July! This guy probably hasn't checked many more cervixes than I have. Boy, did he blow it! Boy, did I blow it—I know when I see an active labor patient; why didn't I get someone else to check her?* As it turned out, the baby did fine, no harm was done, but we had erred. My first response was to laugh about the father yelling, "The baby's in the bed, the baby's in the bed!" But later that morning, as I described the scene to the OB chief, he kindly but firmly reprimanded me. According to him, I was at fault because I was the experienced nurse and the resident was brand-new at his job. I should have double-checked his exam before allowing the patient to leave (even though at this hospital, nurses weren't permitted to do cervical exams).

Stung, I apologized and accepted responsibility for the bad call. Afterward, I fumed over having the blame placed on me: I was the nurse, not the doctor! I didn't have the legal authority or the credentials to diagnose the patient. I had knowledge of and experience with laboring women, but to say that I was responsible for the resident's decision was wrong, unfair—and not unusual. The nurse is frequently held accountable for medical decisions that are not hers to make. But in this case, I was filled with remorse when I thought about the events of the night. I hadn't been watchful of the patient; I hadn't paid attention to my own gut instincts and considerable experience, but had blithely, if unknowingly, allowed a completely inexperienced doctor to make a bad call. On top of all that I hadn't even been sharp enough to realize the date and its implications.

The worst, if humorous, part about the whole story was that this poor husband had driven his wife across the city, a good forty-five-minute drive, to bring her to us. Then he'd driven her home, as we had instructed him. When she went off in the ambulance with the baby, he didn't know where the medics were taking her and assumed it was back to our hospital, so he drove back to us! His wife was across town in another hospital, so he had to drive back across town for the fourth time! Boy, did I feel bad for that man. What a terrible night for him and one he could never forget, since it was his first child's birthnight!

I was able to laugh about it only because the baby was okay. But, God, what if the baby hadn't been okay? What if it had been born with the umbilical cord around its neck? Or meconium—fetal bowel movement in the amniotic fluid—a possible sign of distress, potentially lethal if the baby breathes it in? How could I laugh at the misery of those two frightened young people, alone in their apartment with their child being born and no one at all to help them? Bad business, Susie, bad call. I had let them down and put them at risk; unknowingly, unintentionally, to be sure, but I certainly had erred.

Over time, I learned to identify a physician's level of experience by simple observations of behavior. In the beginning, as I've noted, the doctors were all "doctors." After a year of work I knew that the guy who couldn't keep his eyes open while he wrote orders, who looked harried, irritable, and sick, was the first-year resident. The woman who walked in fresh and alert in her military uniform, makeup and hair just so, without the obvious signs of too little sleep, ready to take on the patients and nurses: that was the third-year resident. The second-year man fell somewhere in between: he looked more rested, more in control, but usually acted so relieved to have survived first year and was so obnoxious to the current first-years that his self-confident aplomb came across as a little suspicious.

It bothered me to watch a young man or woman go through the first year. The demands on these new doctors were horrifying, and the toll taken on their bodies and psyches was great. Many of their patients were high risk. They had to cope not only with normal laboring women, but also with seriously compromised pregnancies. They were a part of a team, to be sure, but this year was their crucible: they had to prove, through doing it, that they could handle the stress, the workload, the complications. Most of them became so irritable that it was difficult to work with them. Each reacted to the stress in unique ways: one resident always felt ill. He pushed the nurses unmercifully, demanding that we wait on him, bring him coffee, Motrin, ice packs for his head; he wanted us to give him massages, or to let him sleep. He whined about our questions and snapped at us when we didn't meet his expectations. He would walk around the unit at night, holding a perineal ice pack—a sanitary napkin with ice in it—to his forehead, moaning about his headache.

One night I called him to check a patient. He grumbled into the room looking dazed with sleep, slipped on a glove, and sat down on the bed. He muttered to the patient to "assume the position" and slid his two fingers into the woman's vagina. Then he turned away from the patient. Standing across the bed from him, I couldn't see his face. I waited. The patient waited. The doctor sat there, staring at the wall. Now I have witnessed med students, residents, and interns fall asleep while assisting in surgery, actually dozing off while holding a retractor in someone's sliced-open abdomen. But I had never seen anyone fall asleep while examining a cervix. I questioned him: "Dr. Rouster?"

"Just a minute," he replied, his fingers still in the patient's vagina. We waited. He sat, staring at the wall. A minute passed. Then another. I started to speak when I saw his shoulders begin to heave. *Oh shit, what now? Is he crying?* I wondered. "Just a minute," he mumbled, fingers still inside the woman's vagina, his shoulders convulsing. "You can do this later," I offered, still not sure what was happening, feeling increasingly uncomfortable about the patient and her husband, who looked at me with bewilderment. "I'm, I'm, arghh," the doctor groaned, as he vomited. I rushed around the bed, reached down, and physically removed his hand from the patient's body. I lead him from the bed to the sink, where he threw up again. He had taken a double dose of Motrin for a headache on an empty stomach and was threatening to vomit the entire time he was in the room! I moved him out into the hallway, apologizing to the patient, mortified that this doctor had actually sat there with his fingers in a patient's vagina for a good four minutes before I removed him from the scene. It made for some hilarious laughter later as the story was recounted to other residents moaning about first-year nightmares, but it was grossly inappropriate behavior and most embarrassing for me and the patient.

The worst thing that happened to these young doctors was the steady erosion of their ideals and their ability to be compassionate with patients. Many of them gradually slid into active resentment of patients. They became angry with the patients for needing them, for expecting them to provide care. The patient became the bad guy—the one who woke them at night when they were desperate for some sleep, who went into labor at three in the morning, who was wrong to need certain lab tests in the middle of the night, or a cesarean, or a cervical check. The patient wasn't cooperating, dammit! The nurses only made it worse because we wouldn't leave the doctors alone; we made them get up, write orders, make decisions, deliver babies, take phone calls. But the patients were really the problem to these residents.

Without consciously realizing it, doctors grow adept at expressing their frustration and hostility toward the patient by couching their words in an accusatory manner.

> *Your cervix isn't dilating.*
> *You're not responding to the medication.*
> *You're not contracting efficiently.*
> *You're not pushing hard enough.*
> *You're bleeding too heavily.*
> *You haven't urinated in the past several hours.*
> *Your temperature is too high.*

Explanations or complaints voiced in this way place the blame squarely on the patient. Few physicians realize the impact of these word choices. By saying to the patient, *you're not contracting efficiently,* instead of *the uterus isn't contracting efficiently,* the doctor makes the patient responsible for circumstances over which she has no control, simultaneously absolving the doctor from responsibility. Most patients accept the criticism, some even apologizing for the failure of their bodies. On occasion, a sharp patient will throw the words right back at the doctor: "Oh, sure!" said one of my laboring mothers. "Insult me! Make me the bad guy because my cervix is floppy! Hah! No way are you going to hang that one on me!"

Passive-aggressive behavior is exhibited toward the patient by exhausted, frazzled residents. Common behaviors include: failure to introduce themselves, avoiding eye contact, ignoring questions, answering questions curtly and too briefly, heaving great sighs of impatience, and even stripping off gloves and stomping out of the room. I have witnessed physicians, residents and attendings both, lose their tempers and bark or even shout at a patient who they feel isn't cooperating. Once, a young resident was trying to push the lip of the cervix back past a baby's head during a contraction. The mother had just received a narcotic to help with her pain and wasn't really all there. When the resident pushed on the cervix, the mother moaned and tried to withdraw her body from the probing fingers in her vagina, squeezing her legs together. It was a perfectly understandable action, given the pain involved and the woman's drugged state, but the resident flew into a rage. She flung off her glove as she screeched at the woman: "Now you listen to me! You have to do what I say! I don't care if it hurts! I don't give a shit if you don't like it! You're going to do what I say, do you hear me? Do you understand me?" Jolted out of her drugged euphoria, the patient nodded her head tearfully, apologizing for not being a good patient.

At a private hospital where I worked after leaving the military facility, I was appalled by the behavior of two of the residents. This hospital had a clinic population of indigent women whose care was provided by the residents. The patients were usually uneducated and non-English speaking. These two residents, both of them female—which made it worse, as far as I was concerned—looked upon the clinic patients as their own private curse. They complained and moaned about their patients, behind their backs and to their faces. Frequently, clinic patients would arrive on the labor deck without calling ahead, presumably because they didn't speak English and possibly because they did not have telephones. The residents abused them verbally for not calling and complained loudly that they "never followed instructions, they just keep getting pregnant, and they don't do what we tell them to do." Verbal abuse was accompanied by neglect during labor. Several babies were delivered by the nurses as these residents stalled and dallied around the nurses' station or stayed in bed instead of responding to their beepers.

One night a young woman arrived unannounced on this unit complaining of cramping and pressure in her pelvis. She wasn't sure of her due date, estimating she was about twenty weeks. Tired and upset that she hadn't called before coming in, the resident began questioning her about her prenatal care right at the desk in the presence of the unit secretary and the nurses. The woman hemmed and hawed, reluctantly explaining that she lived in a shelter and had not obtained prenatal care. The resident excoriated this woman:

"Don't tell me no care is available. You could have gotten care if you really wanted to. Don't you care about your baby? Why didn't you get help? It's there; you just had to ask for it and then show up for your appointments."

The woman became defensive and hostile, not an ideal way to begin investigating the source of her pain. She was a skinny little girl, really, with bad skin and dirty, scraggly sandy hair. Malnourished, the only meat on her frail body was her swollen belly. When we put her on the monitors, we were unable to find the fetal heartbeat. Ultrasound eventually revealed a dead fetus. The woman freaked out: she suffered at least two psychotic episodes during the next twenty-four hours as we induced her labor. She was completely uncooperative, frequently wracked with sobs when she wasn't loudly denying that her baby was dead. The residents washed their hands of her when she refused to lie still for cervical exams. The anesthesiologist threw up his hands in defeat after five attempts to insert an epidural, which failed because she refused to hold still long enough. She delivered her dead fetus in the bed, screaming and scratching at our hands as we tried to assist with the delivery. She kept putting her hands on the baby's head, trying to keep it in her body, as though to deny the reality of it. I put on my schoolteacher voice, held her bony shoulders, and spoke very firmly to her: "You must stop pushing our hands away. Your baby is coming out. You must let us get the baby. Keep your hands away. Do as I say. I know it hurts, but it's almost over, so let us help you."

Fortunately, the resident on duty at the time of delivery was one of the compassionate few. The patient fought him when he tried to check her vaginal canal and cervix for lacerations. When she began to hemorrhage, he agreed with me that we should take her back to the delivery room and "snow her"— put her to sleep—before we tried to check her. She fought like a tiger, tiny, bony little thing that she was, requiring three of us to hold her down until the anesthesiologist could put her under. When we lifted her legs into the stirrups, we were able to clearly see her genitals for the first time; she was covered with herpetic and syphilitic lesions.

This was an extreme case. A homeless, destitute woman came to us for help, and through her behavior made the giving of that help an onerous task. Nonetheless, she was a human being in need. Her socioeconomic status, her belligerence, her refusal to cooperate should not have affected the care we gave her. I wondered how much of her hostility and acting out was a direct result of her initial confrontation with the resident. Already shamed by her homeless status and her lack of prenatal care, to be so fiercely and publicly vilified by the resident certainly must have added to her guilt about her baby's death. Her behavior after that verbal bruising surely wasn't surprising. I was ashamed that I stood by and allowed the resident to speak to her in such a way, that I didn't take the resident to task for it later. I gave the patient every ounce of compassion and gentleness I could muster to compensate for the surly, judgmental behavior of others, but ended up feeling we hadn't done enough.

Not all residents are bad guys, of course, but nurses tend to remember unpleasant experiences with doctors and forget all the times they see physicians performing well. Doctors are expected, by everyone, to know their medicine, to act with decisiveness, compassion, and sensitivity to the patient and the nurse. When they fail to do so, they are judged harshly. Fatigue, mistakes, errors in judgment, memory lapses, even clerical errors are noted by the patient frequently and by the nurse almost always. Indifference and rudeness add to the condemnation of a doctor and if that doctor berates the nurse, however justly, he becomes an enemy to be scorned and ignored whenever possible. Nurses and doctors both have long memories and will invariably hold the other at fault for a long time if there is an incident over which they disagree. Nonetheless, many of the residents I worked with were impressive young physicians.

Learning their trade on the wards and in the operating rooms, stressed for time and with all the urgent demands upon them, most of them still managed to maintain an equilibrium that deserved credit. I watched one young man, Dr. Martin, move from internship through his third year of residency with a gracefulness that awed me. He was twenty-five or twenty-six years old, single, and an exercise enthusiast. Bicycling and running kept his slight figure athletically trim. He had thick, straight, black hair; smooth olive skin; a sensuous mouth and deep brown "bedroom eyes," as we nurses described them. This young doctor rarely exhibited any evidence of irritability or frustration, was unfailingly polite to the nurses and patient with the patients. He went through the rigors of first-year residency with inspiring resiliency and very little of the characteristic whining and complaining.

One night we had a woman deliver precipitously in the labor bed. From her labor room, I yelled for a doctor as I scrambled to unwrap the precip tray—a tray with sterile emergency instruments and linens. Dr. Martin was at the desk with the second-year resident, Dr. Johns, his immediate superior. They both came at my call and throughout the following half hour I marveled at Dr. Martin. Rattled by this unexpected event, Dr. Johns fumbled for gloves and instruments, while Dr. Martin quietly leaned over the bed and delivered the infant, suctioning, clamping, and cutting the cord, all the while gently encouraging the mother with his calm voice. By the time Dr. Johns was ready to intervene, Dr. Martin had completed the delivery, examined the mother for tears, and was assisting me in cleaning up the bed. All this was accomplished in a tiny room packed with two doctors, two nurses, and a med student, the mother on the bed, and her husband at her side.

Early in his training, Dr. Martin recognized that the nurses were resources for him. He surprised me the first time he asked my opinion about a patient; in my then limited experience, doctors rarely did such a thing. I became accustomed to working with him as a colleague. We were a team, discussing a patient's options and treatment, planning together how we would care for her. It was easy to suggest alternatives to him and he respected my ability to communicate effectively with patients, often leaving it to me to explain a planned treatment or to verify the patient's understanding of her care. I never felt constrained about speaking out during his conferences with patients; he encouraged me to add my comments and clearly appreciated my help with difficult or noncompliant patients. When we were on together, I always felt more relaxed, knowing he would respond immediately and politely to my calls, and that he really knew his medicine. Frequently I would ask him to explain a particular maneuver, technique, or treatment. We learned from and complemented each other.

Another excellent physician in training was a young woman, Dr. Sage. Tall, big-boned but graceful and gorgeous, Dr. Sage was an amazingly serene doctor. She was unfailingly courteous, even when she was furious. She had outstanding skills and a gentle bedside manner. Her patience with demanding laboring mothers was renowned. She went through her own first pregnancy in her second year of residency and experienced a difficult labor and a crash cesarean. Her remarks about understanding what it was like impressed me. She always seemed to empathize so well with her patients, unlike most female residents, who were still childless. I was gratified and surprised that she examined every aspect of her own experience for ways in which she could be more responsive to her future patients.

One night Dr. Sage was assisting a medical student with his first delivery. The three of us were in the delivery room together with the mother and father. The baby emerged without any problems. After accompanying the infant to the nursery (in the father's arms), I returned to a quiet delivery room. Dr. Sage and the medical student were waiting for the placenta to be expelled. I stood at the table by the woman's leg and chatted quietly with her about her delivery, as I half-listened to Dr. Sage's instructions to the medical student: "It can take up to an hour for the placenta to come out, although usually it happens within twenty minutes. You just hold onto the cord, don't pull or tug on it, just keep a little gentle traction on it. You'll know it's coming when you feel it go slack and see a gush of blood."

Sure enough, there was the blood; the cord lengthened and I saw the beginning of the placenta swelling in the vaginal introitus. I turned to my papers to record the time of delivery and then swung around, startled as Dr. Sage asked me: "Where is the anesthesiologist? Is he still on the deck?"

I saw her fist gripping something just inside the vagina. The placenta was in the bucket on the table. What was she doing? "I don't know. I'll see," I answered as I headed for the door. Dr. Sage calmly informed me that she needed him *now*: "I have an inverted uterus here and I need him to put Mrs. Gaster to sleep so we can relax this and get it back in the right way. Get two units of blood up here stat and have someone call Dr. Wheatly on his beeper. He's downstairs."

"Okay," I replied, ducking outside to relay her orders. Within ten minutes, the patient had been put to sleep; two units of blood were on hand; the attending physician, Dr. Wheatly, had poked his head into the DR for a report; and the uterus was back in place. Dr. Sage had held it clamped tightly in her fist until the anesthesia relaxed the mother enough so Dr. Sage could push her fist into the bag of muscle and turn it right side in again. Because of Dr. Sage's smooth, calm control over the situation, I had no idea until after the fact what a potentially dangerous, life-threatening event an inverted uterus could be. In this condition, the uterus actually turns inside out: bleeding from the exposed, raw placenta site can be difficult to control. The risk of lethal hemorrhage is great. After restoring the uterus to its appropriate configuration and position, Dr. Sage quietly continued instructing the medical student in the episiotomy repair.

Three days later, against all statistical probabilities, we had another inverted uterus. Inversion of the uterus is so rare a complication that few obstetrical people see more than one in their lifetimes. This time, all hell broke loose. The first-year resident hollered for his backup, anesthesia, blood. Within seconds there were ten people falling over each other in the DR, scrambling for IV tubing, instruments, medication. The patient's blood pressure dropped so precipitously as she hemorrhaged that a "code" was called. Two anesthesiologists struggled to intubate, to insert a breathing tube into the patient, while everyone shouted at everyone else. Not a participant, I stood back out of the way and marveled at the difference in the two cases. Dr. Sage's coolness under fire had made all the difference in the world. She knew what was happening, how dangerous it was, and precisely how to deal with it.

In a civilian teaching hospital, I had the privilege of working with one resident whom I called "God's resident" because he was so outstanding. For me, Luke will always be the ideal against which all other residents are measured. This young man, not yet thirty, was unsurpassed in his compassion, his courtly manners, his patience, and his clinical skills. He never lost his temper with nurses or with patients. He always minded his manners, speaking softly and politely, no matter what the circumstances. He never seemed to be in a hurry and listened to the most inconsequential requests or questions with complete attention. His presence on the unit had a calming effect, as if everyone relaxed somewhat knowing he was there and could be depended upon. To top off his perfection, Luke was a tall, remarkably handsome man, projecting a quiet strength and virility that sent nurses and patients alike into the dithers.

One evening a teenager came in to L&D complaining of premature contractions. She was thirty-four weeks into her pregnancy. When we put her on the monitors, an ominous fetal heart-rate pattern emerged. With each contraction, the baby's heart-rate would drop into the seventies and eighties, recovering slowly and long after the contraction had ended. These decelerations, with their late resolutions, frightened every one of the nurses on the unit. As we watched them on the central monitors at the desk, I called the attending physician to come immediately to see the strip. Such fetal activity can only be regarded as nonreassuring, so I began to put into motion the preparations for an emergency cesarean, calling the anesthesiologist, the scrub tech, the blood bank, and the nursery, and gathering up the appropriate documents.

The attending arrived, looked at the strip, spoke briefly to the young mother, but to my astonishment failed to take any action. I watched two more prolonged decelerations. I knew we were doing everything we could therapeutically to improve the fetal tracing. We had the girl on her left side, head tilted down to take any weight off the umbilical cord and she was receiving oxygen through a face mask. We were scrambling to get a history, get an IV started, and get blood samples sent to the lab and blood bank. A urinary catheter with a collection bag was resting on the bed, waiting to be inserted into her bladder. A surgical prep kit, which would be used to shave her abdomen, was in hand. Three nurses were hovering over the girl, ministering to her as rapidly as possible. We could all see that this tracing called for a crash section. The attending looked at the strip again and asked me to have the resident do a fetal scalp blood sampling to measure the baby's oxygenation status.

I had already paged Luke, needing him on the unit for the C-section. He appeared and I rapidly briefed him as we opened the scalp sampling kit. He inserted a long cone into the girl's vagina, swabbed the baby's head, nicked it with a tiny blade attached to a long plastic handle and held the glass capillary tube against the infant's wound, collecting the blood into the tube. The readout from the pH machine verified that this baby was probably in crisis. The pH was 7.20. Anything above 7.25 is an acceptable indicator of adequate oxygenation; 7.20 suggests possible acidosis or insufficient oxygenation. Luke hurried to present the evidence to the attending, whose response was, "Well, let's repeat that in twenty minutes."

Luke and I looked at each other with incredulity. It is standard operating procedure to wait twenty minutes and then repeat a suspicious scalp pH, but this wasn't suspicious. Combined with the continued and increasingly more prolonged fetal decelerations, plus the fact that there was no variability—fluctuations in the heart rate, usually an indication of fetal well-being—this pH was an ominous signal. This baby was in danger of going down the tubes before our eyes.

The attending was a physician known to have difficulty with emergency cases. He was reasonably competent under normal circumstances, but tended to paralysis when rapid decision-making and fast action were needed. This night was no exception. To my great relief, Luke quietly and politely asserted himself:

"I don't think we should wait twenty minutes. The baby needs to be delivered right away."

The attending replied, "Can you deliver the baby within four minutes?"

"Yes, we can," Luke said.

"You're sure? You're sure you can get the baby out in four minutes? You promise?"

"I promise!" he insisted.

"Well, okay then, let's do it," he said.

I couldn't for the life of me figure out why it was so important to the attending to extract a promise of a four-minute delivery. I knew that a baby needed to be delivered as rapidly as possible once the mother was given general anesthesia, as this mother would be, since the anesthesia could profoundly depress the baby. But this baby was already in trouble and was being further jeopardized by the physician's reluctance to proceed. *Thank God for Luke,* I thought as we whisked the girl to the OR, already prepared for the cesarean she should have gotten twenty minutes earlier.

I stood by to assist the neonatalogist with any required fetal resuscitation efforts. In less than four minutes the baby was passed to us. This baby was essentially dead. A tiny female fetus, she had been soaking in meconium for so long that her skin, her eyeballs, even her underlying tissues were stained green. She also smelled awful, a sign of probable infection. She had obviously been in distress for some time, probably hours before her mother had appeared on the unit. She was nothing but a bag of bones. Her skin hung on her skeleton like folds of loose soft leather; there was no muscle mass to her at all. Her head looked like a skull covered only with green, parchment-thin paper.

In the race to reach her through her mother's abdomen, Luke had inadvertently sliced the baby's cheek with the scalpel. An inch-long incision laid bare her cheekbone; the thin tissue above the bone was green-tinged. She had a very slow heart beat, less than forty beats per minute, and no other signs of life. We resuscitated her, sliding a tube into her trachea and forcing oxygen into her lungs. As soon as she was successfully intubated, the baby was rushed to the neonatal intensive care unit. There she would be stabilized and probably treated with antibiotics, for surely there was some kind of infection present. The cut on her cheek was of very low priority considering that she was as close to death as possible, even with all the technology and medicines we were using on her.

After the surgery was completed, I left the operating room, limp with sweat and the aftereffects of adrenaline. All I could think of was how glad I had been that Luke was the resident on call that night. Without his quiet authority and insistence on immediate surgery, that baby might have died as we watched and waited for the attending to make up his mind. I was filled with sadness over that little girl. I couldn't help but wish that her mother had stayed home another hour so that she might have died quietly within her mother's womb, rather than be dragged forth literally under the knife to a future fraught with high-tech invasions of her body, with little hope of any life, much less a life without permanent disabilities. But I was extremely proud of the nursing staff and of Luke, in particular. He had simply impressed the hell out of me, and I told him so, as soon as I saw him return from the recovery room.

As I complimented him on his skill in handling the situation, his eyes filled with tears. I realized he was berating himself for the scalpel cut on the baby's cheek.

"Oh, Luke, don't, for God's sake, don't do a number on yourself about that! You were doing the best you could under very trying circumstances. Getting the baby out as fast as possible was far more important than a small cut on her face."

"I know. But damn! I just hated seeing that I'd done that. I should've been more careful."

"God, Luke! We probably didn't do that baby any favors by delivering her alive anyway. When I think about how close we came to having her die on us right here, it gives me the willies."

"Yeah. I couldn't believe it when the attending said we should repeat the pH! You know, Susie, I don't think we made much difference to that kid anyway. It's obvious she was in trouble long before, at least hours before her mother arrived here. We just kept her from dying *in utero*. God, it's hard!" His eyes filled again as he turned away from me.

I held his arm briefly, thanking him again for being there and for his good work. I felt his pain and was glad for it. That sensitivity was one of the main attributes that set him apart from his peers, that made him an outstanding physician. I only hoped he would be able to sustain his compassion through the years of training and practice ahead, for he certainly exemplified the very best in a doctor.

When I took my first job at a private "civilian" hospital, I was amazed at the differences in the physicians. Unfortunately, over time, my opinion of many private attendings took a profound nosedive. The first contrast clearly lies in the economics of being a physician. All obstetricians are stressed: babies don't arrive just during office hours and being on call takes a big toll. But the physicians in the military medical system are not in private practice. They work for the government. All the financial costs of providing care fall on the government, not on the individual doctor. Likewise, the military doctors are paid a salary, so the number of patients they care for is financially inconsequential. While their patient load may be heavy, their primary concern, ideally, is to provide quality care. But private attendings have practices to maintain in order to meet their expenses and realize a profit: volume is important to them.

At the military hospital, I didn't have any serious difficulty interacting with doctors. As my years there went by, my clinical understanding of a patient's management became more sophisticated. Eventually it was possible to discern whether a plan of treatment was in the patient's best interest or was ordered to spare the physician unnecessary effort and/or time in the hospital. In most cases in the military hospitals, the residents were in house during their call hours. There was no great advantage for them to delay a treatment, such as Pitocin augmentation of a slow labor. On occasion, a delaying strategy might be employed during the wee hours of the night, to afford the residents a few hours of uninterrupted sleep. In the case of private attendings, however, I soon learned that patients' labors quite frequently were manipulated for the convenience of the physician.

Working nights as I did, it didn't take long to discover that most of the obstetricians, with a busy day of office hours beginning first thing in the morning, would do whatever was possible to avoid having to come to the hospital during the night. Nurses routinely examined the mother, ran a monitor strip on the baby, and called the doctor to inform him of the mother's status. If the mother wasn't in active labor as far as the nurse could determine, the physician would instruct the nurse to send the patient home. This practice, while understandable, troubled me greatly. There is no doubt that experienced L&D nurses are probably more qualified than many doctors to evaluate the progress of a labor. They spend all their hours, day in and day out, for years, reading monitors, palpating contractions, assessing a woman's behavioral changes, examining cervixes. They have had far more physical, clinical contact with mothers in labor than all but the most senior obstetricians.

It wasn't that I questioned the nurses' ability to evaluate a labor patient. It was that when she did that, legally the nurse was leaving herself open for all kinds of risks. To see a patient, evaluate her, and send her home without a physician even seeing her monitor strip was in effect practicing medicine and not within the scope of the Nurse Practice Act, the law delineating duties and actions of nurses. To do so on the authority of a verbal instruction given over the phone further compromised the nurse. Every nurse knew at least one story of a doctor who denied ever giving instructions over the phone. Most physicians relied heavily on the clinical knowledge and experience of the nurses at the hospital; expected the nurses to provide them with trustworthy information about their patients; and graciously allowed for occasional misjudgments, since everyone in obstetrics will make mistakes about the progress of a labor. But when a patient is sent home and delivers there, or a patient has a distressed baby upon her return to the hospital and perusal of the earlier monitor strip reveals that potential problems were present before she left the hospital—in other words, whenever there is doubt as to the proper medical management of a patient—many doctors will not hesitate to point the finger at the nurse, just as the nurse points at the doctor. It's ugly, it's human nature, but it happens unless the nurse is rigorous in her refusal to make decisions that are not legally hers to make.

There were doctors at this private hospital who religiously met their commitments to patients. They would call the desk to tell us a patient was coming in, arriving themselves within minutes of the patient. They would remain in the hospital for the labor, staking out a chair in front of the TV or a bed in one of the on-call rooms. These doctors spent time with their patients and remained in the hospital after a delivery to be sure the patient was stable. They often suffered for their efforts: responding to an office full of patients after being up all night made for some bad days. But they recognized their responsibility to the patient in the hospital and were reluctant to leave their care to others.

These doctors reminded me of my own gynecologist, a physician who had so impressed me that I became his patient when he retired from military service. He was supervisor of the obstetrical residents at the military hospital where I'd worked previously, but occasionally he took on a private patient. When that patient went into labor, he was there with her, present for almost the entirety of her labor, joking and chatting with her, calmly allaying her fears, working to make the experience a pleasant one. When he left the military to set up his own office, he chose not to continue his obstetrical practice because he knew he couldn't meet his office hours and still provide this kind of personal time and attention for an obstetrical patient. He misses delivering babies, but is unable to relax his own professional standards.

Unfortunately, the majority of the civilian doctors I interacted with did not have such rigorous standards. Indeed, from conversations with many L&D nurses, I've learned that it is common practice for nurses in private hospitals to practice medicine for physicians too reluctant or too busy to come in. Even the doctors in group practices usually exhibited a strong aversion to being in the hospital during their patients' labors. The physician on call would rely on the nurses, delay coming in until the last minute, and express outright anger if he or she was obliged to stay any longer than necessary. I can't tell you how many times I've seen a doctor leave the delivery room before the mother is even off the table, returning to his bed or the office without leaving orders or being sure the patient is stable. There were innumerable nights when a physician had to be called multiple times before the nurses could convince him to get out of bed to deliver a baby.

The most outrageous examples of this reluctance to come in were physicians who refused to come in for a fetal demise. On several occasions when I had patients who were being induced to deliver a dead infant, their doctors neglected to see them personally until the delivery. Sometimes the tiny premature fetuses were delivered by the nurse and a resident, the doctor giving telephone orders for the patient's care. Without exception, these patients were angry and hurt by the doctor's failure to attend them. When I remonstrated with one physician, he coyly feigned innocence, saying he was unable to understand why the patient was upset, or why he should come in: "The baby's dead. What do I need to be there for? Call me when she's ready to deliver."

Physicians in this hospital were willing to cover for one another if a doctor didn't make it in time for a delivery. Many times I had to ask a physician if he would do another doctor's delivery. The doctor's needs were met, but the patient was left in the lurch. It just isn't right for a couple to engage a particular obstetrician for their prenatal care, only to have a complete stranger deliver their baby. Even allowing for unexpected emergencies, for traffic complications, for unanticipated events that might prevent a doctor from getting to the hospital, there is no excuse for physicians who juggle their schedules too closely.

Doctors who had no partners were the hardest pressed. One patient on our unit spent most of the day in labor while her doctor was at his office five minutes away from the hospital. The nurses monitored her progress, checking her cervix and keeping the doctor informed via the telephone. When she was ready to push, the doctor was called. "I'll be there in a few minutes," he informed us.

This was the patient's first baby. We nurses knew she had some pushing to do, so we weren't worried about the doctor making the delivery. Her husband, however, went off the wall when the doctor hadn't arrived after fifteen minutes. "Where the fuck is he?" the father fumed. "We paid him good money to take care of this. Why the fuck isn't he here where he's supposed to be, goddammit! I want that son of a bitch to get his ass here, now! This is inexcusable!"

In between pushes his wife tried to calm him down. I said nothing, in my heart agreeing with the man. If the doctor can't provide the service the patient contracts for, he shouldn't take the patient. Or, if he's in private practice alone, he should make it very clear to the patient, early in her prenatal visits, that he won't be present during her labor, that nurses will be providing her care as long as she and the baby are stable. It smacks of arrogance on the doctor's part to take on patients without bothering to tell them how he attends his deliveries.

When this doctor finally arrived, he examined the patient, instructing her to push while he felt her cervix. She did so, bearing down so effectively that she sprayed the doctor with urine from his chest down to his knees! He left the room to change. Fifteen minutes later he still hadn't returned. Now the husband was really fuming! "Jesus Christ! How long does it take to change your clothes? Did he go home to change? Even a woman can get dressed faster than this!" I felt sorry for the woman, having this anger pollute the atmosphere as she strained to push out her first child. What a way to begin, with a father in a fury, red-faced and cursing. I just kept quiet, not wanting to aggravate him any further.

Doctors employed by a group health maintenance organization had the same difficulties being available to their patients. Even though they were scheduled to be in-house during their call hours, many of the HMO doctors would not respond promptly to nurses' calls. Sometimes they were so busy with a large number of patients that they couldn't come when we needed them. There was an unspoken rule among these doctors not to call in their backups except in situations of absolute dire need. As a result, there were nights when one doctor attempted to care for six to ten laboring patients without any help. This resulted in the nurses doing a delivery or calling for a section based on telephone exchanges with the doctor. Several times a patient had to wait hours for a surgical delivery because the doctor wasn't available. Trying to get these HMO guys to come to the unit when their call hours were almost over was a real battle. If they anticipated a cesarean, many of them would stall for a couple of hours until their relief came on to take the case.

One night I paged an HMO physician for a delivery just ten minutes before his shift was over. Over the phone he told me to tell the mother not to push. I called him back a couple of minutes later, informing him that the mother was unable to blow through the contractions and I needed him *now*. Again he instructed me, "Tell her not to push." I was furious. The doctor was only downstairs, in the on-call room. The mother had had more than one baby already; she was going to have this baby quickly. As I called a third time, the baby was delivered by the nurse. The doctor strolled onto the unit about ten minutes later, chatting with his relief physician. I was so angry that I wrote an incident report. Refusing to come upstairs for the delivery jeopardized the mother's and the baby's well-being and put the nurse in a risky legal position. What if the head had come out and then we had shoulder dystocia, in which the delivery of the shoulders is difficult? What if there was hemorrhaging after the delivery, or a prolapsed uterus? How does one justify a serious vaginal or cervical laceration because the physician wasn't present to perform an episiotomy or to control the delivery of the head?

Several weeks later, the physician explained to another nurse that he had been feeling very ill and had a bad case of bursitis in his elbow that night:

he didn't think he could manage another delivery. I refused to accept this second-hand excuse. If he couldn't do his job, he needed to call in his backup. It was that simple. Telling the patient not to push is just not acceptable. The patient shouldn't be expected to meet the doctor's needs. The patient shouldn't be expected to fight her body's activities because the doctor doesn't want to make an effort. I can't bear this kind of attitude!

The physician makes an implicit contract with the patient. It is accepted and understood by both parties that the patient will follow the doctor's instructions for her prenatal course while the physician will monitor her pregnancy, protecting her and her baby from any possible problems, to the best of the doctor's ability. The doctor will be present for the delivery and will do everything to ensure a good outcome. Doctors don't hesitate to scold a patient who isn't being careful during her pregnancy. If she misses appointments, or gains too much weight, or doesn't get enough bed rest if she's at risk, the doctor will let her know without any question that she's not being a good patient.

But when the doctor isn't being a good doctor, it isn't considered to be the same thing. The doctor blames the patient, labeling her a "problem" patient. The dissatisfaction the patient may have about her care is ignored. There is a silent agreement among many physicians to deflect their own responsibility onto the patient; to affect amazement when the patient is angry about being neglected; to assume that the physician knows best and is acting in the best interests of the patient, when in reality he is acting in his own best interest. The arrogance implicit in this attitude is obvious; physicians have been socialized in their training to believe that they are somehow better than those they serve. The doctor-patient relationship ceases to be reciprocal: the doctor has all the power on his side, short of the threat of a malpractice suit from the patient. Doctors assume that it is their right to dominate this contractual agreement and that the patient is being ornery if she expects more than he is willing to give. Astoundingly, most patients buy right into this attitude. They think their doctor is "just wonderful" if he's there to catch their babies, not acknowledging that he has neglected them during their labors or that their care in actuality is provided almost solely by nurses.

Occasionally, I've found the behavior of some physicians in front of their patients downright disgusting. One private attending spent the early evening waiting in the doctors' lounge while his patient labored. He made hourly trips to her room to check her cervix, muttering his frustration with her progress as he did so. The doctor had made it very clear to all of us that he wanted to be home by midnight. After about four hours, not an overly long period of time for the first stage of labor, she was fully dilated and ready to push. It was 11:30. With her first push the baby's heart rate dropped to the nineties, but returned immediately to its baseline level of about 130. This deceleration was a normal one, frequently seen during pushing when the umbilical cord is briefly compressed. The rapid return to baseline at the contraction's end is a reassuring sign.

However, the physician saw two such variable decelerations on the monitor in the lounge and came striding down the hall past the nurses' station.

"Fetal distress!" he bellowed. "Fetal distress!" He examined the woman vaginally and then resumed his yelling:

"Fetal distress! Fetal distress! We're going back for a forceps delivery stat! Call peds! I want Simpsons on the table stat!"

"Okay," I responded, as I dialed the pediatrician's number and watched the tech scurry to the delivery room to put out the Simpsons forceps. As the nurses rolled the patient's bed into the hall, the doctor yelled at me again: "I want Simpsons on the table!"

"It's being done now," I replied. As the woman was moved through the doors to the DR suite, he hollered at me again: "Call the peds and get Simpsons on the table!"

I came toward him, grabbing a paper hat and mask on the way. "It's taken care of, Doctor, the pediatrician is on his way." *Jesus, what is with this guy?* I thought. *Does he think I'm deaf or what?* In the delivery room, as the woman was being positioned on the table and washed down by one nurse, another nurse checked the fetal heart rate. It was audibly strong, in the 130s. As I checked resuscitative equipment on the baby island, I was flabbergasted by the physician.

Striding back and forth beside the table, he gowned and gloved as he crowed loudly,

"Yes, yes! Just last month, after I saved a baby's life in the same kind of situation, the father told me I was just like Superman! He told me in the office that I really impressed him when I saved his baby, that I was Superman! That's what he said, Superman!"

The anesthesiologist piped up, "More like Ratzo Rizzo, I'd say!"

I guffawed! I couldn't help it. I was so stunned by this doctor's behavior; how dare he talk so cavalierly about saving a baby's life without any thought for how he might be terrifying the mother and father. To me, this guy was a blatant megalomaniac, shouting out his own praises. The anesthesiologist's remark just set me off. I couldn't hold back my laughter and obvious disgust at the doctor. Surprised, he looked at both of us with reproach, but thank goodness he shut up. The baby, of course, was perfectly healthy, even after being subjected to a probably unwarranted forceps delivery. The doctor was out of the hospital before the woman had reached the recovery room—by midnight, of course.

Similar examples of physician insensitivity abound. A woman who had just given birth to a baby with birth defects so serious the baby wouldn't survive was having her episiotomy repaired right after the delivery. She kept crying out with pain, complaining about how much it hurt. The doctor continued to stitch without offering more pain medication, brushing aside the mother's complaints with the casual comment, "Oh, if you had a live baby to take home, I bet this wouldn't bother you so much."

A nurse came to me one night as I was finishing up a delivery, to ask me for assistance in her patient's room. "She's pushing and the doctor is just sitting in there, in the way, and I can't pay attention to her and get all the supplies ready for delivery." I followed the nurse into the room, introduced myself to the mother, and began to open supplies. The doctor was sitting in a rocker near the end of the bed, talking sports with the woman's husband. The woman was naked from the waist down, feet up in stirrups, genitals exposed, straining with effort as she pushed with her contractions. For twenty minutes she pushed, the nurse encouraged her and I readied the room, working around the doctor's chair. He never so much as acknowledged the mother's effort and was oblivious to the inappropriateness of his behavior. He just sat there, chattering away about basketball, glancing now and again at this woman's naked vulva. It was so tactless, so insensitive, and so insulting I wanted to kick him in the balls. Tight-lipped with fury, the other nurse and I were almost literally steaming with outrage as we went about our work. I was reminded, painfully, of my own labor and the doctor who so casually puffed on a cigarette while I contended with my contractions.

In marked contrast with this physician, whom I could never take seriously again, was an obstetrician whose devotion to his patients reaffirmed my faith in the art of doctoring. Slight of build, with large brown eyes and beautiful hands, Dr. Andretti was not only easy to look at, he was also quiet and reassuring, touching his mothers with gentle hands he was careful to warm beforehand. He was the only doctor I ever saw actually assist his patient throughout the pushing stage, holding up her legs, applying warm compresses to her perineum and calmly encouraging her efforts. He was extremely careful in cutting episiotomies. Instead of just whacking through the stretched perineal tissue with a pair of large scissors, he did almost all the cutting inside the vaginal canal, so that external stitching and its concomitant discomfort were minimized. I absolutely loved working with him. Deliveries were peaceful, serene events with the two of us working in tandem. His attention was always focused on the imminent arrival of a new family member and the excellent job the mother was doing—even if she wasn't—providing an appropriate aura of celebration and joy to the environment.

Dr. Andretti's bedside manner and constant concern over his patients, his insistence on top-quality care, and his obvious clinical skills made other physicians look even worse in comparison. I had heard a lot of stories during nursing school about doctors who acted like assholes, who screamed at nurses and residents, who threw instruments in the operating room or tantrums at the nurses' station. I made a silent promise to myself that I would never allow a doctor to shout at me or treat me badly. I was too old and had worked too hard to get my nursing credentials to be treated like someone's servant. In the military hospital I hadn't been confronted with any such offensive behavior.

After my first year at the military facility, I thought I should move to a civilian hospital for better pay and benefits and a more luxurious environment. After less than two weeks at that job, I scuttled back to my military friends after observing a civilian physician heap verbal abuse on both nurses and patients. No way was I going to put up with that kind of treatment! Or so I believed then.

Unfortunately, standing up to a doctor in a temper was far more difficult than I had imagined. It was three years before I got my first taste of offensive physician behavior. This particular physician, Dr. Furison, was an older man, in his late fifties, with many years of experience under his belt. He was a tall, loose-limbed man, wrinkled, freckled, and bald. Every interaction I'd had with him had been casual, yet professional. For the most part, the other nurses enjoyed his company and respected his work.

But after several long and demanding hours on the unit one night, Dr. Furison lost control of himself. He went into a vitriolic tirade about the lack of attention to details, the missing instruments and equipment he needed, and the overall poor management of this unit. As manager and charge nurse that night, I was the recipient of his ire. While many of his complaints were justified, his ill-tempered criticism of me was not. Much to my dismay, I was intimidated by his rage and had no idea how to respond other than to apologize quietly and do what I could to calm him down. I felt demeaned by the experience and further ashamed of my inability to defend myself, or at least to tell him not to yell at me that way. It was one of several incidents that revealed my abhorrence of emotional confrontations and my desire to appease, no matter the cost to my own self-esteem.

Another night I had a patient who was unable to stop making loud, harsh grunting sounds when she pushed. Try as she might, she just couldn't contain the growling noise of her effort. It didn't bother me too much. I remembered my own involuntary grunting when pushing out my son. Somehow the noise seemed to help her move the baby. It was similar to the sounds weightlifters make when hefting several hundred pounds. The only problem with this woman's noise was that it was difficult to communicate with her during her pushing. Accordingly, my voice was raised as I counted and encouraged her. Between the two of us, the decibel level was pretty impressive!

When the baby began to crown—when the fetal head emerges through the vaginal opening—I walked out to get Dr. Furison. I had the room set up for a birthing room delivery since by all criteria this was a prime candidate for such a birth. When I approached the doctor, telling him she was crowning and we were set up for the delivery, he lunged forward at me, his face beet-red with rage. He thrust himself right into my face, spitting on me as he shouted:

"I will *not* deliver an out-of-control patient in the labor room! I will *not* tolerate this lack of control! You get her to the delivery room and you get her to be quiet, do you understand?"

I was so stunned I just did an about-face and obeyed his order to move the patient. In the DR he yelled at me about the setup of the room, the slowness with which the tech and I positioned the woman on the table, and various other grievous faults. Finally I stood next to the woman, palpating her contractions and trying to focus on her efforts, offering quiet encourage-ment for her pushing. Her husband joined me in this activity. The patient was still unable to push without a final loud grunt. The doctor let all of us have it:

"That's *enough*! Everybody in this room just shut up! It sounds like a chicken coop in here, all of you yelling at each other! Now listen, Mrs. Cantly. I will *not* tolerate your lack of control! You keep your mouth *shut* and you do what I tell you to do when I tell you, or I'm not delivering this baby! Do you understand me? Do you?"

The patient turned to me. Her eyes filled with tears, which trailed down her cheeks. Her husband stood stiff with anger by her side, looking at me with absolute fury in his face. I looked back at the woman, fighting my own tears of impotence. The baby was delivered in absolute silence. I dried him, tagged him, and wrapped him without speaking, unable to trust my ability to maintain control over my urge to cry. As I placed him in his mother's arms, we were able to greet him gently, the three of us admiring him to-gether. Dr. Furison finished his repair and had the audacity to thank me for my help as he left the room.

I was devastated by this experience. This was a lovely couple, having their third baby. They had been pleasant and cooperative throughout the brief labor. They wanted to enjoy this birth since it was to be their last baby. We had worked well together, establishing an easy rapport. Mrs. Cantly was not at all out of control when pushing, she was just noisy about it. Dr. Furison hadn't bothered to come into the labor room to see for himself how well she was doing. He dashed the couple's hopes for a birthing room delivery for absolutely no reason at all except his apparent inability to keep his temper and be tolerant of her particular style of pushing. His anger and insults in the delivery room completely and irrevocably changed the nature of this child's birth. This baby came into a room filled with negative emotion, his mother in tears of shame, his father furious, the nurse trembling with outrage, the physician on a tear. The whole thing was inexcusable.

I was further shamed by my cowardice. I couldn't get into a fight with the doctor right there in the delivery room, in front of the patient. Calling him on his insulting behavior would have only exacerbated an ugly situation. But I was never brave enough to convey my outrage to him in private. I let him get away with it. All my avowals of outrage about doctors who behave badly and promises never to allow myself to be so treated were the bluffs of a coward.

I am still struggling to learn how to confront a physician who acts inappropriately. It takes thoughtfulness and a cool demeanor that I find difficult to summon when I am angry. Gradually I have begun to develop the skills necessary to engage in such confrontations without tears or aggressive words, but each incident demands that I think carefully about what I want to change in the doctor's behavior, what is in the patient's best interest and how I can convey my unhappiness without feeling intimidated or demeaned, and without putting the physician on the defensive. My selfish inclination in such situations is to rigorously avoid any confrontations even as I steam inwardly over the injustices I've witnessed. Childishly, I try to place the blame on the doctor, furious at having to deal with an adult who acts like a toddler.

But it isn't just the doctor who is at fault. I hate that my interaction with the patient is jeopardized by conflict with the doctor. I feel shame when I do less than the best for my patient in the interest of keeping the peace with a doctor. I may not be able to change his behavior, but I have a responsibility to my patients and myself to at least call him to task when he is abusive. Nothing is more debilitating than when I have to battle my personal reluctance to take a stand and be assertive. This is an arduous task for a woman brought up to be respectful of authority figures, and it seems like I am rarely up to it.

Even after years of work, this shortcoming in my personality continues to haunt me. Late in my career another incident occurred that absolutely enraged me. A woman came to our unit almost fully dilated, in hard, active labor. She was rushed into a birthing room by her nurse while another nurse and I scrambled for equipment and materials for the delivery. The three of us, all experienced nurses, were working quietly and rapidly, efficiently preparing for the birth with ease and organization. The woman was hollering for an epidural as her primary nurse applied the fetal monitors to her belly and obtained baseline vital signs. The other nurse started an IV as I prepared the infant warmer and pulled gloves and sutures for the doctor.

All the while we kept encouraging the mother, explaining how very close she was to delivery. Within ten minutes of her arrival in the room, she was fully dilated and the baby was descending down the birth canal without any pushing efforts on her part.

"Look at that! We can see the baby's head during the contraction! You can push if you want to! You're almost there!" we explained as we broke down the birthing bed, removed the bottom half, placed the woman's feet in stirrups and washed her vulva with antiseptic solution.

"I can't push! It hurts too much! Oh please, get me the epidural!" she begged. Her doctor entered the room, saw the baby's head showing during the contraction and tried to soothe the patient.

"You're really close, Lillie. Just a little bit more," she advised.

"No, I can't stand it. Please, Doctor, please can't I have the epidural?"

"Sure you can, honey, sure you can," the physician replied. Turning to us, she asked us to call the anesthesiologist and then left the room. We three nurses looked silently at each other, an unspoken agreement in our eyes. This woman was so very close to spitting out this baby that all three of us knew just a few more minutes were all that we needed. Paging the anesthesiologist, waiting for his return phone call, collecting epidural supplies and getting it administered could take fifteen to thirty minutes minimum. So we stalled. I prayed silently, "*Just stay out of the room, Doc. Just leave her with us and we'll get her through one or two contractions and this will all be over and she'll be fine. I'm not even sure we have time to get an epidural in!*" Two of us bent over her, exhorting and cajoling:

"Come on, Lillie, push with this one! The baby's head is right there! We've got our fingers on it. One or two more contractions and you're done, we promise!" Her husband looked at her bottom and added his voice to ours. The baby was right there.

"No, no, I can't! It hurts too much!" she cried, just as the doctor reentered the room. "Oh, Doctor, please, I can't stand this pain," she sobbed.

"You don't have to," she murmured. "Where's the anesthesiologist? Let's put this bed back together and get the epidural," she instructed us, before making her exit once again. The woman screamed and thrashed through another contraction and then looked around at all three of us. Our faces and our silence betrayed us.

"What's the matter? Did I make the wrong decision? Do you think I'm wrong to ask for the epidural?" she questioned. Stung with remorse that I had revealed my thoughts, I apologized.

"No, Lillie, you're not wrong to want the epidural. It's just that you're so close, it would only take a couple of solid pushes to get this head out. We just want to help you do this, but I know you can't really be reasonable about a couple of contractions if they're hurting you so much. I'm sorry, Lillie. The anesthesiologist is on the way."

I couldn't believe it. The bed had been broken away; she had her feet in stirrups; the baby was crowning! One or at most two more contractions and she would be over the pain. An epidural now? I understood her distress: she just wanted relief. But she really didn't realize how very close to delivery she was, even though we told her. She just wanted the pain to be taken away.

Well, we put the bed back together. The doctor, back in the room again, stretched out Lillie's legs, patting and stroking her. The anesthesiologist arrived and inserted an epidural while the doctor held the mother's legs together. Within fifteen minutes she was comfortable. But, guess what? Now she couldn't push because she couldn't feel anything below her ribcage, and the baby had slipped back up the vaginal canal a bit when the doctor had extended Lillie's legs and when she'd rolled over for the epidural. For thirty minutes her primary nurse "pushed" her, until the doctor finally called for the vacuum extractor and the baby was delivered with suction. Lillie thanked the doctor effusively for the epidural. As soon as the baby was taken to the nursery she sat up in bed to apply fresh makeup and don a silk negligee.

Lillie was the only patient for several hours that night, so most of the L&D nurses were sitting out at the desk, ready to assist us if we needed any more help. They watched with bulging eyes of incredulity when I came out of the room to fetch the vacuum machine. I just shook my head at them as I wheeled it into the room. When the delivery was finished, all the paperwork completed and the mess cleaned up, I came out to the desk. Leaning over one of the nurses' shoulders, I hissed, "That's just not right! It's not right! That baby would have been born in no more than ten minutes if that doctor had just stayed out of the room! There's no excuse for this! Look at all the added expense: anesthesiology fees, equipment and meds fees, fees for a vacuum delivery, not to even mention one word about the attendant risk to the baby with an epidural and a vacuum! An hour to do what could have been done safely and rapidly in ten or fifteen minutes. But no . . . the doctor hears her crying and doesn't want her patient to be in pain, even for a few minutes, so she holds everything up, instead of just getting in there and making the lady push. I can't stand this! There ought to be some way to complain about this! That vacuum delivery just wasn't necessary. Damn!"

One of the nurses looked up at me and said wearily, "There is a way to complain. You can bring up your objections to the complaint committee for doctors and nurses."

"Oh yeah, how do I do that?" I asked.

"Guess who's a member of the committee?" she replied. Yep, it was that very doctor. I gave up.

This incident is an excellent example of the continuing conflict between physicians and nurses. This doctor was a good doctor: she knew her medicine and was a caring, competent physician. Her response to the patient's distress was understandable. She had the authority and means to stop the pain and didn't hesitate to do so, I assume because she didn't want one of her patients to go home thinking the doctor had allowed her to suffer. Such an attitude might lose a paying patient for the doctor's practice. Obstetricians get a good deal of pressure from their patients to manage childbirth with a minimum of pain for the mother. It's almost a conditioned response in many older physicians to order medication or anesthesia at the first sign of discomfort in the patients. This doctor simply made a decision to take away the pain and deal with the consequences of that decision—prolonged pushing, vacuum delivery—after the patient was comfortable.

As it certainly should be clear by now, nurses don't like to have their patients yelling with pain, either. But in this case, we nurses knew, without any doubt, that ten minutes of intermittent pain would result in a delivery: the patient just needed to be helped through those few minutes. However, we didn't have the authority or the power to accomplish that result. The doctor held sway, even though her decision meant delay, added risk to the mother and baby and a considerable increase in cost.

Undoubtedly, we should have handled the situation differently. One of us should have had the courage to take the doctor aside and persuade her to give us just a few more minutes with the mother before we called the doctor in to deliver the baby. Maybe, if we weren't working so rapidly and putting so much effort into trying to calm the mother, and if we hadn't been so surprised by the doctor's insistence on the epidural, and if we hadn't be trained to always defer to the physician, we might have thought of confronting the doctor.

Even in hospitals where nurses are treated with respect by the physicians, where nurses are members of a team of caregivers, there is still the underlying, unspoken rule that the physician is the final authority. Nurses may have the training and experience to manage a patient's care appropriately and competently, but nurses don't have the legal right to prescribe treatment or medications and must always have a doctor's order to validate the care they provide. If there is a conflict in opinion about a patient's care, the doctor's wishes are the final prerogative. Nurses spend an inordinate amount of time persuading doctors to accept the nurses' evaluation of the patient's needs. I can spend hours with a patient and have a very good idea of what she needs, only to be blocked by a physician's preference for some other kind of treatment.

A physician's personality obviously plays an enormous role in patient care and in the conflict between doctors and nurses. Doctors who view nurses as their personal servants and patients as their source of income are the worst, from my perspective. Physicians like these behave as though it would be foolhardy to ask a nurse for her opinion about a patient. They issue orders, becoming abusive if the orders are questioned, refusing to even consider that the nurse might have a legitimate concern. I can't tell you how many times I have saved a doctor's ass by questioning an order. This is expected of me, legally and by the doctors themselves. Wrong medications, wrong dosages, or routine orders that aren't thought of by the physician get picked up by the nurse, who must then call the doctor for a correction, frequently being subjected to irritable responses and sometimes nasty tongue-lashings from the doctor. I could also tell you about the times I have been reprimanded for *not* reminding a doctor to write a needed order.

Working with older doctors who have long-established routines can sometimes be unbearable. Doctors like these seem to feel threatened by new nurses who don't kowtow to their wishes and who volunteer unsolicited suggestions about patient care. Such a physician was a courtly gentleman who drove us nurses up the wall. Dr. Meadows was always exquisitely dressed. Even when he wore scrubs, he exuded fastidiousness: his scrubs came not from the hospital linen service, but from home, freshly laundered and pressed. He was of medium height and lean, with overly long arms and large, gnarled hands. His thinning gray hair was professionally sculpted to hide incipient balding. The leathery, creased skin of his tanned face betrayed the hours he spent on the golf course. Every time I saw him, I was transported by a vision of him elegantly attired, sipping mint juleps on the verandah of an antebellum plantation home.

In a paternalistic fashion, Dr. Meadows obviously cared for his patients. Always speaking softly and patronizingly to his mothers, he showered them with praise and overly long hugs after their deliveries. But Dr. Meadows was twenty years behind the times. He treated his labor patients as if they were seriously ill, dependent little things that needed a God/father to tend to their woeful hurts. Every patient of his received an epidural, whether she needed it or not: "You wouldn't want to suffer anymore, would you, darlin'? The pain is going to be terrible!" he would say. After every delivery, he ordered hefty doses of narcotics to be given through intramuscular injection, regardless of the patient's need or desire for pain relief. This infuriated us nurses because almost all vaginally delivered mothers simply do not require narcotics. A couple of Tylenols or a mild analgesic pill is all that was necessary, while a narcotics injection knocked the mother out for hours. When I had to give these injections, I could just forget about the mother keeping the baby in the room, encouraging family bonding, or breast-feeding.

In effect, these injections delayed everything involved with the mother's recovery. Postponing the start of breast-feeding inhibited breast-milk production. The baby had to be bottle fed, which frequently led to difficulties in adjusting to the mother's nipples. The mother felt drugged and sick for hours and often believed she was far more ill than she actually was. The narcotics hampered her ability to get out of bed to empty her bladder, requiring the use of a bedpan and often necessitating a catheterization, which put her at risk for a urinary tract infection. Postpartum recovery and infant care instructions from the nurses had to be delayed until the drug wore off sufficiently for her to comprehend what we were trying to convey. It was ridiculous. Dr. Meadows's regimen delayed his patients' recovery and added expense and time to their hospitalizations, not to mention how it added to the nurses' workloads.

We nurses had to resort to surreptitious methods to circumvent Dr. Meadows's orders. Whenever I had one of his patients, I quietly informed her that he had ordered narcotics for her, which meant that I was required to give them to her. Explaining how they would make her feel and how they could interfere with her recovery, I offered an oral medication for pain if she wanted it. I assured her that Dr. Meadows was only concerned about her comfort, but that it was very rare that a newly delivered mother required such strong medication, adc'ing conspiratorially, "He's a little stuck in his ways." Every time I spelled it out like this, my patients refused the injection and even helped me keep it secret from Dr. Meadows. A few of the nurses just went ahead and gave the narcotics, rather than go through all this subterfuge with the mother and risk the doctor's wrath, but all of us were pissed about it.

Because of his old-fashioned, sexist perception that women were weak, dependent, and sickly, Dr. Meadows also interfered with their breast-feeding efforts. Despite all scientific evidence to the contrary, he firmly believed it was wrong to allow a mother to nurse for more than five minutes on each breast during the first twenty-four hours. He insisted on regulated, four-hour feedings, rather than on-demand feedings based on the infant's appetite. We nurses all had extensive training in breast-feeding theories and techniques. We had a lactation specialist on staff who was a walking encyclopedia on breast-feeding. No matter how much any of us argued with Dr. Meadows, he stubbornly refused to listen to us, writing orders defining precisely how we were to teach the mother to breast-feed. These orders were in direct opposition to the hospital's own documented policies. Once again, I skirted around the edges of his orders, getting the mothers who wanted to nurse longer or on demand to insist on it. I could document this in the nurses' notes, making it the patient's preference rather than part of the nursing instructions.

After the year of working as assistant nurse manager, my second nursing job, I quit, burnt out by the problems on my unit and for the most part thoroughly disgusted with many of the doctors. Working then as an agency nurse at various military facilities, I was once again involved with in-house residents. My initial patience with residents had worn thin. The eagerness with which I greeted new residents and the pleasure I derived from helping them learn their profession was diminished by a sense of futility. As a new, unknown nurse, I had to reestablish my credentials, clinical skills, and trustworthiness with these doctors. They had no way of knowing that I was an experienced

L&D nurse. Watching them fumble and struggle with patients and decisions was far more exhausting than it had been when I was new and didn't know any better.

With each new class of residents the nurses have to start all over. Routines, procedures, documentation, the physical location of equipment and supplies, all the myriad details of providing good care on a unit have to be learned by the new doctors. While they're learning, the nurses have to exhibit extraordinary patience or be labeled as troublemakers, as noncooperative bitches. Once a nurse has clinical experience, it is difficult for her to stand by and watch a new doctor make mistakes, waste time, or unnecessarily hurt his patient. The advantages of receiving care in a university setting or a residency program is that the doctors are in-house, more readily available when needed. They also perform as a team; since several doctors make joint decisions about care, patients are not at the mercy of just one physician, who may not be competent. But there are disadvantages. Each rotation of residents reassesses the treatment and progress of the patient and more often than not, changes orders that the nurses have been following. The patient doesn't get continuity of care and the nurses are caught in the middle, trying to do the best for the patient with conflicting or countermanded orders and instructions.

The other aspect of residency programs that concerns me is the emphasis on technology. Much of what a resident learns about obstetrics he gleans from other residents. If the supervising physicians do not make a concerted effort to demonstrate different routines and techniques, the residents can't learn them. Most of the residents I work with today are almost completely dependent upon the technology and equipment of their profession. They don't know how to deliver care without electronic monitors, complex machines, special lights, and specific instruments. They give all their attention to the guidelines and specific treatment plans from their textbooks and lectures while failing to learn how to pay direct attention to the mother. A labor graph *must* be adhered to, so a mother who may labor and deliver just fine without extraneous interference is subjected to unnecessary interventions.

An example might be the way epidurals are performed. In a private hospital the staff anesthesiologist usually does the epidural. Ideally, he has finished his training and is experienced in his craft. But a residency program in anesthesiology has protocols and rules of treatment that must be followed. This means that a mother will be required to wear four ECG leads, an oxygen mask, and a blood pressure cuff for the duration of her labor, prohibited from eating or drinking anything, have countless blood pressure and neurological checks and position changes. She may be denied pain relief if the anesthesiology resident believes it is too early or too late in her labor for an epidural. She may have to remain in bed and on the L&D unit for several unnecessary hours after delivery until the anesthesiologist releases her to the ward. All of the rules are based on sound medical practice, but the lack of flexibility is an added, unwarranted stress.

This occurred one night with a patient whose labor was being induced. Elsbeth's baby had such severe anomalies (defects) that it was absolutely certain the infant would die soon after birth. The baby's brain hadn't developed: ultrasound revealed a fetal skull empty but for the brainstem. Over a period of weeks, Elsbeth had been counseled extensively about her baby and repeatedly assured that every effort would be made to keep her as comfortable as possible during her labor. I was impressed by her strength as she began this labor, tied to a bed for the duration until she was delivered of her first-born, a nonviable baby. The director of the obstetrics program and the chief resident had taken great personal interest in Elsbeth, giving her and her husband more time and support than was usual.

The beginning of Elsbeth's labor was uneventful. She and her husband, Brett, were able to talk with me about their baby, their loss. Although Elsbeth was in her late twenties, she looked like a young teenager. Petite, shy, and soft-spoken, she made me think of a timid dormouse. I can't remember what Brett looked like physically, but I'll never forget the anguish in his face as he asked me whether a brain transplant was possible for their baby.

As labor progressed, the narcotics I had been giving Elsbeth were ineffective in alleviating her pain. She asked for the oft-promised epidural. Unfortunately, the two doctors who knew her so well had departed, leaving in charge a resident who had had no personal interaction with this young woman. I told the anesthesiology resident she was ready for the epidural. He nodded, busy with another epidural. He had already interviewed the patient, counseling her about the epidural. Much to my dismay, he stopped me in the hall fifteen minutes later to tell me he couldn't do the epidural because the doctors were afraid it would slow or stop her labor: we'd have to wait until she dilated to four or five centimeters.

This really upset me. Elsbeth was only dilated one to two centimeters; it could be hours before she made it to four centimeters. The narcotics weren't helping. Here I was in a tiny little room, holding her hand, rubbing her back, making her breathe in a controlled manner, while this young woman twisted and moaned with pain, drawing her legs up in that bicycling movement indicative of serious pain. There was absolutely no reason not to give her the epidural; we were stimulating her labor artificially with drugs and we would go on doing so, whether she felt the contractions or not. There was no danger to the baby; it might even be already dead. We weren't monitoring it at all. The single most important task we had in providing her care was to help her get through this agonizing emotional experience with as little physical discomfort as possible. What difference did it make if the epidural slowed things down? She was going to have a dead baby to bury after her labor; to me it was ethically wrong to deny her whatever relief we could provide.

As I began a slow burn, I made myself pause, take a few deep breaths, and think how I could best obtain the obstetrical resident's cooperation. Asking politely if I could have a few minutes to talk alone with him, I explained my concern:

"I'm really caught in the middle here, Doc. Before he left, the OB chief gave me explicit instructions that this woman was to be kept comfortable and to be given an epidural as soon as she asked for it. The patient is expecting this to happen. It's been promised to her. Now she's lying in there, in some heavy-duty pain, contracting every minute, and the anesthesiologist tells me you don't want to slow her labor with an epidural. I need some help understanding this."

He shook his head. "It wasn't me. I don't even know this patient. The anesthesia chief is the one who said no to the epidural. Let's check her cervix first."

Back to the room I went to hold Elsbeth's hand, trying to explain the delay, really upset over this young woman's pain. It was so unnecessary. A half hour passed before the resident checked her cervix and told the anesthesiology resident the epidural was okay, even though she hadn't dilated any more. Another half hour passed while we waited for the anesthesiology resident to confer with his chief again and convince him the epidural was appropriate. During this time I made up my mind that I was going to raise hell if she was denied relief. I told the charge nurse that I'd give the doctors fifteen more minutes to decide and then I was going to call the OB chief. This could have been a disaster for me in terms of my working relations with the residents, but I didn't care. I fought internally with my own inherent timidity while I tried to comfort Elsbeth through the pains.

Fortunately the anesthesiology resident was completely sympathetic to Elsbeth's need and my concern, and managed to get permission to do the epidural. Another twenty minutes passed before my little patient stopped hurting. I was infuriated by this incident. The anesthesiology chief made a decision over the telephone without ever bothering to consider the emotional ramifications of denying pain relief to this patient. He knew she was giving birth to a baby with lethal anomalies but he focused only on the guidelines and policies for performing an epidural. Without communicating directly with the obstetricians, he made an obstetrical decision that required lengthy consultations, caused me tremendous emotional upset, and forced Elsbeth to endure two hours of unnecessary excruciating pain.

In any number of clinical procedures, the nurse is caught between attending to the patient and meeting the demands of the doctor. In private hospitals I've had to ignore the patient's needs because the doctor expects me to wait on him. For instance, a physician comes into the labor room to administer an epidural. I can't stand next to the woman and ensure she maintains control during her contractions while holding still for the epidural. I can't hold her feet with one hand and lean into her face to comfort and encourage her and explain each step. I have to open the epidural tray, set out the medications, hand the doctor his gloves, throw away his garbage, document his dosages and her blood pressure and pulse. I have to tape up the catheter, clean up the debris, and reposition the patient after the doctor has inserted the catheter. I'm not nursing the patient, I'm assisting the doctor, who is perfectly capable of performing all those tasks himself, but doesn't because he's the doctor, he's busy, and he needs to see another patient.

In the residency programs where I've worked, the residents did all this stuff themselves, freeing me to concentrate on the patient. Imagine my surprise after leaving the military residency program for the private hospital to discover that graduated doctors, physicians who have finished their training, are somehow unable to do a vaginal delivery without considerable assistance.

In the residency program, I assisted the doctors only by tying their sterile gowns for them and getting equipment that wasn't readily available, like a pair of forceps or clamps. All the usual instruments and equipment were already laid out in the delivery room. After the delivery, the residents cleaned up their own mess. They were gowned and gloved, already messy from the delivery, so it made sense for them to throw the instruments in a basin, put used needles into the needle bucket, wash the patient's vulva, and gather up the paper drapes and place them in the garbage. While they did this, I could assist with initial breast-feeding, clean up the infant warmer, unstrap the monitors, and so forth.

In the private hospitals where I've been employed, everything necessary for a delivery is prepared beforehand, usually by the nurse. The doctor washes his hands and enters the room. A scrub tech or the nurse hands him a towel, ties his gown, adjusts his light or stool, and then hands him each instrument as needed, from the table right beside his arm. After the baby is delivered, the physician sutures the episiotomy, offers "congrats" to the patient, and leaves the room to do his charting. The nurse or scrub tech washes the patient, cleans up the instruments and the garbage, and takes the stool, instrument table, vacuum machine, infant warmer, light, and scale out of the room. Now I'm not suggesting that the doctor should "do the dishes," but does a hospital really have to provide a full-time scrub-tech staff to hand instruments to a doctor who has two hands himself? This is expensive. Having a scrub tech or another nurse present during a delivery is enormously helpful to the primary nurse, of course, because that second pair of hands permits her to attend more closely to the mother and baby. But having a scrub tech just to attend to the physician absolutely amazes me.

I've had innumerable doctors actually stand at the bedside and wait for me to open a pair of gloves for them before doing a cervical exam. This is one of those subtle power messages: the doctor is perfectly capable of opening his own gloves, but expecting and waiting for me to do it affirms his dominance. It's amusing, because I really do enjoy helping physicians work. I don't have any problem at all with making a procedure a little easier or smoother, and I routinely go out of my way to save them steps. But if I have to attend to the doctor when the patient needs my attention more, I get irritated with this learned helplessness. *Open the goddamned gloves yourself, for chrissakes! My hands are busy getting this patient turned over or cleaned up or whatever!*

Such situations are problematic for nurses because most hospitals are dependent financially on the patients admitted by private medical practices. If the doctor who sends numbers of patients to a hospital is unhappy about how nurses and other "underlings" carry out his wishes, the hospital runs the risk of losing that doctor's patients. In one hospital in which I worked briefly, the physicians were gods: they decided each and every policy in the place. Not one nurse or nursing representative sat on the hospital's policy board; any and every nursing action had to be approved by the doctors, up to and including the nursing documentation forms that the nurses used with every patient.

I'll never forget my incredulity as I sat in an orientation meeting at that hospital listening to the director of nursing. She spent five minutes talking to us about our professionalism and how significant we were in health care. Then she spent fifteen minutes laying down the rules about doctors. "If a doctor wants a fresh cup of coffee, you will get it for him. If a doctor wants you to follow him on rounds and carry the charts for him, you will do so. You will stand up when a doctor enters the room and you may never, never address a physician by his first name. We expect you to show appropriate respect for our doctors because they bring money into this hospital: you don't." Is it necessary to say that I didn't stay at that hospital very long?

I find myself wondering, "Who am I working for? The doctor or the patient? The hospital or the patient? It's a balancing act always, and it's rarely balanced. My job definition states that I am supposed to carry out the doctor's orders. I'm also supposed to protect the patient from harm, teach her what she needs to know about her condition, and provide whatever care she is unable to provide herself. So I scuttle back and forth trying to do my best for both. Physicians who treat me as a team member, who encourage my participation in the patient's treatment, who ask for and listen to my input on problems with patients and acknowledge my contributions with a simple thank-you, get the best I can possibly give them. Physicians who don't also get the best, but I sure don't like or respect them.

As time passes, I have learned to diminish my expectations of doctors. I try to make allowances for actions and decisions that bother me, reminding myself of all they are forced to juggle by this crazy system of medical care.

But even as I do so, I am increasingly wearied by the daily conflicts, however small, between doctors and nurses and doctors and patients. I am exhausted by the effort required to cooperate in the giving of care, by the callousness, indifference, arrogance, and lack of courtesy exhibited in the behavior of so many physicians. It always feels like I'm walking a tightrope, trying to excuse or ignore the small issues, while being brave enough to go to battle for my patients on the big ones, and maintaining a sense that I can work as part of a cooperative team in giving care to our patients.

The most significant therapeutical maneuver that I employ is to recall each of the good doctors, the men and women who have taught me my craft, who have demonstrated in so many small ways their knowledge, skills, and compassion for their patients. Remembering the times when doctors have interacted with me and my patients in just such a positive way helps carry me past the tiresome and ugly experiences. Those doctors who truly practice the *art* of medicine are inspiring examples of how to do it right. I am grateful for the opportunity to work with them.

Chapter Seven

ON-THE-JOB TRAINING

Nursing school was finished. Nursing boards were taken and passed. It was time to find a job. I spent the summer following graduation sorting through belongings, holding a huge garage sale, having real estate agents parade through my house with prospective buyers, coming to terms with the abrupt collapse of a year-long relationship with a man I'd loved too foolishly. My ex-husband and I, along with his second wife and our children, had been engaged in family counseling for the past year as we tried to decide how I might leave this city in which we had lived for thirteen years to start a new life, without greatly damaging the two children. It was a wretched year as I came to grips with my need to break away from my old life, and wrestled with the terror and guilt I felt at placing my needs above those of my children.

I wasn't a housewife anymore: for four years I had been an impoverished single mother, a student, a woman driven to find a meaningful way to earn a living. Elegant dinner parties, trips to Europe and the Caribbean, designer clothes, shoulder-rubbing with intellectuals and academics—these were all long gone without much ado or regret. But selling the house, giving away the furniture, leaving behind the home, neighborhood, and city I had lived in longer than any other place during my life—this was wrenching. Worse, by far, was the anguish I felt for my children. There was no question about what was necessary for me, financially, emotionally, and psychologically. I needed to sever, finally, the still-present invisible threads of dependency on my ex-husband, to be geographically and psychologically on my own.

I had a nursing license now, a reasonable means of support—for the first time in my life, at age thirty-eight—and no intention of ever being financially dependent again. Unless I changed my name, if I worked in any hospital in this city, I would forever be perceived by the medical community not as myself but as the sister of one of the most powerful and well-known physicians in the area, my older brother. I wanted to be free—free of the past, of my ex-husband and my lost marriage, of the house and friends we had shared, of my family ties—free to explore this expanded self I had become: single woman, nurse, professional, wage-earner. But I did not want to be free of my children. Above and beyond all else, they were my core, my essence, my meaning, my duty, my reason for being alive. I had planned to take them with me when I left behind my past, never imagining any life without them in it. They came from me, they were a part of me and I of them, and I felt we belonged together as long as they were children.

But they also came from their father, and when I laid out my plans to move away, to a new city, new job, new life, he said, "No." So while I worked to complete my schooling, we spent a year in therapy, together and singly, negotiating terms of custody, trying to meet everyone's needs. The final solution was a compromise: the children would remain with their father and his wife for one year, while I established myself in my new environs. I convinced myself that this arrangement would be the least traumatic for the children and would allow them the opportunity to deepen their relationship with their father without my interference. Until now I had been their primary parent, the constant in their lives, while their father skirted around the periphery, held off by my casual, yet visceral maternal possessiveness and his own wariness about his ability to parent. In my heart, I was devastated.

All of this, this extraordinary emotional upheaval, was not unique to me and my family. Women everywhere in my world grappled with the same issues and conflicts. The struggle to balance individual needs with those of others was just part of being human, of living in Western society with all its clamoring demands for achievement, financial success, self-fulfillment. But no matter how common the situation, my gut reaction to it was only mine. No intellectual, rational acceptance of the reasonableness of this plan for my family can ever erase the grievous torture of leaving my children behind. Caught in a maelstrom of change, I finally capitulated to the argument from therapists and my ex-husband that this was the best plan. Exhausted and numb, trying to convince myself that I knew what I was doing, I acquiesced under the pressure of conflicting desires—to be my own person, to have my children with me, to do what was best for them.

My house sold, children left with their father, ricocheting between wild spasms of blubbering tears and seizures of euphoria, in a car stuffed with cherished houseplants, I survived a long hot drive to my sister's apartment in a new city, where I would camp out until I found employment and a place to live. Want ads were perused, a résumé written, and phone calls for interviews completed. A physician friend suggested I interview at a military hospital where nurses were sorely needed. I laughed: me, a child of the sixties? An antiwar protester? Work for the military? For people who wore uniforms and saluted each other? I decided to use the military hospital as my practice interview, never seriously considering the idea of joining the Civil Service, that maze of bureaucracy known for its mindboggling inefficiency and arcane policies and procedures.

I was interviewed by an officer, the director of the critical care floor, in this large medical center, where the labor and delivery ward was located. I wouldn't have known she was a senior officer if she hadn't told me, even though she was in uniform. My one private intentional act of defiance against the "war machine" was never learning to read military insignia accurately, and I occasionally addressed a commander or captain as an ensign, much to their indignation and my perverse glee. Of course, I always humbly apologized—"as a stupid civilian I just couldn't keep these ranks straight in my head!"

This officer led me down long hallways to the L&D unit, leaving me with another officer who was a midwife and the head nurse of both L&D and the antepartum and postpartum wards. We chatted: I told her about my prepared childbirth teaching and my late entry into nursing school, and she told me about being a nurse-midwife and her own recent first baby's birth at age thirty-eight. She gave me a tour of the unit. I tried to ask intelligent questions, but not taking this interview seriously, I was in such a carefree state of mind that I felt like I was just visiting, having a good old time talking childbirth practices with this nice woman. To my surprise she took me to the employment office and told people there to sign me up: she wanted me. With incredulity, I asked her, "Why? How do you know after just an hour? How can you assess someone so quickly?"

"Well, you have some background in childbirth and I like your attitudes about how it should be. Going back to school and doing so well is an indicator of your ambition and your abilities. And, I don't know, you just project yourself as a very competent, confident person. You're mature, you've had two kids, you're not the run-of-the-mill twenty-one-year-old new graduate."

I was pleased by her words and utterly astounded by her assessment. Me, confident and competent? I didn't know how to do anything clinically. I knew a lot of theory but I had only given five injections and changed five sterile dressings in nursing school—and made countless beds. I'd never drawn any blood, or worked with any IVs, much less started one. I had written volumes on the nursing process and nursing care plans; I had a great research paper under my belt. But taking care of a real patient, being responsible for her care during labor and delivery, starting IVs, giving medications, reading monitors—all by myself? You've got to be kidding!

I told her I'd be in touch and went on to my "real" job interviews. Again, I was offered a job on the spot at three different hospitals, to my growing delight. Much to my dismay I discovered, however, that labor and delivery nursing was considered a specialty and that very few hospitals were interested in hiring new graduates with no experience. L&D nursing was a much sought-after position; as a result most hospitals only hired experienced, in-house nurses. The pay offered to me by the military hospital was laughable: $17,000 a year with lousy benefits, compared to the $23,000 with outstanding benefits offered by a prestigious university hospital for a job doing neurosurgical nursing.

I was torn. I wanted to have a little money, after four years of severe penny-pinching and huge student loans. I didn't know what to do, couldn't make the decision; salaries and benefits and shifts and patient/nurse ratios swirled around in my head. My physician friend cleared the air for me real fast.

"There are two questions here, Susie. One is money. What was your annual income when you were married?"

"Around eighty thousand dollars a year. Why?"

"What was your annual income for the four years after you were separated and divorced, while you were in nursing school?"

"Fifteen thousand dollars, before taxes."

"So, you know you can make it on seventeen thousand. The first question is, how important is money? The second question is, what kind of patients do you want to work with? Neurosurgery patients or women in labor?"

The answer was immediate, a foregone conclusion. The entire reason I'd gone into nursing was to be involved with the birth process. I smacked myself on the head, knocking out the confusion. I was very fortunate the officer at the military hospital had offered me a job. She went out on a limb in doing so, realizing she would have to train me in basic nursing skills in addition to specialty nursing. If I didn't take her offer, I'd have to spend at least a year doing med-surg nursing and then have to hope for an opening in L&D. I *hated* med-surg! I'd been poor as a child and as a divorced woman. I had student loan payments for the next ten years, but I'd incurred those loans so I could be an obstetrical nurse. In short order, I took the job at the military hospital.

After a week of orientation—filling out endless civil service forms, getting lost trying to find different offices and meeting rooms, sitting through orientation talks, including one on the Communist threat and the necessity of being wary of spies, and of wearing for the first time the military-issue nursing uniforms that were designed for Dolly Partons rather than small-breasted women such as myself, I finally found myself on L&D for my first shift. I dressed in green scrubs. *Oh, thank goodness I don't have to wear that awful white uniform,* and carried my clothes and purse to the nurses' station since I hadn't been assigned a locker yet. I met a number of people, whose names refused to lodge in my brain, and listened to the mumbo jumbo of morning report, pleased that I could interpret at least a few of the acronyms flying around the room. "AROM, UCs, FHR, IM, IV" I could handle, but what was "IUPC, FSE, NSVD, VBAC?" The nurse assigned to be my preceptor was, of course, on leave for two weeks, so the head nurse told me she would show me the ropes.

While the hospital was immense, with more than a thousand beds, the labor and delivery unit was tiny, buried within the bowels of the critical care floor, with nary a single view of the outside world. To check the weather or glimpse the sky, we had to go into the patients' rooms on the adjoining ward. There were only five labor rooms, each a cramped, windowless little cubbyhole, painted institutional green and jammed with a complicated narrow metal hospital bed, one ratty, worn armchair, and a rolling supply cart topped with an electronic fetal monitor. A large trash barrel squatted underneath the built-in sink at the foot of the bed. A closet, stacked with supplies, occupied the space next to the sink. A heavy door concealed a narrow shower stall and a toilet. Getting a woman out of bed to use the bathroom required inordinate dexterity and agility: there was a space of only about two feet between the bedside and the wall nearest the bathroom door. I quickly learned it was easier to manueuver the woman, her monitor belts, and IV lines and pole out of the bed on the side farthest from the bathroom, where there was at least enough room for two people to stand side by side.

These five adjacent rooms opened onto the main hallway of the unit, facing the nurses' station and one of the four delivery rooms. Further down the hall were scrub sinks and storage rooms. A four-bed recovery room with an adjoining half bathroom was located on a secondary hallway branching off from the main hallway at the nurses' station. The unit's none-too-clean floors were industrial-strength linoleum, heavily yellowed with years of accumulated buffed and rebuffed wax. All the walls in these common areas were tiled, off-white, dented, and scuffmarked with black smears from gurneys careening back and forth from the delivery rooms. Announcements, instructions about personnel actions and medical emergencies, duty assignment sheets, phone number lists, doctors' beeper and office numbers, even lengthy typed instructions on how to handle a telephone bomb threat, and various other papers cluttered the walls and desk surfaces. A large white board hung on the wall between the first two labor rooms, directly facing the nurses' station.

This board was the census board, the epicenter of the unit, for on it was written the identities, condition, and status of the patients. Name, age, room number, gravidity, and parity—number of previous pregnancies and births— dilation and effacement, anesthesia and/or medications used, intact or ruptured membranes, risk factors—each notation sketching a portrait of our patients. At a glance, anyone working there knew immediately how busy or slow the shift would be. We could anticipate potential problems and mark the progress of each patient through the unit. We could locate various staff members, whose names were scribbled next to their assigned patients. The board was our starting and ending point. We gathered around it for a report at both ends of our shifts, listening to the charge nurse run through the data, adding comments or telling stories about our patients and our activities. Rarely did any of us get through even an hour without looking at the board, performing a continuous assessment of the unit's activity.

Across from the board, the nurses' station consisted of a freestanding desk unit on which squatted five fetal monitor video screens, two telephones, telephone directories, policy and procedure manuals, and miscellaneous memos, directives, reports, and circulars. Three or four delapidated rolling desk chairs and stools crowded the space behind this desk. Their torn Naugahyde seats were held together with dirty, peeling surgical tape; armrests were scarred with graffiti and sported a patina of ground-in oil from the countless hands that relaxed or fidgeted upon them. Against the wall opposite the larger desk, the chairs could be rolled to another built-in desk, complete with third phone, more of the same papers and reports, and gray plastic patient charts. A tall, stainless-steel cupboard was squeezed next to this desk. This cupboard held medications, monitor equipment, a small refrigerator in which to store pharmaceuticals requiring low temperatures, and the narcotics box—a double-locked, two-shelf container wherein controlled drugs were kept.

In addition to all the essential accoutrements of our work—papers, phones, charts, manuals—these two desks were repositories for pizza boxes, Styrofoam takeout containers, mugs, cups, soup bowls, napkins, crackers, purses, stethoscopes, blood pressure cuffs, paperback books, magazines, pens, paperclips, tape, syringes, needles, and so on, ad nauseam, the clutter and junk of all the people who worked and moved through the unit every day: doctors, nurses, aides, janitors, medical students, administrators.

This confined area served as our conference room, our work station, our recreation area, and our refreshment lounge. During the next four years, this nurses' station, along with the corresponding one a hallway away on the postpartum ward, was my home-away-from-home. I cleaned it, sorted through its debris, and trashed it innumerable times. Along with everyone else, I worked and rested, argued and discussed, cried and laughed within its borders. It became as familiar and comfortable to me as my own kitchen. It was where I became a nurse, and I loved and hated it simultaneously.

The four delivery rooms of the unit varied in size, but all were similarly equipped. A bulky steel delivery table occupied the center of each room. This table was actually a complex device. There were handles and platforms and stirrups and pedals that could be manipulated manually or electrically to adapt the surface for a variety of medical/surgical options. It took me forever to learn how to operate these tables, a task complicated by individual idiosyncracies in each. Every room also contained a rolling bank of emergency equipment and monitors for the anesthesiologists, a fetal monitor, a mobile infant warmer/resuscitation island, two or more stainless-steel carts and tables for equipment and instruments, suction and oxygen equipment, portable and fixed lights, IV poles, a baby scale, and built-in floor-to-ceiling supply cupboards. The rooms were colorless, stark, and unwelcoming.

No one could be mistaken about the function, the utility of these rooms. They were designed for practical, efficient, methodical, medical activities. Warmth, color, vitality, and hospitality were provided by the people who functioned in these rooms. Empty of people, they were intimidating, almost hostile with their gleaming surfaces, their complex machinery. It never ceased to amaze me that these rooms, and all the other delivery rooms I would work in, could be the place where new life began, where great drama, excitement, fear, joy—the full range of human emotion—occurred. The very starkness of these rooms, the undeniable coldness, battled with the biological, human activities enacted within their walls. No matter how familiar these rooms became to me, or how accustomed I grew to their forms and functions, I have never lost the rueful sensation that in them I am occupying a perverse, alien country, at odds with who I am and what I am doing.

The sounds of this bizarre, busy place—the hum of flourescent lights, harsh in their glare; the clicking and beeping of monitors and IV pumps; the rattle of gurneys rolling through the halls; the clangor of ringing phones; the sighs and moans of laboring women; the cheering laughter of participants in a birth; the swishing of the massive double entryway doors—combined with a distinctive odor to epitomize my workplace. There is nothing more immediately evocative and recognizable to me than this smell: a blend of alcohol, industrial cleaners, ammonia, antiseptic soap, plastic wrappers, blood, feces and vomit, freshly laundered linens, Chinese takeout, pizzas, and burnt popcorn!

After report on that first day, everyone wandered off to take care of patients, read charts, check orders, count narcotics. I sat stunned by incomprehension: *Well, now what am I supposed to do?* A young man in scrubs strolled up to the desk where I sat. *Was he a doctor? A medical student? What?* Dressed in blue scrubs like my own, he was slender, just over six feet in height, with well-muscled arms and broad shoulders that tapered elegantly down to a slender waist and, as all the women on the unit concurred, a sexy butt. He had deep-set green eyes, a mischievous grin, and fine black hair, short-cropped military style. Leaning nonchalantly against the desk, he inquired, "Hi, who are you?"

"I'm Susie Diamond, the new nurse. Really new. I just graduated from nursing school and I don't know anything."

"Hey, great! I'm Nick, I'm a paramedic here. We'll teach you all you need to know, don't worry. It's nice to have you. We need some more nurses around here."

I sat there grinning at him stupidly, wondering why there were paramedics on L&D. He confessed later, sheepishly, that he called himself a paramedic because it embarrassed him to identify himself as a licensed practical nurse in the military. I had no idea at that moment how significant this man would be in my professional growth, but I was grateful for his friendliness.

The rest of the day passed in a cloud of confusion. The head nurse kept forgetting me. She'd give me some little task to do or suggest I read the SOPs (the policies and procedures manuals) and vanish, leaving me as bewildered as I'd been when I first came on the Deck, as the L&D unit was called.

Over the next week, I wandered around, familiarized myself with the unit, learned some names and faces, tried to fathom the reams of papers that comprised a patient's chart, and attempted to understand the jargon and nicknames on the unit. It was a foreign country with its own exclusive language, customs, rituals, and rankings, both medical and military. Each time I found myself unsure of where I was supposed to find a certain item or how to perform a certain task, which was every time initially, I looked for Nick.

> *What is an IMED?*
> *Where is the scrub room?*
> *What does she mean, "do the dishes"?*
> *What is a Dinamap?*
> *What is a FSE?*
> *How do I "set up for internals"?*
> *How do I "break down the table"?*
> *What does "setting up a room" mean?*
> *What is a "dial-a-flow"?*
> *Where is the lab, blood bank, OR, parking office?*
> *How do I use a Doppler?*
> *Show me how to "do the exam room."*

I asked Nick endless questions. I followed him around, watching what he did, listening to what he said, learning like crazy. He was always available to me. He answered all my questions, no matter how obvious or how often I repeated them. So much information was flying in my face that my head hurt at the end of the day. My brain literally felt scrambled. I'd listen to an explanation from the head nurse without comprehension and then search out Nick to explain it again. He watched out for me, finding what I needed before I could get frustrated in the search, while making sure I learned where to find it again. Before he started a task, he'd invite me to join him.

"Come on in the delivery room, I'll show you how to break down the table. Come with me, I'll show you how to clean the postpartum room. Here's how to put on a monitor. Here's how to read the strip. Let's go through this internals setup again. Watch out now for your sterile procedure, you don't want to contaminate the openings of the tubes."

The best part of the first days was going into the delivery room. The head nurse walked me through two or three deliveries, explaining what my duties were, giving me pointers on how to organize my time and tasks, and how to watch for untoward events, like a baby that wasn't real responsive at birth or a mother who was bleeding too much.

"Look at the baby when he comes out, Susie. If he's waving his arms and his legs are kicking or pulled up tight and he's crying, he's going to be a good baby. If he's limp and blue, get ready to really stimulate him. . . . Hear that sound, Susie? That's the 'gutter' sound, like rain rushing down a gutter. When you hear that, you've got a mother who's hemorrhaging, bleeding a lot more than is acceptable."

I loved being a part of it: helping push the bed through the door, getting the woman positioned on the table, drawing up medicine into syringes, prepping the perineum, drying off the baby, assigning Apgars, putting on identity bracelets, filling out the papers, crowing with delight over these new babies, praising their mamas and daddies, holding them in my arms. I was there— a real member of the team, contributing, helping, not just standing by as an observer.

I learned. The staff was wonderful to me. The other nurses gave me time and explanations, most of them friendly although harried. They watched me and waited while I learned the job, forming their opinions about me as I slowly began to contribute to the unit. The head nurse gave me miles of space and time to take it all in, process it, and begin to organize all the thousands of bits of information I needed to know to be a good nurse. The casualness with which she answered my questions disguised her considerable clinical knowledge and expertise. I never ceased to admire her patience with the residents and interns. It was hard for me to understand how she could tolerate their fumbling attempts when she knew so much more than they. She never pushed me, never criticized me, never gave me more to do than I could handle. A good bit of the time I think she forgot me, leaving me in the practiced, capable hands of Nick.

He held my hand literally and figuratively for three months, walking me through every task, every procedure, with patience and a tremendous willingness to teach for which I was terribly grateful. He never seemed to be in a hurry, even when everyone else was flying around frenetically responding to emergency lights or hustling a patient to the delivery room for a crash C-section. Nick just ambled along, flipping his bandage scissors around on his forefinger, like a gunslinger tossing his pistol, always arriving at the emergency scene at the same time or before all the other scurrying people. Although I studied him whenever I wasn't one of the scurriers, I never could figure out how he accomplished this! There was a lithe, unconscious grace in all his movements, sort of catlike. This feline grace, combined with his unflappable self-possession, exerted a calming effect on everyone around him, even when they were angry with him. It was as if here, in this sterile modern environment, the spirit of an Indian hunter or woodsman of old was embodied within the slim body of this young man. I later learned that my fanciful images of him were not off-the-mark: hunting was his most highly favored off-duty activity.

For me, always too serious, woefully lacking a sense of humor as I concentrated fiercely on learning my work, the most enjoyable aspect about Nick's tutelage was his droll and ever-ready wit. He joked and teased everyone as he went about his work with a effortlessness that belied his skills and his complete mastery of the work of the unit. He knew how everything worked and how to fix it if it didn't. He knew everyone from doctors to housekeepers and did a lot of hugging and clowning around during the day, maintaining a sense of fun through emergencies and harried shifts, playing practical jokes, and entertaining the patients and staff during quiet hours.

Because I was allowed so much leeway in my orientation, each day was an adventure. I went to work eager for the next experience, looking forward to the laughter and friendliness, observing with fascination the interpersonal dynamics of the staff. My preceptor returned from vacation to begin giving me intensive training in obstetrical skills. She was experienced and adept at clinical instruction. She taught me a great deal about time management, setting priorities, and correct documentation. She had excellent clinical skills and was obsessively organized, a trait in which I was woefully lacking. We enjoyed each other, but I had some difficulty with her habit of gossiping about other staff members. I decided very early that I wanted to form my own opinions about the people with whom I worked and had to insist on several occasions that my preceptor not fill me in on various items of interest about co-workers.

I have never been a person of much discretion or privacy. If someone asked me about myself, I told them whatever they wanted to know. In the past, this openness frequently resulted in intimate exchanges of personal history and led to some important relationships for me. People would confide to me the most personal information, allowing me to offer comfort and advice, apparently because I had been so open with them. I was to learn the hard way that on a hospital ward such guilelessness was dangerous, exposing me to malicious gossip and cruelties I couldn't have imagined as a housewife. I had no preparation for the subtleties of the competition and territorial posturing among nurses, doctors, unit secretaries, and other hospital staff. I approached everyone in the same way: I needed and wanted to learn everything about my workplace. Everyone's work was of interest to me. I pleaded ignorance and asked politely about every task: how do you do this, why do you do it, what is the purpose and thought behind each activity. Most people helped me willingly, even though some laughed about my ignorance behind my back.

I leaned on everyone, but most especially on my preceptor, the head nurse, and Nick. These burgeoning friendships did not go unnoticed by my fellow workers. Not surprisingly, I found myself being identified as a teacher's pet, since the head nurse made herself so available to me. It never occurred to me not to go to her with questions. I used her knowledge and her skills without realizing that some of the nurses thought this practice unusual. They were bent out of shape because I jumped rank when I went straight to the head nurse. My preceptor had her own enemies, who automatically became mine, without my knowledge, when my friendship with her developed. And there were several people who were blatantly jealous of the attention Nick gave me. They resented the obvious fun we had together. Several of the nurses felt it was inappropriate for me, a registered nurse, to consort so obviously with an aide, which Nick, an LPN, was. It was beneath my rank to do aide work, like setting up delivery rooms or washing the "dishes," the instruments.

This was confusing to me and it took me several years and too many conflicts to learn to be more discreet, to be careful of gossip, to guard what I said about my personal life and my interactions with co-workers. The intricacies of working relationships, the territorial infighting, the concern with and jockeying for rank and position were fascinating to me at first. Eventually, I found it insulting, demeaning, irritating, and ugly. But in the beginning, I didn't know how to be guarded.

It was hard. I wasn't prepared for the emotional impact of gossip about me. It hurt my feelings and made me cry, much to my embarrassment. It affected the way I interacted with people. It took a toll on me, gradually souring my enthusiasm, my love for my workplace. I hated having to watch what I said, how I behaved. I hated having to guard against possible misinterpretations of my actions. Worst of all, there were times when I behaved just as reprehensibly, indulging in gossip and fault-finding.

But I was defiant about my friendship with Nick, even after a friendly caution from the head nurse. He had taught me too many things, spent too much time with me for me to pull rank and dismiss him as an aide. Nick was absolutely the best clinical instructor I had ever had. He didn't have a nursing degree, but he was without question a nurse, par excellence. His clinical skills came from years of work in a cardiac care unit and then L&D. He loved to teach; he was a natural at it. All he needed was an eager student, which I was, and he was off and running, demonstrating, instructing, performing, guiding with such obvious pleasure that learning from him was a joy. My first IV was an excellent example of his masterful teaching.

It was hospital policy that anyone who would be starting IVs had to spend a day in the OR prep room being taught the procedure before they could do IVs on their units. Scheduling difficulties had made it impossible for me to take this mini-course during my first three weeks of work, so Nick made me a fake arm. Taping an inflated rubber glove to an armboard, he attached a piece of tube underneath the glove to simulate a vein. He showed me how to rig the IV bag and tubing, how to flush the line, how to set up the tape, the adhesive bandage, the Betadine ointment, the tubes, syringe, and needle for the blood samples to be drawn after getting into the vein. I practiced with the fake arm under his watchful eye, as he talked me through one complete insertion. Then he made me go through it again, describing to him what I was doing each step of the way, and why.

A couple of days later, a patient needed an IV. My head nurse told me to do it. I reminded her that I hadn't completed the required training in the OR. Nick drew me aside and asked me if I wanted to try anyway. When I agreed timorously, he approached the head nurse for permission, which she laughingly gave.

"Sure, go ahead, if Susie wants to."

"Oh my God, I don't think I know how to do this!" I sputtered, as Nick led me to the IV cart and began pulling out all the items I needed.

"Yeah you can. You did it the other day on the dummy. Piece of cake, Diamond! Now put all this together like I showed you."

As I assembled the bag of fluid, tubing, needle, catheter, blood tubes, and starter kit, Nick began telling me a story about his hunting buddy. He chattered away with great animation about an adventure he'd had with this guy up in the mountains. We entered the patient's room, where I arranged the equipment as Nick regaled me with the details of his story, demanding my attention by touching my shoulder to get me to look at him, laughing and asking if I was paying attention. I went through the motions of preparing the IV: pieces of tape cut and waiting, syringe and needle unwrapped and ready, blood tubes and IV tubing within easy reach, tourniquet on, hand squeezed to fill the vein, vein palpated, explanations given to the patient.

Before I knew it, I was ready to insert the catheter needle. Still talking, Nick reached over, felt the vein I was planning to enter, nodded and said, "Go for it." As I stuck the needle into the woman's arm, he kept right on with his story, laughing with abandon at his antics in the mountains. He had deliberately timed the climax of the story with this moment! I felt my face go hot and my heart pound as I pushed that huge needle into the woman's arm and saw the blood return in the end of the catheter.

"Okay, now pull out the needle, put on the syringe, and draw back the blood. That's it. Now take off the syringe and attach the IV tubing, nice and tight. Open the port, see that it's flowing; the IV is going good. Now quickly, before the blood clots, get a needle on that syringe, and push blood into the purple tube first. That's your CBC tube. It has heparin in it to keep the blood from clotting so they can do the count. The other tube you always do second.

That's the type and screen tube. It goes to the blood bank. Doesn't matter if it clots or not. But you don't want to waste time getting the blood into the CBC tube or you'll have to stick the patient again, because it clotted. Now put your Betadine and Band-Aid on and tape up the tubing. Don't forget to take the tourniquet off, you don't want this good lady to lose her arm, huh?"

It was done. I never had time to be afraid or nervous. He made me listen to his story, diverting my attention, never allowing my anxiety to reach a conscious level. We walked out of the room and I jumped on him, hugging him and pounding on his back with exuberant relief.

"I did it! Wow! I did it!"

"Way to go, Diamond!" He laughed and then hugged me.

"You rat, you never stopped talking. You had me so engrossed in your crazy story that I didn't have time to realize how scared I was!"

What a high! Putting a needle into someone's body was the one clinical action that truly frightened me. I didn't hesitate with urinary catheters. I wasn't queasy with surgery or blood and body fluids. Bedpans and emesis basins didn't bother me. But something about sliding a sharp needle into someone's skin, in search of an elusive vein, seemed so invasive, so hurtful that I had been filled with dread about this task. Nick recognized my fear and pulled me right through the process, first by making sure I was familiar with the equipment and technique, and then by being there, talking and demanding my attention while supplying me with his physical presence as emotional support.

I was amazed at his insight into my anxiety and his unerring sense of how to help me overcome it, by making me just do the deed. He employed this teaching technique repeatedly with me, eliminating my fear, stressing the positive, praising my efforts and attempts, making little of my failures. My confidence in my ability to master the clinical aspects of my job soared under his tutelage. With this IV success, I knew I could depend on his support, so I just stopped being anxious about what I didn't know. I relied on his knowledge and his abilities; learning new clinical skills became a breeze.

As I moved through the weeks and months, I realized that clinical skills were actually the easiest aspect of my job. Doing a urinary catheterization, an IV, an injection, preparing a patient for surgery, assisting with procedures—all clinical activities—weren't that difficult to learn. Practice and repetition led to competence and skill. The only clinical area that continued to be of concern was interpreting electronic fetal monitor tracings. Because it is a relatively new technology and because it is an indirect indicator of fetal well-being, fetal monitoring is subject to considerable variation in its interpretation.

I have attended several conferences on fetal monitoring. I have perused monitor strips by the thousands. Watching the display screens is absolutely second nature for anyone working on an L&D unit. Those screens are the only available evidence of the baby's well-being. Whatever activity one may be involved in at the nurses' station, eyes are always turning to the monitors to assess and reassess the baby's status. The mother we can put our hands on. We can see her, talk to her, touch her, do things for her to make her more comfortable, to keep her healthy during labor. The baby is out of sight, beyond our touch, delineated only by this strip of paper, these green squiggly lines on a screen. The difficulty lies in the interpretation. There are no absolutes in reading these strips. We are only making educated guesses about how well the baby is tolerating the impact of labor.

With time I came to believe that experienced nurses were usually more skilled than the doctors in recognizing subtle or problematic strips. Older physicians may have more clinical years of experience than many nurses, but they haven't been watching strips any longer than the nurses, and they only look at their own patients' strips. The nurses look at *all* of them, *all* the time. While in training, doctors are exposed to many strips, with group discussions about the funny ones, but they go into practice where they will only watch their own patients. There are no accepted national standards yet, so one doctor's "late deceleration" may be another's "variable with a late component." There aren't even universally accepted terms for the events noted on the strips.

Nonetheless, many a lawsuit has revolved around these strips and what they purport; because of this, it is imperative that I know as much as possible about fetal monitoring. With all the strips I look at, it still surprises me how little I know, how easily I can be uncertain about what I am observing. It also amazes me that obstetricians don't routinely attend, as do many L&D nurses, conferences and workshops on fetal monitoring. At one conference, 350 people sat in a crowded hotel ballroom for three long days, avidly absorbing information about monitoring. Of all those people, only six were physicians. The remainder were L&D nurses, nurse-practitioners, and midwives.

My first successful experience with reading a monitor strip occurred in my third week of work. The fetal heart-rate tracing looked strange. I didn't know why it was so flat, with extremely subtle drops after each contraction: barely visible little arcs, like a contact lens looks resting curved side down on your finger. I fetched the head nurse: "Come look at this strip. I'm not sure this is anything, but it looks funny to me."

She caught me pleasantly off guard when she informed the entire staff at report that afternoon that "Susie picked up on a series of very subtle late decels." She was proud of me. It became my policy to always ask for a second opinion, a verification from someone else, when I was unsure of a strip. It is my belief that I was able to learn all my clinical skills as quickly as I did because I never hesitated to ask for help. I didn't care if my questions were stupid or if people thought it was silly of me to ask. If something about a patient bothered me, if there was some symptom or behavior that didn't make sense to me, I asked other nurses and the doctors to help. It was too easy to have a baby crash, to miss subtle clues because of other duties. I wanted to err on the cautious side, when I erred.

So I learned and I'm still learning. Labor and delivery nursing is a specialty field. In tertiary care (high-risk) hospitals it is similar to working in an intensive-care unit. While I may be directly responsible for just one patient, I am convinced that good obstetrical care is a collaborative effort. Because there is so much leeway in the so-called science of obstetrics, several heads are better than one in interpreting information and providing care. A good L&D nurse will always be humble enough to rely on her colleagues for help, to ask whether they think she is responding appropriately. Such questions and discussions are learning opportunities in themselves. A good nurse will always avail herself of these opportunities, sharing what she knows, taking in what others know, always willing to expand her awareness of theory and practice in the care of her patients. I've also learned that not a few nurses, out of fear of looking foolish, fail to use such opportunities. People who become arrogant and think they know everything about labor and delivery always get caught in the end!

Every time I found myself feeling smug about how good I was, how competently I performed, something would occur to humble me again. I'd miss a heart-rate deceleration or forget to take a vital temperature, or neglect to inform a doctor of an elevated blood pressure, and then I'd have to deal with the consequences. These little lessons in humility served to keep me sharp most of the time, heightening my concentration and my stress level, but I welcomed them. Caring for an invisible patient, the fetus, and its distraught mother demands close attention. It's not like washing cars or bagging groceries. Much of the job became routine as my skills and knowledge base grew, but I couldn't let my guard down, ever.

A "bad" baby is to be avoided at all costs. It isn't just the fear of lawsuits, although I have recurrent nightmares about being sued. Performance anxiety dreams in which I drop a baby, can't find the right medication, get lost on the way to the delivery room, or fail to save a hemorrhaging patient are standard fare for me. It's the knowledge that something I may have done or failed to do could affect the quality of another being's entire life. Watching a baby go down the tubes on a monitor strip because his mother has a serious infection, struggling to get a baby resuscitated because he won't breathe on his own, fighting to stop a serious postpartum hemorrhage so a mother doesn't have to be transfused, each may result in lifelong consequences. Keeps you on your toes, for sure!

The hardest thing I had to learn about nursing, however, was organization and time management. It has taken me years to reach a point where I am reasonably organized and able to complete my work in a timely, appropriate manner. Most L&D units are understaffed, which means that the nurses will have more responsibility than is actually safe. In addition, the nature of obstetrics is such that lack of organizational skills and the ability to set priorities will doom the caregiver. Babies can arrive with no notice. Mothers can require a surgical delivery with absolutely no delay. Medications must be given within specific time frames. From the minute the patient hits the door, there are tasks to be performed that must not be neglected or delayed. A perfectly benign-looking mother may be a walking time bomb with the elevated blood pressure and protein in her urine that indicate severe pree-clampsia, a potentially lethal disease of pregnancy. If the nurse doesn't check a blood pressure, dipstick a urine sample, and check reflexes right away, that mother may end up convulsing. If the nurse doesn't check the bleeding of a newly delivered mother, she may end up giving that mother a blood trans-fusion. If the nurse doesn't respond to a fetal deceleration on a monitor, a previously healthy baby may be jeopardized.

Sorting out all the details, recognizing what are critical, must-do tasks, working out a system of priorities, was the most difficult aspect of learning my job. When I wheeled a woman into the delivery room, it took me months to get the routine down:

> *Pull the bed into position next to the delivery table. Take a second to turn on the baby warmer. Get the mother on the bed, positioned in the stirrups. Put on the monitors so you can hear the baby's heart rate and get a printout strip going. Pour the sterile water and Betadine into the scrub basin. Don sterile gloves and wash the perineum. Tie the doctor's gown. Draw the Pitocin into the syringe so it's ready. All the while talk to the mother, explain what's happening, what we're doing. Palpate the abdomen and assist the mother with pushing. Be ready at the warmer when the infant is delivered. Be sure the suction and oxygen are on and functioning. In the first minute, dry the baby off, stimulate him by rubbing his back and drying him, remove wet towels, check heartbeat, check respiration, suction if necessary, check muscle tone. Talk to mom and dad while doing all this. Ad-mire the baby out loud. Clamp cord stump and cut off excess, check for three ves-sels. Fill out the baby bracelets and put them on. Do paperwork in between more critical tasks. Push the Pitocin into the IV bag and open the flow regulator. Get a temp on the baby, a blood pressure on the mother. Et cetera, et cetera.*

The first months I was a harried fool in the delivery room, running around frantically, working up a great sweat and panting through a wide-open mouth behind my mask. It seemed to take forever for me to get all the steps down, to be able to anticipate possible needs, to have everything checked and ready. Most of the time, I had help. When Nick and I worked the same shift, the delivery room experience was a leisurely pleasure for me, since he did almost all the tasks. Other assistants varied in their abilities, but usually I was free to concentrate on mother and baby care, leaving nonpatient tasks to the assistant.

My assertiveness blossomed, however, when I spent time in the delivery room without an assistant. The docs would be asking for things—gloves, forceps, fix the lights, raise the table, adjust the stirrups, and so forth—while I was trying to get the fetal monitor on or prepping the patient. It didn't take me long to learn how to say politely, with laughter, "Just a sec! I've only got two hands!" or "I'll be right with you, just let me take care of this." I had to learn what was important and what could wait, and then I had to have the courage to stand up to the doctor if he or she was pushing me unnecessarily. The worst part of all was when I was new to a unit and didn't know where specific items were or how to work the suction or oxygen or the delivery table. It was—and is—mortifying to have a team of doctors waiting for me while I fumbled in drawers or on shelves, looking for some piece of equipment.

The other problem I struggled with in my time-management difficulties was patient documentation. It was hard for me to take time away from direct interaction with the patient to chart what I was doing with her. I didn't want to write down vital signs every fifteen minutes when the patient was crying and writhing in the bed. I just wanted to focus on her; paperwork seemed so unimportant! Having to choose between writing nursing notes or spending an extra fifteen minutes helping a new mother with breast-feeding was torture for me. I made notes on my scrub pants to save time during the critical moments before a delivery or because I'd forgotten to take the clipboard into the patient's room. By the end of the shift you could always tell how busy a night I'd had by how scribbled up my pants were. I thought I could put off some notes until a quiet time, only to discover that I couldn't remember any of the details that needed to be charted and there weren't any quiet times when I needed them.

I managed to master charting on L&D within a few months but any time I worked on the postpartum ward I'd be writing notes for at least an hour after the end of the shift. I watched other nurses and the docs to see how they handled this ubiquitous, onerous task and picked up a few tricks of the trade. On occasion I was distressed to see notes written by a nurse or doctor who had not actually interacted with the patient. Histories and phys-icals were often completed by physicians who copied information in the chart without actually verifying the information with the patient. Several times I watched nurses write completely fabricated notes: one nurses' aide made up entire sets of vital signs for twenty patients without even entering their

rooms. I was disturbed by such actions but I understood some of the underlying motivation.

There is simply never enough time to attend to the patients' physical
needs adequately, provide emotional support, *and* maintain proper documentation. The pages of notes I had written about a single patient while in
nursing school were impossible in the real world. A crisis that might eat up
four hours of a shift would be represented on paper in less than two paragraphs. All the acronyms in medical charts had obviously evolved out of the
desperate need to reduce writing time. I learned to stand at the bedside
carrying on a conversation with the patient while simultaneously writing a
note on her status. I *hate* doing this. It was one of the big no-no's in nursing
school: the patient deserves your full attention, you may miss something
significant in her words or expressions if you're not looking at her, and not
least of all, it's rude! I always apologize when I have to write while talking,
and I make every effort to put down the papers and seek eye contact, indicating my attention and concern whenever possible. But there is simply no
way to avoid the paperwork: it must be done, accurately, succinctly, and as
soon as is physically possible after the care is given. "If it isn't written down,"
a nursing aphorism insists, "you didn't do it!" Just imagining having to
explain in court some nursing note I'd written ten years earlier or something
I remembered doing but didn't document gave me cold sweats.

One of the biggest problems with paperwork, everywhere I've worked,
is the duplication or repetition of information. For one birth I will probably
write the same details—gravidity/parity (number of pregnancies and of delivered babies), age and blood type of the mother, Apgars, weight, date, time
and type of delivery, bracelet number, and sex of the baby—a minimum of
five times, on five different pieces of paper. The mother's history and physical
information is reviewed orally and on paper by the nurse, the medical student,
the doctor, the anesthesiologist, and the pediatrician. The nurse repeats much
of this data to the hospital supervisor—whose need to know I will always
question—maybe to the lab, maybe the blood bank, maybe the chaplain,
maybe the social worker, and definitely the oncoming shift of nurses. To
streamline this plethora of data requires endless hours of discussion and committee work with the quality assurance people, the nursing administration,
the physicians, the nurses themselves—all on one's own time, of course. Then
new documents have to go through a trial period, then a printing, etc. It is
such a stultifying and agonizing process that most units bow to the inevitable
and fumble with the reams of papers that already exist, complaining bitterly
all the while. Eventually computers will relieve some of the paper congestion,
but so far computer use in the hospitals I've known has only added to, rather
than reduced, the workload.

Knowing what to write is a whole other issue. Nurses' notes must be
brief, cogent, and legible, and they must be written in such a way that what

you write can't be used against you in court. Fear of lawsuits taints every carefully written note. If something untoward happens to a patient as a result of the care she is given, it must be documented, but oh so carefully. Never, never give away any data that might be held against you. For example, if a patient suffers a serious vaginal laceration because of the misapplication of forceps, the chart would only indicate the severity of the laceration and how it was repaired, not what caused it.

If a patient is furious about her care and signs out against medical advice (AMA), you'd better hope the nurses have documented information about her complaint. We had a patient leave the hospital AMA after ten days of argument, discussion, cajoling, and placating. Nothing we could say or do seemed to alleviate her anger at the care she was receiving. When nursing administration examined her records, there was no evidence of any of the problems she alleged. All the nurses had carefully documented her physical care—medications, procedures, etc.—but not one had written a note about her psychological status and all that we had done to try to placate her. There was no documented reason for her departure. This left the hospital at risk for a lawsuit. She could say anything she wanted about how we had treated her and we had no evidence to the contrary.

Working on the ward forced me to be organized in a fashion I'd never accomplished in my private life. There were so many tasks necessary to complete each shift, so few hands to complete them, and so much paperwork that I thought I would collapse under the weight of my responsibilities. The first two years I usually worked the day shift. In most cases, I was joined by one nurse's aide and one LPN. It was remarkable how difficult the day could be if I didn't have reliable help. I had never managed anyone before and found it extremely difficult to give orders to another person. I always expected my co-workers to know what to do and to want to do it well. Several of the employees on the unit gave me a heavy load of grief for months before I became more hard-nosed and assertive.

One day, about eight months after I started work, I was reduced to tears by the end of the shift. My two helpers, an LPN and a nurse's aide, had ignored my requests and assignments all day. Both had left me alone on the unit after telling me they had to be somewhere for a military duty. I didn't challenge their right to leave, not realizing it was within my authority to do so.

I was alone for three hours in the middle of the shift. Twenty-four patients, all requiring postpartum checks, teaching, medications, assistance to the bathroom, IV fluid changes, and so forth, and only Susie to answer the call bells and do the running. The head nurse was out for the day. Nick was working on L&D, which was frantically busy all day. There was no one I could appeal to for help. I had charge-nurse paperwork to do, in addition to my charting. (The charge nurse is the nurse responsible for the unit during one shift. She assigns work, directs the flow of traffic, and answers for any mishaps during the shift. She may or may not also be the head nurse, the manager of the unit. Usually charge duties are rotated among the senior staff nurses on each shift.)

At five o'clock, two hours after the end of my shift, I finished my last note in tears, crying with anger, frustration, and exhaustion. I complained to Nick about the unfairness of it all, asking why he hadn't come to my assistance, even though I knew how busy he had been. I had grown so accustomed to depending on him that I was hurt by his inattentiveness. He listened quietly and then taught me another important lesson.

"I saw it happen. I watched you the whole day. I knew you were in trouble and I stayed away," he calmly announced.

"What? Why the hell did you do that? If you knew I was in trouble, why didn't you help me?"

"Look, Susie. You are a good nurse, clinically. You've learned your work well. You are outstanding in your interaction with patients. There isn't anyone on this unit who can compete with you in those areas. But you are a lousy manager."

I was aghast. Nick had never openly criticized me before. He had witnessed many of the mistakes I made as I learned my job, but he'd always praised my efforts and used those mistakes as teaching opportunities.

"Well, uh, what do you mean? Those aides know their jobs. I gave them their assignments. Do I have to baby-sit them to get them to work?" I demanded self-righteously.

"Yes, unfortunately, sometimes you do. With some people you have to be so explicit there can be no question about what you expect. Sometimes you have to write out their tasks and make them come to you when they've finished to check them off. Your problem is that you're too soft. You let people walk all over you. Sure, I could've helped you, but I didn't. I won't always be here. You have to be able to manage your assistants without me standing by to back you up. You have to learn how to be hard-nosed. For example, the nurse's aide didn't have to leave the unit. You are the charge nurse. If you need her for patient care, she can't tell you otherwise. But you have to be firm. Some people will push you, test the limits over and over again, until they learn you can't be pushed around. Your problem is that you want everyone to like you. You expect everyone to work as hard as you do, to care as much as you do. Well, learn this real fast: they won't and they don't. So you have to make 'em do their work right. They won't like you for it, but you aren't here to be friends with them, you're here to get a good day's work out of them. I'm sorry. It was hard to watch you go down the tubes, but you needed the lesson."

I listened. I knew he was right. As a child I had learned, from my mother's example and in the Catholic schools I attended, to avoid confrontation and conflict at all costs. A good girl did not express anger. A good girl did not question authority figures. A good girl did not act out her negative emotions. Until I starting working with other people, I had managed to avoid most situations that called for assertiveness. I was almost phobic about emotional confrontations and was so successful at suppressing negative emotions that I couldn't even identify what I was feeling when I was angry. I did what I was taught at my mother's knee: I cajoled and smiled, acquiesced and apologized. I was a wimp. My marriage had undoubtedly been critically damaged because of this phobia.

When I was newly married, my husband was in graduate school, so I earned our living. I worked for two years as a secretary in an engineering firm. The pay was good, I loved the men I worked for, and did well at my work, but the only other woman at this company was irritated by my presence and easy rapport with our bosses. She began a hate campaign: by the time I resigned my position, the whole office was in chaos—people taking sides, rude insults being exchanged, tears and recriminations souring each day. I was young and inexperienced, but I behaved as abominably and childishly as she, whining and crying to everyone about how unreasonable and nasty she was being. I left under a cloud of pain, sickened by what had occurred, and never realizing that I had a problem. I just ran, desperate to get away from the emotional upheaval.

That was my last job until I started nursing. I handled conflicts in nursing school by writing very articulate letters, which kept the possibility of face-to-face confrontations at a minimum. Now I was repeating the same kind of behavior on the ward—whining and crying to Nick after allowing myself to be abused and mistreated by two people under my authority. God, it was humiliating! But how hard it was for me to be assertive. It took me years to learn how to assign tasks and to ensure they were completed.

I was too soft too often. When the childish behavior of some of the staff infuriated me, I'd rail about how ridiculous it was for me to have to expend time and energy dealing with adults who weren't performing up to par, on top of all my patient care work. I resented the time, effort, and psychic energy it took to deal with lazy, rude employees. I couldn't understand why people didn't just do their jobs, and cut out all the shit. But I didn't want to acknowledge my own contribution to these conflicts. It was too frightening to stand up for myself, particularly when a pissed off employee was spitting in my face. So I complained and cried and couldn't sleep at night, all the while trying to lay the blame for interpersonal conflicts on other people.

These conflicts eventually absorbed so much time and energy and caused such hostility that I was simply floored by them. If one or two employees were unhappy on the job, they could and did wreak havoc on the unit. Arguments, malicious gossip, and downright refusal to carry out a task would all occur. Hours were lost in counseling sessions, writing incident reports, monitoring behaviors—all at the cost of good patient care.

When I began to assert myself after Nick's lecture, I made enemies. I can't begin to describe the toll it takes on my psyche to have to contend with a hostile subordinate who deliberately sabotages my efforts. Before she was transferred to another unit, one particular LPN caused so much trouble that I dreaded going to work. She had nearly all the nurses in a state of complete frustration; she underwent almost daily counseling sessions with the head nurse. One night I was bombarded with patients on L&D. Fourteen women went through the unit in an eight-hour period. Three deliveries occurred almost simultaneously. I had only an aide and this LPN. Somehow she managed to sit at the desk for several hours, ignoring first my requests and then my commands for assistance, lackadaisically attending to little jobs here and there, just skirting the edges of downright insubordination. Eventually she actually refused my demands for help and I wrote her up. My exasperation only intensified when my complaints were ignored because I wasn't a military nurse with rank over her, even though as charge nurse I had the authority to give her orders.

Being a civilian employee in a military facility sometimes made my work more complicated, as this episode illustrates. The staff at this hospital was about evenly divided between military and civilians. Our patients were either active-duty soldiers or their dependents. Quite a few of them were surprised to have a civilian nurse and always asked me why I chose to work in the military.

In some respects, the civilian staff had an easier time: we couldn't be reassigned against our will to another ward, we couldn't be called in for emergency staffing before military personnel, we could call in sick without having to go to "sick call" and be seen by a doctor, we could take more time off for maternity leave than active-duty mothers. When conflicts arose between nurses and doctors, the powerful nursing command structure was available and ready to defend us, unlike at most civilian hospitals where I worked, where the doctors usually had the final authority over such conflicts.

But if a soldier was insubordinate or lazy or incompetent, it was far more difficult for civilian nurses to affect a punishment for that soldier. While in theory, the military nurses' aides and LPNs were under my authority when I was charge nurse, if they were brazen enough, they could circumvent my instructions. I wasn't an officer, I didn't outrank them, and the troublemakers were cunning in their ability to skirt the boundaries of this "artificial" chain of command, knowing their commanding NCOs would be unlikely to take action against them on the word of a civilian.

I still have problems with subordinates. It remains difficult for me to insist that someone improve his performance. I tend to do the job myself, alone, rather than have a patient suffer because a subordinate is lazy or un-motivated or rude. This is a continuing battle for me and one of the main reasons I left a management job after only a year. I have no patience with people who don't care about doing a good job, particularly if their laziness or sloppiness has an adverse effect on the patients. I also have no desire to police such people. I didn't go into nursing to be a baby-sitter. I just want to take good care of my patients. Gradually I've learned to distance myself from people I work with who don't meet my performance standards. I'd rather do more work and do it well by myself, than deal with the conflict and stress of trying to get a lazy co-worker to perform. But I'm still avoiding my fear of confrontation and my lack of assertiveness.

As time passed I did learn enough to hold my own, most of the time. It felt wonderful to reach the point where I could be the only nurse on L&D for a night shift without being fearful. I could trust my skills and knowledge enough to know I could handle the unit. The ultimate compliment came in the form of trust from the doctors. How lovely to hear a resident sigh with relief when I came on and say, "Oh good. Su-sie's on tonight. Now I know I'll be able to get some sleep." The residents knew I would only call them if the need was real, but that I wouldn't hesitate to wake them if I was unsure about something. I enjoyed many nights alone, knowing the doctors were getting much needed rest while I guarded the patients with confidence.

The night shift became my preferred shift because of the autonomy I enjoyed. I didn't have bosses standing over me, watching what I did. I didn't have to worry about all the nursing tasks that occur only during daylight hours, such as admissions for diabetic teaching or surgery, scheduled cesareans or inductions, daily postpartum checks and teaching, linen changes and baths, ambulating patients and changing dressings. Most patients on the ward slept, if we left them alone, and only L&D dealt with unexpected patients. I loved walking to the lab or the blood bank in the middle of the night. The empty halls and the quiet wards were so peaceful, unlike the bustle and hassle of a large hospital during the day.

Of course at night there were many times that I was frantic for un-available help. Getting lab results or respiratory therapy or housecleaning or food could be nearly impossible. At another hospital where I later worked, no housekeeping was available at night: I cleaned the rooms after each labor and delivery, mopping the floors, scouring the birthing beds free of blood and fluids. But somehow the night shift fed my maternal instincts: I was awake and watching over my charges while they slept. It felt good and I sure loved climbing into bed in the mornings while the rest of the world went off to work!

*　　*　　*

Two years passed. I was doing well in my work. My personal life was strange the first year. My sister Katy and I leased a lovely apartment together and enjoyed sharing each other's daily lives. I spent a lot of weekends making a five-hour drive to be with my children, who were doing well with their father, although our separation remained unbearably painful. I dealt with the pain by ignoring it, immersing myself as completely as possible in my work.

The visits with the kids hurt like hell; I felt so estranged from them. They were changing, growing up without me. Rebecca got her hair cut for the first time without me. She started menstruating without me. Michael looked so changed every time I saw him, it felt almost like he was someone else's child. I spent $350 on hypnosis to quit smoking, went a week without cigarettes, and then fell apart after a particularly painful visit with the kids and was soon smoking two packs a day again.

We coped, the kids and I. We spent as much time together as we could. My phone bills were horrendous. When I was with them, I concentrated on having a good time. They were fascinated with stories about my work and we endlessly discussed plans for our reunion. At the end of the year, Katy and the kids and I, along with the dog, moved into a four-bedroom town-house. Michael walked to the public school a few blocks away. Rebecca started junior high. We were together again! I worked nights because Katy was home with the kids while I was at work. In the mornings I'd get them off to school and fall into bed until three in the afternoon when they came home. I'd have the evening with them until I left for work at 10:30. It worked reasonably well, except when they had a doctor's appointment or there was an afterschool activity I had to attend. My children got used to Mom being crabby and looking like a zombie during the day and were wonderfully supportive of me. I wasn't the attentive mother I'd been in their early years: I was working full-time now and that reality was something we just had to handle. It was hard and left quite a few scars, but at least we were together.

The first two years at that first job, I really had fun. We somehow found time to play, in spite of all the stress and craziness of our wards. There's undoubtedly a relationship between working with laboring patients and an intense focus on anything of a sexual nature. Dirty jokes abounded. Old scrubs with holes in them were open invitations for "stripping parties." One nurse ripped at so many torn scrubs that the entire staff ganged up on her. On a quiet evening, she was cornered in a back room and had her scrubs, bottom and top, ripped off by everyone working that night. Many a night we would fill the board with false information, causing the oncoming shift much distress until they figured out that the "patients" were invented.

One night I came on a little early. Evening shift personnel were wandering around, not doing much before report time. I stood at the desk perusing the monitor screens. All the screens were active, with fetal heart rates and uterine activity of five patients in full view before me. As I watched, one baby's heart rate started to drop. No one else on the unit seemed to notice. As the heart rate continued in the low eighties, I ran for the room, pissed off that the evening people weren't paying attention. I hadn't even received report yet and here was this baby crashing on us! I flew into the room to find one of the residents sitting on the bed, holding the monitor against his chest, while another nurse pressed the uterine device to simulate contractions! They howled with laughter as I struggled to calm my palpitations and cursed them good-naturedly for tricking me. The laughter only increased as I went from room to room to find more phony patients! They got me good!

Another day, I answered the phone. A woman told me in a pathetic little voice that "something was hanging out of her vagina." The adrenaline started pumping as I questioned her, while my brain was flying through all the concerns of managing a prolapsed cord until the patient could reach the hospital. If the umbilical cord falls or "prolapses" into the vagina before the fetal head, each contraction squeezes it, shutting off blood flow to the baby, which can cause irreversible damage and even death.

"Are you standing up or sitting now?" I asked.

"I'm standing," she replied.

"Well, lie down and put your feet up!" I instructed her. "Is there some-one there who can get you to the hospital? Can you see what's hanging down? What does it look like?"

"It's sort of gray and looks like a wet rope," she told me. *Oh my God*, I thought. *How are we going to do this? The baby may be dead already.* When the woman started laughing, it took me a few seconds to realize I was the victim of a practical joke. I must have cursed the nurse on the other end of the line for five minutes before I got control of myself. She had really scared me!

One of our nurses was leaving for another job. We wanted to give her a memorable last shift. I brought my camera in. We talked one of the resi-dents, an outrageously good-looking guy, into getting on the delivery table. All the staff donned masks and paper hats and positioned themselves around him on the table. We put his legs up in the stirrups, amid much laughter and teasing about "seeing how it felt," and then called the nurse into the room. Her response was so wonderful that we couldn't resist taking the joke further. I ran down the hall and woke the senior resident: "We need you in the delivery room, stat!" She flew back with me, grabbing for a mask, firing questions at me.

"Who is it? Did someone just walk in? Didn't she call before she came? Why didn't anyone warn me?"

When she came into the room, the "patient" was writhing and moaning on the table. Such hilarity ensued that the rest of the night was spent gig-gling. I got it all on film as a good-bye gift for the departing nurse.

Nick was a big instigator of practical jokes. I learned a great deal about the therapeutic effect of laughter from him. When we did rounds together on the ward, he razzed the patients on the ward unmercifully.

"Time to wake up, ladies! Roll out now! Get up and get showered. You don't want your husbands to see you looking like this, do you? Good lord, girl, look at your hair! Let me see your toenails. What? You didn't polish your toenails before you came in here? Is that a nice thing to do to us?" In minutes he'd have the women simpering and giggling like little girls.

"I just think it's nice to focus some attention on them as ladies, Susie," he explained when I expressed my amazement at what he could get away with. "All the attention goes to the baby, so I want to have them remember themselves and their own attractiveness." I've used this technique frequently since then. It lightens things up after a long night with a crying baby and a sore bottom or belly.

He took particular interest in the long-term antepartum mothers we had on the unit. It wasn't unusual to have a woman stay with us for weeks, even months at a time, if she was at risk. A patient with a placenta previa—a condition where the placenta implants over the cervix instead of high in the uterus—and bleeding episodes, a mother carrying twins or triplets, a premature labor patient, or a mother with prematurely ruptured amniotic membranes, all might be in-hospital residents until their deliveries. If these women were stable, Nick looked for ways to brighten their days. One mother, enormous with twins, he escorted downstairs in a wheelchair. He rolled her out to the grassy slope behind the hospital, ceremoniously seated her on a sheet in the grass and shared a pizza picnic with her. It was the only time she was outside in almost three months. She stretched out on the lawn and waved her arms and legs back and forth, telling him she was making "grass angels."

Mrs. Addison was with us for three months. Her cervix was prematurely dilated. She was having premature contractions on a regular basis. She was in one of the tiny, windowless labor rooms forever, it seemed, lying in a deep Trendelenburg position with her bed tilted head down, to keep pressure off the cervix. She had to use the bedpan lying almost upside down. She also had to eat in that position. IVs ran into her arms continuously in an attempt to stop or at least control her contractions. No privacy. No activity other than watching TV and reading. No windows. No uninterrupted sleep. Terrible food. Frequently harried or impatient staff members. Belts around her belly twenty-four hours a day. After several miscarriages, she wanted to have this child in the worst way, calmly ignoring her husband's and mother's anger over her condition. They felt it was too much to put up with, to try to sustain the pregnancy at such cost to her.

The woman was a saint! I marveled at her fortitude, her motivation, her patience. We talked a lot during the hours I cared for her. Mrs. Addison explained how much she wanted this baby and how she realized she would probably not have another. For someone who had seven siblings and who had dreamed all her life of having ten children of her own, this baby was simply too precious to lose. She didn't mind putting up with all the discomfort and boredom, as long as she could give this baby another day or week or month of gestation time within her. "It's only a few weeks out of my whole life, after all. Is that too long a time to invest in a baby's life?"

One day I walked into her room and was startled out of my skin! There in that tilted bed lay tiny Mrs. Addison. Stretched out full-length next to her, his arm under her head, was Nick. "I just wanted to see what the world looked like from this angle!" he explained as she giggled helplessly in his arms. "Now don't be telling your husband you were in bed with another man!" he solemnly admonished her. I sat down in the chair, helpless with laughter, simply delighted by his lunacy.

A few days later Nick and I took Mrs. Addison for a "stroll" outside. This was an enormous undertaking, first necessitating lengthy discussions with the head nurse and the OB chief to obtain permission and then requiring considerable muscle to move the bed and the IV pole with three heavy IV pumps attached. Off we went to the elevator and the ground floor where we pulled and pushed Mrs. Addison around the entire hospital. It was the only time in three months that she had been outside of her tiny, windowless room. Nick pushed the bed and IV pole, teasing and laughing with Mrs. Addison whose eyes were devouring the green of the lawn and trees. I was frantic: What if she started contracting while we were doing this? What if we caused more cervical dilation? On the second trip around the building, Nick looked at me and asked, "You're not having much fun, are you, Diamond?"

"No, I'm not. I'm sorry but I'm just too nervous about this."

"Okay, it's probably time to go back in anyway," he answered. He leaned down over Mrs. Addison and whispered loud enough for me to hear as he grinned reassuringly at me, "Next time we'll leave this worrywart Nurse Diamond upstairs, so we can have us a good long stroll out here!"

She delivered finally, a healthy baby whom she named after the resident who had supervised her care. She returned to the unit, baby and a glorious homemade cake in hand, to thank us for our work. It was wonderful to see her upright and walking, beautifully dressed and made up, back in control of her person and her life. I could laugh with her then about Nick's playfulness and my nerves during her walk around the hospital.

After two years of working with me, Nick was reassigned to a new unit. His last day on the ward was Valentine's Day. Everyone had gathered at 0700 for morning report: six nurses, three aides, three medical students, and three residents, all of us by some weird fluke, female, except for Nick. As we stood around the board, listening to report, Nick ambled away from us. A nursery aide approached him down the hall a little ways from us. He started whispering to her and she began to laugh loudly and push at him, "Go on! You are not!" she hollered, interrupting report as we all turned to see what all the noise was about.

"Oh, yes I am!" Nick chortled. "Just watch me!" With that, he turned to face all of us women, pulled the string of his scrub pants and dropped them to his ankles in one fluid motion. Then he stood there grinning as he swiveled around, back and forth, modeling his white boxer shorts, which were adorned with large red hearts and the words I'VE GOT A HEART ON! You never heard so much screeching and hollering from a gaggle of women! As we convulsed with laughter, the doors to the unit opened and through them walked the assistant chief of obstetrics! Nick didn't even flinch; he just kept on modeling his underwear! What a send-off he gave himself and all of us!

In those first two years, I learned the importance of a sense of humor on a hospital ward. Teamwork is critical on any unit. Nurses and doctors need to be able to depend upon one another, to know they are not working alone. Praise for work well done, group discussions of problems—not fault-finding and blame-laying—and shared emergencies go a long way in dissipating the stress of an active L&D unit.

Humor changes the environment radically. Laughter over mistakes, teasing, and joking all help move the hours along and reduce the sense of working continually in a crisis situation. I wasn't consciously aware of the value of humor until several people left for other work assignments, Nick included, and I began to realize that whole days had gone by with a minimum of laughter.

As I moved on to other hospitals and other L&D units, the lack of humor became more glaringly apparent. I had to consciously remind myself to be playful, to tease and praise and laugh with my co-workers and my patients. I had to be willing to occasionally look like a fool in the eyes of my co-workers while playing with patients in order to lighten the atmosphere of a tense labor room. My sense of humor wasn't as free-flowing as Nick's; I had to work on it. But I continue to utilize laughter and joking as often as possible because the therapeutic effects are so obvious.

Another gratifying aspect of my first years as a nurse was the opportunity to teach others. When a new class of nursing students hit the unit not long after I began work, I empathized so strongly with them that I couldn't do enough for them. I remembered my own fear, my own insecurities so recently past. I encouraged them, praised their efforts, belittled their mistakes, thanked them profusely for their help and did as much hands-on demonstrating of patient care for them as I could.

I also welcomed new medical students eagerly, taking them around the unit, showing them where things were, how to chart, how to start IVs, how to assess a monitor strip. I explained my interactions with patients to them and tried to demonstrate effective methods of communication with a patient. Most of them watched me closely, and I knew I was making an impact on the development of these doctors-to-be. That was really important to me; I reveled in the opportunity to shape more caring, compassionate, and sensitive physicians and nurses. The extra time and effort required could sometimes be onerous, but in the beginning I didn't mind.

Eventually, however, I reached a state of exhaustion that prohibited much of this teaching, and drained most of my enthusiasm. But back then, I remembered my own fears before I knew much about labor and delivery and I recognized how invaluable my training was by Nick, the head nurse, and other contributors. I knew I owed it to new people to give some of that learning back to them. The time of exhaustion, of burnout, was still in the future.

Chapter Eight

A FAMILY'S TRIUMPH

REPORT: Mrs. Tyler—23 y.o. WF, multip, 40 wks. Admitted to L&D at 1810. Ext monitors x2 applied, IV ofD5 1/3 NS started in L arm c̄ 18G angio cath. FHT's WNL, reactive. VSS. Membranes intact. At 2045 pt AROMed, fluid clear, internals applied. Ctx q 3-4 min. Ctx continue thus through the night. Pt √ed at 0140, cervix 6 cm. Pt tolerating ctx well, FHT's OK, good BTBV. Husband at bedside, providing support. 0500—cervix still 6 cm, Pitocin started at 1 miu. Pt experiencing N&V. Ctx q 3 min, good variability. Pt given Stadol 1 mg/IVP for pain. Ctx q 2-3 min, strong intensity. 0615-mother requesting epidural. Cervix 7 cm. Pit 4 miu's at 0800.

As mentioned in the previous chapter, the above report is an example of typical nursing documentation. If written in English, it would fill two to three pages! While obviously unintelligible to the layman, telescoping sixteen hours of Mrs. Tyler's labor, the report told me what I needed to know to begin my morning at work.

Mrs. Tyler was having her second baby. She had an IV and external fetal and uterine monitors were strapped to her belly. She and her baby were normal according to outward indicators—her vital signs and the baby's monitor. Her membranes had been artificially ruptured and internal fetal and uterine monitors were applied. She was contracting and dilating adequately, until 0500 when Pitocin was started to augment her labor. Some nausea and vomiting was experienced; a narcotic was administered to ease her pain. At 0615, she wanted an epidural and was turned over to my care.

It started up like most slow days on L&D: I'd been working for just six months as I began this shift. I had only the Tylers in labor, which meant I could spend more time than usual in the labor room, assisting them. In their late twenties, they were a strikingly handsome pair. The young man, Mark, was tall, good-looking, and well groomed, with clipped dark hair and an athletically trim body. The mother, Marie, an attractive redhead, sat up in the labor bed with her makeup intact and her hair somehow still carefully arranged, hardly giving the impression of being in labor and lacking a night's sleep. She was counseled by the anesthesiologist for an epidural and our first interaction involved that procedure. By 0800, she had obtained relief via the epidural and relaxed visibly, focusing her attention on me. We talked; I went through my usual routine, verifying that she and her husband understood the monitors, interpreting some of the information they'd received from the physicians, answering questions and reassuring them both. We developed an easy rapport from the beginning. I asked my standard question: "Are you looking for a boy or a girl?" Unknowingly, this touched off a lengthy discussion that was of great significance later.

"I don't really care, as long as it's healthy," Marie replied, a frequent response from many expectant parents. I murmured my approval, "Yeah, that is what's important, after all." A flat statement erupted from her quiet husband, Mark, startling me with its force:

"I've had bad dreams all through this pregnancy."

I chuckled, reassuring him that nightmares or really weird dreams were common in a pregnancy. I told him about dreaming that I had given birth to a puppy when I was pregnant. Unsmiling, he shook his head and said, "No, I've had nightmares that this baby is a monster."

Instantly alerted to an unusual fear in him, I began to question them, trying to elicit more information so I could understand the origin of this fear and respond appropriately to his concern. As we talked, it appeared that both of them were frightened about the possibility of an abnormal baby. Some couples have similar intense anxiety, but nothing was said by either of them to indicate a possible reason for their concern. I asked them if there was a history of any problems in the family. Mark replied that no, they were just concerned. Their first child, a boy named Matthew, was three years old. He was hyperactive, "a handful" according to Marie. They didn't tell me then that Marie was a physical therapist, which might have been partly responsible for their feelings.

Empathizing with their obvious distress now that the topic was being openly discussed, I told them of my experience with my best friend, whose baby had spina bifida. Marie and Mark gave me their full attention, almost hanging on my words, as I spoke softly and with obvious emotion about the impact of that baby's handicap on her family, of how awed I was by my friend, as I watched her not only cope with this unexpected trial, but grow and mature to a strength and power I doubted I could find in myself.

Silently, I began to berate myself then for talking about such a subject and breaking my own rule: never tell horror stories to a pregnant or laboring mother. I felt deep chagrin over my big mouth and worried about speaking inappropriately. Attempting to assuage their fear and my own guilt, I apologized bluntly and honestly. "I'm sorry. This is not something I should be discussing with you at this particular time, while you're in labor. Sometimes

I'm not too tactful. Just remember that you're young, healthy, you've had good prenatal care, and you have no reason to think your baby's going to be anything but beautiful, like both of you."

"No, that's okay," they both assured me. The conversation drifted to a more superficial level, and nothing more was said about their fears. To this day, I rebuke myself for yapping away inappropriately about a handicapped infant. But I also wonder if that conversation wasn't a crucial one for this couple.

Around noon, we moved Marie to the delivery room. She had progressed rapidly in five hours, and was pushing effectively now. The baby's head was visible on the perineum and delivery was close at hand. In between her pushing efforts, Marie was excited, looking around the room, asking questions, telling Mark to take pictures "so we'll have a record of where the baby is born." Mark was noticeably nervous, but I attributed his behavior to normal fatherly jitters.

Nick and I were doing our nursing tasks, attaching the fetal scalp lead to the monitor, drawing up the Pitocin, prepping Marie, and positioning her legs in the stirrups. The obstetrician, Tony Trevino, was his usual cheerful, irreverent self, joking and encouraging Marie as she pushed. The anesthesiologist stood at the head of the table, making sure the epidural was providing sufficient perineal anesthesia. Two pediatricians were checking equipment at the infant warmer. I had called them to the delivery, per our protocol, since there had been meconium, or baby feces, in the amniotic fluid when Marie began to push. Because of this sign of potential fetal distress, they would be taking responsibility for the baby at birth, leaving me free to deal with the paperwork and provide emotional support for the parents during these last few minutes.

Marie kept pushing and at last the head was out. Dr. Trevino suctioned the infant's nose and mouth. Mark was all over me, touching my shoulder and asking, "Is it okay? Is it okay?"

"The baby's not out yet, Mark, relax!" I scolded, laughingly.

Now he was almost hopping from one foot to the other, trembling with nerves. I moved in close by Marie's leg, in front of Mark, and watched the baby slip out. I saw a flash of torso and buttocks and then Tony was clamping and cutting the cord, holding the baby, head down, in such a fashion that her body was hidden from our view. Opposite me, behind Tony, Nick was watching silently. "What is it?" cried Marie.

"It's a girl," Tony answered, too brightly.

"Is she okay? Is she okay?" Mark chanted, moving back and forth beside the table.

"Calm down, Mark, calm down," I said as Tony turned his back to us, swiftly passing the baby to the pediatricians. Marie was laughing and crying simultaneously, "A girl, a girl, I want to see her, is she all right?" Mark's agitation had become so extreme that I was alarmed.

"Give the peds a chance, Daddy. They'll tell us how she is as soon as they can."

I hadn't heard a peep from the baby yet and was beginning to wonder about her myself. I stepped up to the warmer and knew immediately that something was very wrong; the peds had the infant completely wrapped in towels except for her head. Normally, the baby is left uncovered under the radiant heaters while they do their initial assessment. I walked back to Mark, whose fright was now full-blown, and held him by the arms, trying to calm him.

"Settle down, Mark, settle down."

With their backs still turned away from us, blocking our view of the baby, the peds called out, "She's a little cold. We're going to take her to the nursery to warm her up and check her over." As they left the room swiftly, Mark slumped in on himself and muttered abjectly,

"Something's wrong, I know something's wrong."

"Cut it out, Mark." Marie laughed. "You're beginning to make me nervous." Tony, I realized, was ominously quiet. I looked questioningly over my mask at Nick. Almost imperceptibly he shook his head. I saw great pain in his expressive eyes before he lowered his face, breaking eye contact. He turned and slipped quietly out of the room. This unusual act made me realize that whatever he had seen had affected him deeply.

Now it was completely silent in the delivery room; Marie on the table, Mark at her side, Tony repairing the episiotomy. I realized I was holding the baby's identity bracelets in my hand.

"I'm going to run these bracelets to the nursery, Tony. I'll be right back."

Just outside the door, Nick was waiting for me, his unmasked face filled with pain. He hesitated as though uncertain about what to say. He swallowed and touched my arm:

"Wait, Susie. Before you go in there you need to know the baby is bad. Something's really bad. She has no arms and her legs are all wrong."

"Okay," I snapped, shocked, and stumbled blindly into the intermediate nursery and to the warmer surrounded by pediatricians and nurses. There she was, a cherub-faced, pink little girl, waving two half-arms with no hands or forearms. She had no legs, just funny little feet sticking out of what? Her buttocks, her thighs? I didn't stand and stare. I didn't allow myself any time to comprehend the enormity of this event.

"I have her bracelets," I said inanely, waving them in the air, grief-stricken as I realized there was no place to attach them; they wouldn't fasten on the stumps of her arms and there were no ankles. Someone quietly instructed, "Just put them down in the corner here." I turned to go but suddenly remembered something I felt the peds needed to know before they brought this infant to her parents.

"Her daddy told me he had nightmares during the pregnancy that the baby was going to be a monster."

"Well, she isn't a monster! We'll certainly have to make that really clear!" one of the peds answered emphatically.

Fortunately, Mark didn't ask me anything when I returned to the delivery room. I don't think he even knew I had been away. I was busying myself with paperwork when the door opened and two or three pediatricians walked in with the baby.

"Well, Mrs. Tyler, you have a beautiful baby girl. She appears to be very healthy. Her head and her torso are just perfect, but I'm sorry to tell you, she's got some serious problems." The doctor stood with the baby in his arms about two feet away from the table. I stood beside and to the rear of Mark, gently holding his arms above the elbows so I could catch him if he passed out. Nick had slipped into the room with the pediatricians. His face blanched, Mark looked as if his worst fears had just been realized. Marie, ramrod stiff on the table, barked hoarsely, *"What?* What's wrong with her?"

"She has no forearms, or hands, and no legs."

"Oh no! Jesus Christ, no!" Marie shouted violently. "What do you mean, no arms? Oh Mark, Mark, *oh no!*" Mark held onto her arm and buried his face against her shoulder. I continued to hold onto his arms. He stepped back as the pediatrician said, "She's a lovely baby, cute as a button."

"Oh, give her to me!" The words spat out of Marie's mouth as she reached both arms for the baby. Mark stood dumbfounded as she enfolded the baby in her arms.

"I can show her to you if you'd like," the pediatrician offered.

"No! I don't want to see it. Not now, not later! Oh my God, Mark!" she wailed. The blanket around the baby fell away slightly, momentarily revealing an unfinished arm. "Oh Mark, look, honey. Oh my God. Oh my God. No, I don't want to see."

"We've found through experience, Mrs. Tyler, that it's easier for parents after you've seen her; the reality is usually better than the fantasy," the pediatrician said quietly.

She held the small bundle silently for a moment more and then said, "No. Give her to her father. Let her father hold her." She thrust the baby into Mark's startled hands. I eased him onto a stool. He held the infant in his arms, rocking back and forth, searching the baby's face and moaning incoherent, soft little cries. I had my hands on him through all of this and now clasped him around the shoulders, whispering nonsense words to him and the baby.

"She's beautiful, hello little one, look how alert she is, oh Mark, look at her watching you with those big eyes."

Somehow it felt important to maintain body contact with this young man, as though my touch, the closeness and solidity of my own body could keep him anchored in this space. It seemed as if he would simply dissolve into a cloud of grief. Marie lay on the table watching him, a solid shape of rage, her anger intermingling with his sorrow until it was almost tangible in the room.

After a few minutes, Mark handed the baby mutely to the pediatricians, who left the delivery room. Mark and Marie held onto each other as she talked, frantically, angrily:

"We can't keep her. We have no money. We can't take care of her. You've got to understand. How could this happen to us? We can't keep her. I have to work full time because Mark's unemployed. He's got to go to college. We can't manage this baby *and* Matthew!"

Tony, Nick, and I were quiet, letting her talk. "I can't even cry, I'm so angry. Why? Oh Mark, oh God, *why?*"

I've thought of that time in the delivery room repeatedly, of how incomprehensible the whole scene was. There they are, two young people moving through a universal rite of passage, doing it according to Western ritual. She lies elevated like a sacrificial animal on a hard, cold steel table, legs held aloft in the air, draped with sterile blue paper, plastic tubing infusing bottled fluids into a vein in her arm, a catheter inserted into her back and taped in place, machines and equipment all around her, a male physician seated on a rolling chair positioned between her wide-spread legs, her genitals exposed, cut and bleeding under the harsh delivery lights. Her husband is rendered strangely impotent by the circumstances and his lack of medical expertise; dressed in foreign blue scrubs, his face covered by a mask, his hair by a paper hat, allowed only to stand at her side as an observer of her physical travail.

Under the eyes of complete strangers they must confront one of the most profound events they will ever experience, the birth of their child. And these parents are not given the normal rewards for tolerating the alien nature of a hospital birth. They have no relief or satisfaction after completing the strenuous work and bearing the pain of childbirth. There is no cheering staff, no awe, no thrill at seeing and hearing a new human being take her first breaths. There is no joy in this room.

These two young adults have just been handed what is probably the most serious challenge of their lives. They have been altered irrevocably, in the few moments it takes to delivery a baby, far more than most parents are with the advent of a child, for their baby is not normal. For the rest of their lives, they will be confronted daily with the reality of a severely handicapped child, and it is here, in this cold, sterile, unforgiving room, surrounded by strangers, that this new reality smashes into them.

> DELIVERY ROOM NURSING NOTES: 1120: Onset of 2nd stage. To DR via litter @ 1230. Connected to fetal monitor: FHT: 132. Hibiclens scrub to perineum. NSVD of viable female infant over ML epis by Dr. Trevino @ 1245 c̄ epidural anesthesia. Spont del of placenta @ 1250. Repair of episiotomy & third degree lac c̄ 3.0 suture. EBL: 375, Infant's weight: 7-2. Apgars: 7/9, per peds. Parents initial reaction to infant: Infant born s̄ lower arms & legs. Parents held infant in DR—Mother asked to hold—in shock, anger. Meds in DR: 20 U Pitocin, reinj epidural.

As Nick and I moved Marie to the recovery room, she announced angrily that she didn't want to see or be with anyone. I told her I would limit the number of staff in and out of the room and try to give the Tylers as much privacy as possible. Marie lay on her side, with Mark sitting on a stool drawn up close to the side of the bed. They were clinging to each other, foreheads almost touching, murmuring quietly, but falling silent each time I entered the room or neared the bed.

After I got Marie settled and checked her bleeding and blood pressure, I left them, returning to the nurses' station for the first time in a couple of hours. One of the nurses pulled me aside and plied me with questions about what had happened. I tried to tell her about the birth, the baby, but couldn't find the words. Now it was hitting me hard. Nick appeared; he must have seen the delayed shock in my face. Speaking quietly, he moved toward me: "You look like you need a hug," he said as he put his arms around me. I hid my face against his shoulder and realized I was trembling.

"Oh Nick, it's so bad."

"I know. That poor baby, that poor little girl." I hung onto him, needing the comfort his hug gave me, until I could pull myself together and return to the recovery room.

The pediatricians were in the room, questioning Marie and Mark about their medical histories. When they left, Marie said, "We don't want anyone to know, Susie. We don't want any calls. Please don't tell anyone anything, not anything. I want to talk to someone about adoption proceedings, please."

I was taken aback and struggled to hide my gut reaction to her words. Assuring her that no information would be given over the phone, I tried not to convey my dismay at their desire to give up their child. I knew, in those few minutes in the recovery room, how I was going to deal with this situation.

I felt strongly, and with a clear certainty, that it was not my place to interfere with their responses to this catastrophe. It was not my business how they dealt with their baby, and it was not my job to tell them what they should do about the baby or how they should feel or how they should act. I recognized that this was the Tylers' business, and theirs alone. No one else—not me, not anyone—had the right to interject their feelings or attitudes or judgments. I told Marie and Mark that I would be their advocate; I would do whatever I could to help them through the next few days, find the right people for them to talk to, and guard their feelings as best I could. I asked them to use me, to lean on me for support, information, and help, and to inform me if anyone on the staff gave them a hard time. I spoke quietly and nonjudgmentally, convinced that I must never impose my own feelings or beliefs on this couple.

A little later, I caught Mark as he passed the nurses' station.

"I'm going home for a while: I need to check on Matthew and the dog needs to be fed," he explained. I searched his face as I drew him aside and spoke to him briefly. He had been silent since the baby's birth; Marie had done all the talking. Now I wondered what thoughts were careening around in his brain. He stood before me, haggard and pale, a look of total incomprehension on his face. I held his arm and looked at him squarely in the eyes, trying to convey my concern.

"Mark, are you sure you can drive? You've been up all night, and you've had a terrible shock."

"No, I'll be all right," he replied quietly, ducking his head.

"Mark, maybe this isn't the right time to say this, but I'm worried about you. You need to talk, to let out your feelings. Marie is voicing hers without any trouble, but you're silent. I know you're in a state of shock now; it's difficult to believe that this has happened, but please, Mark, don't hold it in too long. It'll fester and make everything worse. I'm a good listener, if you need a shoulder." My eyes burned suddenly with tears; I wanted so badly to mother this boy, who had become a victim of fate before he could possibly be ready for it.

"Please pay attention to the traffic. Don't let your mind wander, okay? And try to get some sleep before you come back. Marie will be in good hands, okay?" He tried to smile at me and stumbled away down the hall. I couldn't bear thinking of his lonely drive home; couldn't imagine what he was going to tell their son about his new sister, so I shut my mind down and returned to the recovery room.

As I took her vital signs and helped her to the bathroom, Marie was quiet, listening without hearing as I told her how to care for her episiotomy, about her bleeding, her breasts. She lay back in the bed and spoke quietly into the darkened room.

"What can I do, Susie? I know what you said about your friend and how strong she grew. But Susie, listen, I don't have that strength, I just don't. I know what my life would be like if we keep Erica: trips to physical therapy, doctors, braces, all that goes with a handicapped child. I just couldn't do it. I know myself and I know I couldn't do it. Matthew is wonderful, but his needs are great and he demands more time than I can give him, even now. How can I possibly handle this baby, too? It tears me up because the most important things in the world to me are my marriage and my family, and I know what keeping this baby would do to my marriage, to Mark, to Matthew, and to me. It would destroy us, I know it would. I can't lose Mark."

I listened, dumbfounded, wondering how she knew all this, so soon after the baby's birth. Had she known she might have a handicapped baby? I didn't know she had worked with handicapped people, so I marveled at how organized her thinking was, how well she was able to articulate her fears. I was surprised just to hear her call the baby by name: she was bonding with the baby even as she planned to give her up. Lord help her!

Marie looked away and was silent briefly. Then she whispered softly, brokenly, "I lose either way. God knows how this will affect Matthew and Mark. If we give up the baby, it'll wreck my marriage, and if we keep her, it'll wreck my marriage."

What could I say? How could I offer her advice? I only knew that I mustn't try to smooth things over, or deny her feelings, or say anything as stupid as "I'm sure everything will work out." I straightened her covers and offered the only words I could come up with.

"This is so hard, Marie. I am so sorry. Just take it one step at a time. You don't have to decide anything now, this minute, or even tonight. Try if you can to rest now. You worked so hard during your labor and didn't get any sleep last night. Try to rest a little. One thing at a time, okay? I'm just outside the door if you need me."

I went home not long after this exchange, leaving Marie huddled in the darkened recovery room, talking to the neonatal clinical nurse specialist and the social worker about her baby and the chances of having her adopted. I drove in a mental fog to my aunt's house to have dinner with her and my children. When I walked into her house, I wrapped my arms around both Rebecca and Michael. Perplexed by my silent, intense embrace, they stood cooperatively as I stroked their arms down to their fingertips, marveling at my good fortune, bewildered by the fate that had given me whole, sound children while handing an armless, legless infant to that young, innocent couple. After we had driven home and they were both asleep, I stood beside their beds and thanked God that I would never have to experience what Marie and Mark were going through this long, endless night.

REPORT: 0700: Mrs. Tyler following nl PP involutional course. Used sitz bath & heat lamp x2 last night. She & husband looked at, held &

cried over infant. Father fed baby last night. Appropriate grieving behaviors noted.

It pleased me to know that Marie had wept, that she was beginning to express some of her grief in addition to her righteous anger, but I was surprised to learn that the Tylers had kept the baby in their room, caring for her during the latter half of the night. My boss assigned me to "special" them for the shift, which meant I was not responsible for any other patients. I entered their private room curiously. Marie was performing her morning ablutions; Mark sat on the cot looking sleepy, like an oversized, newly awakened child. The baby was not in the room.

We exchanged good mornings and I talked briefly with Marie about her postpartum recovery. Then she sat on the edge of the bed, and said quietly but emphatically:

"Listen, Susie, we need you to understand something. You need to explain this to them out there. We can hear them talking and we know that everyone thinks it's significant that we had Erica in here last night. That we're taking care of her, you know. But that doesn't change things. We love her, and we want her to get the best of care while she's here, but we are not going to keep her. We can't. We just can't afford it—financially. Please make that clear. We need to see the social worker. We want to talk to the orthopedist and the neurologist, too. Okay?"

"Okay," I answered. I looked at Mark. "You're real quiet, Mark. Is there anything you want to say, or ask?"

He shook his head, "No, we just want the best for Erica." I told them I would call the social worker and do my best to find out when the physicians would be in to talk to them.

When I found the social worker, we conferred briefly in the hall and then went into the room to talk with Marie and Mark. I remained for the interview, determined to fulfill my duties as their advocate and to make sure they understood what he told them. His style of interviewing was tentative, as though he was skirting the issue and uncertain of how to discuss their child. Both Mark and Marie gave me questioning looks as the social worker delicately probed their feelings about adoption. Finally I entered the conversation. Reiterating what I had heard, I summarized the social worker's questions and the Tylers' firm desire to look for placement for the baby. The Tylers concurred, "Yes, that's what we want."

The social worker left after promising to see what he could do, and the Tylers and I heaved sighs of relief. Just then, the nursery nurse brought Erica into the room. The baby was wide awake, her large, slate-colored eyes exploring the surroundings with a visible, intelligent curiosity.

"May I hold her? I haven't had a chance to yet." I picked up the tightly wrapped infant and sat down in the armchair, laying her out on my knees so

I could look at her face. Marie sat next to me, her body rigid and straight on the edge of her chair. Mark stood in front of us, watching. Erica's eyes were wide open; her facial expressions appeared to respond to my voice and my own expressions. "Hello, little one. Oh, you are very alert, aren't you? And you're so lovely. Yes, you are really listening to me, aren't you?"

"You can unwrap her and look at her, if you want to," Marie said. Her voice was muted, her words strangled.

"Oh, good, may I?" I replied as I began to unwrap Erica.

"You don't have to if it bothers you," Marie added. I knew immediately that I was being tested. She wanted, needed to see how I would respond to her baby's deformities. Indeed, she was testing herself; she was quiveringly stiff beside me.

"No, it's okay, Marie. I want to see what you've got here, Erica." I smiled and talked to the baby as I undressed her. She had a pretty little face, button nose, cupid's bow mouth, smooth and creamy skin. Her head was covered with soft reddish brown hair. I stroked both of her arms, baby-soft yet firm, but inexplicably terminated at the elbows. No forearms, no pudgy baby wrists, no grasping, waving hands or fingers. As I held Erica's fore-shortened arms, she moved them easily and with apparent strength. "My, you are strong, little girl. Look at you, waving your arms around!" Moving down her body, I felt her chest and belly, her torso straight, well-fleshed. Then I examined her legs, such as they were: a bit of flesh, like the beginning of a thigh, that abruptly became a foot, normal in shape, but having only two toes. Both arms and feet were perfectly symmetrical.

Focus on what is normal, on what she does have, I told myself. "God, Marie, she's so alert and so cute. Look at the way she's watching me. She looks so wise, like she knows a lot more than a newborn is supposed to!"

"I can't do it, Susie," Marie blurted. "It's okay when she's wrapped up. But I can't take her out and walk down the hall with her. I can't stand it. I don't want people to see. I have all these cute little dresses, but I can't put them on her." It was too soon; she was still in shock. She couldn't see past the stumps of arms, with the matching dimples where elbows should have been. She couldn't see what the baby did have, only what she was missing.

I acknowledged her feelings, refusing to argue with her. "I know, Marie, I understand. This is just shitty."

She couldn't know that I really did empathize with her. I had never had to face a reality such as this. My children were exquisitely normal. But I flashed back to a day, years earlier, when I had been forced to face similar emotions. Heavily pregnant with my son, I had walked onto the neuro ward at Children's Hospital to see, for the first time, my best friend's new baby. We'd gone through our pregnancies together and I wanted to be with my friend now, after her daughter's surgery to enclose the myelomeningocele (a central nervous system hernia) that protruded from the small of her back.

I remembered walking into the room, seeing this baby, asleep on her belly, a thick dressing on her back, stricken with shock that she looked just like her mother. Standing there, with my son kicking in my swollen belly, looking at this child, I finally comprehended, with brutal clarity, that she was paralyzed from the hips down, for life, for always. There was no cure, no one could fix it. This was the way she was, and would remain, forever. Thankful that my friend wasn't in the room, I turned and fled the hospital. I found my car and drove in a panic to my husband's office. When I walked in on him, he saw the catastrophe in my eyes. I collapsed in his arms, near hysteria with outrage over this baby, and terror for the one I carried unseen beneath my ribs. I wanted my friend's baby to go away, to cease to exist, to never be, because she was imperfect. She wasn't the way she was supposed to be, I lamented as I shook with tears and terror.

Now I sat next to Marie, holding her malformed baby on my lap, reliving that time, and all the times with my friend when I had to fight—for my friend, for her baby, and for myself—my aversion to the way that little girl moved, looked, and acted. My heart went out to Marie as I recognized her pain, her irretrievable loss. I couldn't fault her feelings, her need to reject her baby. I could perceive the sense of outrage, of betrayal that her body had produced this severely limited child. Erica had no hands. She had no legs. No fingers to grasp things, no thumbs to suck, no knees to scrape. How could I judge Marie or fault her reaction? Had Erica been mine, I would have been howling with rage, keening with grief.

So I held the baby and acknowledged Marie's anger, Mark's pain. We looked at Erica and then at one another. I accepted the anguish in the parents' eyes and let them see mine. All the while this baby watched me, lying alert and very much there on my lap, waving her arms and making funny little faces, endearingly. When she was wrapped up, she truly was a lovely baby. Her face projected awareness, her delicate features responded to my voice and my expressions. I couldn't help but be convinced that there was a wise little being there in my lap, a new person soaking in everything around her, learning in leaps and bounds about her new world; doing so quite cheerfully, with heartbreaking innocence.

During the three days that I interacted with this little girl, this conviction persisted and grew, and I repeatedly drew her parents' attention to her obvious awareness of us. Erica's personality was vividly there, from the beginning. In addition, there was an essence or aura about her that was undeniable. I wanted to believe that this child was special, that there was something extra in her to counter the absence of normal limbs. Years later I still hold that belief in my heart, that the spirit within that tiny newborn body was special, and would affect others in the same strong way throughout her life.

Later that morning, Marie told me that she and Mark had talked to their parents; they had told them the truth about Erica and their families were loving and supportive. Marie said her mother had offered to adopt Erica and care for her, but she had refused the offer: "We couldn't do that. We just couldn't." Marie's mother arrived that afternoon. After meeting her, I turned away in pain as gently and quickly as I could. She held Erica tightly in her arms, pacing the room with tear-streaked cheeks, crooning to her granddaughter.

The following day passed in a blur. Mark, Marie, and I talked and seethed with frustration as we waited for reports from the neurologist and orthopedist. The Tylers wanted to know if Erica had any internal problems and what her future might hold in terms of activities of daily living. Would she ever be able to walk? What kinds of prostheses would be available? Where could she get treatment?

Mark followed me when I left Marie's room at one point, and asked me diffidently about an exposure he'd had two summers earlier to possibly toxic material.

"I was working in a paint factory, so I was exposed to a lot of chemicals. Do you think that could be what caused this?"

"I don't know, Mark, I don't think so, but let's ask someone who might know." The OB chief was walking down the hall toward me, so I collared him then and there. He leaned against the wall and spoke softly to Mark, reassuring him gently that his exposure to the chemicals was unlikely to have caused Erica's deformities. I ached for the young man's fear, remembering my friend's endless questioning whether something she had done had caused her daughter's spina bifida. I knew these questions would haunt Mark and Marie for years to come.

The social worker appeared and informed me that he had a family interested in adopting Erica. He wanted me to reassure him that the Tylers truly wanted to place Erica, since this family had adopted other handicapped children, and had "lost" the last severely handicapped child they had planned for. He didn't want to get their hopes up if the Tylers weren't serious. Filled with joyful thanks that such people existed in the world, I went with him to tell the Tylers. He asked them again if they were sure, and then told them about this family.

Mark and Marie asked him questions: Where did the family live? How many children did they have? How could they afford to care for so many? Would Erica be well-cared for, and would they love her? The social worker described a large family, with sufficient income and a clear record of devotion to several adopted children, both normal and handicapped. He explained that the family believed in open adoption and wanted Erica's parents to bring her to them, to meet them, and to visit whenever they wished. I watched the hope grow in the Tylers' eyes and saw the relief flood their faces, as they began to believe that maybe this horror might be lifted from their shoulders in a loving way, that their little girl might have something of a love-filled, normal life provided by people who were equipped to do so. They gave the social worker permission to call and finalize the arrangements with relieved certainty that this was what would be best for their baby. When he left the room they hugged each other and me, all of us grinning through tears. When I left, they were calling the airlines to book a flight to the adoptive family's home.

That afternoon Marie's mother and Mark's sister brought Matthew to visit his parents. He bounced around Marie's room, touching everything he could reach and asking strings of questions. Slender and sturdy, he had Mark's coloring and was a handsome little boy. After I asked Marie if I could talk with her relatives privately, we sat together in the visitors' lounge. Attractive and well dressed, both were stricken with grief. I used the opportunity to praise Mark and Marie, to describe how they had behaved with dignity and grace during a long difficult labor. I emphasized the importance of recognizing their accomplishment, and not letting it be diminished by the uncertainties of Erica's future.

They were both highly concerned about Marie's emotional state, murmuring fears that she would break down. They told me of their confusion about the decision to have Erica adopted, and were almost inarticulate as they tried to express their complex feelings. Marie's mother told me that her father would be arriving in the morning, and that she didn't know how that was going to be. "Marie's daddy is everything to her." We didn't push the subject; I really just wanted to give them an opportunity to ask questions and to air their feelings. Both women assured me during the course of our conversation that they wanted to help Marie and Mark however they could. Their love and concern was obvious, as was their pain and fear that whatever they did might not be the right thing.

I spent hours on the phone that night, talking to my sister and to Nick. I needed to express my feelings as well, to mull over what was happening and how I was interacting with the Tylers. I felt even more fiercely as the days passed that Erica's future was their decision, and only theirs. I was angry about some of the talk I'd heard from staff members at the hospital. One of the pediatricians had been heard to comment angrily that the Tylers "had to take what God gave them." An intern doing her pediatrics rotation kept talking to them about Erica's care "when they take her home," resolutely refusing to acknowledge their decision to have her adopted. I knew in my heart, as I explored it all with Nick, that whatever decision was finally reached by these two young parents, their pain would be enormous and they would be irrevocably altered by their decision. I also was convinced that no one had the right to impose, overtly or otherwise, their judgment or their beliefs about what was best for this baby. Only Marie and Mark would end up taking her home or handing her over to someone else to care for her and shape her into the human being she would be. Only her family would carry the burden of that decision and the resulting emotional scars for the rest of their lives, not the pediatricians or obstetrician or orthopedist or neurologist or social worker or the nurses.

The next day was a long one. The airline tickets for the trip to the adoptive home were purchased. Marie was recovering well, with the expected exception of a sore bottom, and we spent some time focusing on the normal postpartum concerns: how to care for her breasts, her episiotomy, when to resume sexual activity, etc. It was therapeutically relaxing for all three of us to talk of these things, letting the larger issue of the baby rest for a bit. They were beginning to once again focus on their plans for Mark's college education and Marie's career, and they were feeling more in control. However, I could sense the agitation in Marie, just beneath the surface, as she waited for her father to arrive. She was a little too bright, a little too together, smiling and chatting about this and that. I could tell that this wasn't going to be easy and I tried to help her prepare for it, but she brushed my concern aside: "Oh, my family wants to support us in whatever decision we make, and they will. I know they will. This is just so much better for Erica."

The orthopedist finally appeared and reported that Erica was a healthy normal infant, with the exception of the missing limbs. He assured them that with much physical therapy and many prostheses over the years, Erica would probably be able to ride a bike and even dance. I could feel Mark's mood lighten as he listened. His hopes for his daughter's future were beginning to grow; I could see it in his face and his posture.

Quietly then, they asked the doctor about any potential causes for Erica's condition. Without hesitation, he answered: "Oh, it was something that you ingested; either something that you ate or breathed or absorbed from the environment. A drug or a food, or something. We know developmentally when the malformities occurred, but there doesn't seem to be anything from your pregnancy history that sheds light on what the teratogen might have been. You might want to do some research into the water in your area or whatever."

Both of them grew very still as he nonchalantly gave this explanation. Marie seemed to close in on herself for a few seconds, but Mark turned and looked straight into my eyes with a look I'll never forget or understand. I don't know if he was thinking about his job in the paint factory, or if he realized something Marie had eaten or taken had been the cause, or if he was just blown away by the doctor's words. I didn't ask, then or later, even though I was incensed by the doctor's insensitive, callous explanation. It was too late now; nothing I could say would ameliorate the impact of those words, or the responsibility, however unknowing, for Erica's losses. We never discussed it further.

Marie's father arrived. I greeted him and stayed away for a while. Around

2:30, I entered the room, and was formally introduced. He was a thin man, dressed in a suit, with beautiful hands whose long, tapering fingers made me think of a pianist or surgeon. A tailor and immigrant from Eastern Europe, he had a heavy accent and a shy demeanor.

Tensions were high in the room; I could feel the distress. My arrival had interrupted their conversation; Marie's mother started fussing with her purse, moving about the room as if looking for the exit. I asked permission to talk with the grandparents, and receiving it, hustled the two older adults down to the dayroom.

There I reiterated my pride in their children, focusing my attention on Marie's dad. I could see that he was struggling with his emotions and I acknowledged how painful the situation must be to him.

"Could we talk about how you feel about all of this? I'd like to help in whatever way I can."

"I have to say that I don't like this adoption business at all," he said. He went on, struggling to find the words, fighting tears, his face twisted with emotion, his hands opening and closing on each other in his lap. "I don't think it's right," he said.

"Have you told Marie how you feel?" I asked.

"No, she doesn't think. . . ." He gestured toward his wife.

"Wait a minute," I said. "What do you mean?"

Marie's mother said, "We're afraid to push this at all with Marie. She's been through so much, it doesn't seem right to have to make this decision now. What will it do to her? It might push her over the edge. . . ."

I leaned forward, with a sense of urgency, wanting them to know how strongly I felt about what I was saying. "Listen, please, you need to talk with her now. I get a very strong sense of how loving you are and how you want to support these kids."

They nodded in agreement. "Yes, whatever they decide, we'll be there for them," Marie's mother asserted.

"But," I went on, "you need to accept right now that whatever decision they make, it's going to hurt. If they give up the baby, it'll hurt the rest of their lives. And if they keep her, not only will it be very hard, and Marie knows better than one would expect that raising Erica will be hard—"

"Yes, she knows. Because of her work," her father interrupted.

"Okay, but believe me, you won't be helping either of them if you don't talk to them, with them. They need to know how you feel. Worrying about whether Marie's going to break down isn't the point; you just can't put off the pain. You can't protect her from the reality of this. I think it's shitty that this important a decision has to be made in so little time, but it's not going to be any easier two weeks or two months from now. I'm telling you, I know from personal experience that if you really want to be there for them, you have to communicate with them now. You have to share your feelings. It's okay to be angry, or disappointed, or sad, but they have to know how you feel."

I paused, took a breath, and asked, "I'm going to ask you straight out, what is it that you don't like about this adoption? The family she's going to, or Marie and Mark's reasons for placing her, or what?"

Marie's dad leaned forward and told me tearfully, "I know my daughter. I know her well and I know what she's capable of. I just feel that if they do this thing, it'll be the biggest mistake of their lives. They won't be the people I'd want them to be, I hoped they could be." He was trembling; I ached for him.

Something clicked inside my head. I realized that in spite of the shock of his granddaughter's condition, in spite of his grief and concern for his daughter, this man was thinking about larger issues. He wasn't concentrating on getting through the next few days or weeks, he was worrying about his daughter's character, her strengths and weaknesses, and her growth as a human being. I silently bowed my head to him in respect. His innate dignity made me feel honored to know him, however briefly.

For the first and only time, to give him some space to recover, I indulged myself and told them how I felt, with tears and quiet passion in my voice. "Can I share my feelings about this with you? This is Susie talking to you, not Nurse Diamond, okay? Personally, I think that everything that happens to us happens to us for a reason. That we choose our lives and our parents, and that everything we choose and do because we're supposed to learn something from it. I think this beautiful baby, with all she's missing, happened to Marie and Mark for a reason. Call it anything you like, karma, or fate, or a test from God, or a gift from God, but I think this is their big test, and how they react to it will affect how successful they are as human beings. So I hear you, sir, I hear you."

Marie's mother leaned forward and implored me, "Will you tell them that, Susie? Please tell them how you feel. They really care about what you think, they look up to you."

"No, ma'am. I'm sorry. I can tell you, but no way would I ever tell them how I feel. I know that sounds heartless, but I don't have any right to tell them. *I'm* not taking that baby home. *I'm* not giving her up for adoption. *I'm* not the one who has to live with this decision day in, day out, for the rest of my life. I have no right to intrude; no one does, outside of family. You are the people who will bear the costs of whatever they decide; you will be living with your children's pain and loss and grief. So *you* need to talk to them. Not me. It's simply not my place."

I could see Marie's father's relief; he settled back in the couch and squared his thin shoulders. I finished: "It's going to be hard, today, and a year from today, but if you love those two kids and truly want to help them, be honest. Tell them how you feel and why you feel that way. They know you love them and want to help them. Please tell them. If you truly think giving Erica up for adoption is wrong, they need to know, because you can't help them if you're blaming them.

"If I've said the wrong things, I apologize. I'll help in whatever way I can." I stood and shook his hand, hugged Marie's mom and made my exit, emotionally drained, exhausted, and afraid that I had interfered. Still, I felt right about our conversation. I went home and kept my fingers crossed that somehow my words would help, or at least not hinder, the delicate negotiations that I knew this family would be engaged in for the rest of the evening. I almost held my breath that night, wondering what the outcome would be.

When I joined the Tylers in the morning, Marie smiled at me. "Susie, you're going to think we're crazy. Sit, we have something to tell you. I know you're going to think we're nuts, but we changed our minds. We're going to take Erica home with us."

I smiled. My heart leaped up inside as I said, "You had a talk with your father, huh?"

"Yeah, we talked a lot. Daddy was pretty upset, but it's okay. We think we've been trying to make a decision too fast, to get it over with. I don't know how well this will work, but we want to take Erica home and see how we manage for at least a couple of weeks before we do anything drastic." She was smiling, a bit sheepishly, and trembling with unshed tears and her fear of the enormity of it all.

"How do you feel about this, Mark?" I asked, as always trying to give him the opportunity to voice his own feelings. He stood up with a bounce in his step and said, "Oh, I think it's okay. I want what Marie wants. Listen, I've been thinking about this and I've figured out a way that Erica can use a pacifier. See, I'm gonna get a strip of velcro and attach a pacifier to it, and then it can be around her arm, see, like this, and she can get it into her mouth without needing hands, see like this!" He was grinning, more animated than I'd ever seen him, gesturing and shaping the idea with his hands and arms, demonstrating the design as he explained. Joy flooded me; the day before this young man had told me about his dream of studying engineering, and that he'd always been interested in biomedical engineering. Now he shyly explained that he intended to pursue that field, so "maybe I can come up with some ideas that would help Erica."

We celebrated in that room that morning. I rejoiced for the Tylers, for their parents, and for the baby they were taking home, the baby they were not relinquishing to someone else, at least for now. And I rejoiced silently for myself because I knew, with quiet relief and unabashed pride, that my words the day before might have given Marie's father permission to talk straight to his daughter. At least I hadn't messed up; I had validated his right to reach out to his daughter when she needed him to do so. I knew what they were in for; I understood how hard it was going to be. I had learned some of that over the years, watching my friend and her daughter triumph over spina bifida. But I had faith that they were going to meet this test and pass it with flying colors. The first step had been taken—now there were no barriers between this couple and their families. I was humbled by their courage and felt privileged to have participated in this extraordinary time in their lives.

I held Erica and talked directly to her, telling her how special I thought she was, how I wanted her to be a good girl and bring her parents joy. Mark took pictures of me with the baby, and of Marie and me with the baby. I hugged Marie and told her I knew how scary it was and that I thought they were very brave. I asked if I could make some calls for them to find what resources were available to them in the community. We exchanged phone numbers and addresses and I promised to call them at home as soon as I had any information. We said good-bye, but I knew our relationship wasn't over yet. I was determined to help them however I could; God knows, they were going to need help. Curiously, I have no memory of their departure from the ward.

NURSES' NOTES: 1500: Pt left hosp ambulatory c̄ d/c instructions, husband and infant!

That evening I called the Easter Seal Society and asked if they could help me find someone to assist the Tylers. They referred me to a group called PAC, Parents of Amputeed Children. I spoke to a gentle-voiced man who was the president of this group, silently wondering what tragedy had led to his presidency. I explained Erica's situation, asking if he could be of help. He told me, "I'll call them. I'll take it from here." Marie called me several days later to report that PAC's president had arranged a consultation with several doctors at Children's Hospital, had given them information about Shriners' Hospital's services, and had introduced them to a young mother and her son, who was eighteen months old and had the same limb reductions as Erica. Marie said they sat and watched this baby play with a ball on the floor: they had been amazed at his abilities. She also said the mother had been left alone by her family after the baby's birth, and hadn't had any outside help for nine months, since she hadn't known where or who to call.

Five months later I received a letter from Marie, a letter filled with joy. Erica was growing normally, had been without any illness, and brought Marie and Mark great pleasure. Marie thanked me for being with them during their time of crisis, insisting that my presence had made it possible for them to make the right decision. She wrote of how glad they were that they had kept Erica, of how devastated they would have been otherwise.

Two photographs were enclosed in the letter. With her brother hanging on the crib rail and grinning at her, a round-faced, dimpled-cheeked three-month-old baby girl smiled out of the photos at me. She was surrounded by stuffed animals, a mobile hung over her crib. Her smiles lit the pictures; her eyes sparkled. My kids looked at the pictures and laughed at this baby's beautiful happiness. "What a gorgeous baby!" my daughter said. Both of my children completely failed to notice the absence of limbs, although Erica was dressed in an adorable little sundress that did not hide her lack of proper arms or legs. I read the letter, laid my head down on the kitchen table, and cried with unrestrained joy. The Tylers had made a good beginning. The life ahead of them would be difficult, fraught with unusual tasks and painful events, but their commitment to their child was solid and the happiness they derived from her presence was undeniable. It was a good beginning.

A year later I received another letter. Marie wrote that Mark was doing well in college and that she had a good job and help with the kids at home. She reported on Erica's progress; the little girl had been fitted with artificial arms, was receiving excellent care, and couldn't be held down. She was crawling everywhere and learning to talk. Matthew had adjusted fairly well. They took Erica to church every Sunday and planned to enroll her in a day-care center so that she could spend time with other children. They had met other families with children like Erica, and she and Mark had learned that there is always someone with more problems than their own. Family and friends had been completely supportive. Marie reiterated how glad they were about their decision not to have Erica adopted and described her as the "best baby in the world."

With that letter were two more snaps of Erica. In one she sat on a couch next to her brother, with her daddy's baseball cap on her head, dark curls spilling out from under the cap, her eyes still shining, dimples like parentheses enclosing her big grin. In the other, she's on the floor in front of a Christmas tree, surrounded by gifts and wrapping paper, beaming at the camera. She is a stunningly beautiful little girl.

Chapter Nine

MOTHERS AND FATHERS

One night, about five years into my career, I took care of a young woman who was unmarried and planning to keep her baby, or as we sometimes call such women, a "single parent, keeping" (SPK). Her boyfriend was with her, but I was informed in report that he was not the father of the baby. I had little to do with this nineteen-year-old girl. Her membranes had ruptured and we were giving her a few hours to go into labor spontaneously before we intervened to induce it. The monitors indicated a healthy baby and intermittent, mild contractions. I encouraged her to sleep and made hourly visits to her room to take vital signs and assist her on her trips to the bathroom.

She was pretty, with a young, smooth, fresh-looking face. I particularly noticed her satiny blond hair, which glistened with health and lay straight and silken about her face, framing her clear, slightly flushed cheeks. She was very quiet and withdrawn, barely responding to my remarks or my activities in her room. She betrayed little emotion, even when I gently questioned her about how she felt. Denying pain, she refused offers of medication to help her sleep and appeared reluctant to engage in any form of conversation. As a result, I was quiet, not talking any more than was necessary.

In the early morning, the resident instructed me to begin a Pitocin drip to stimulate her labor. As I set up the IV pump, I reviewed with the young woman what the Pitocin was supposed to do, how she might feel as the contractions became more intense and more frequent, and what her options for pain relief were. She made some remark about being afraid of epidurals and being afraid of having much more pain. I finished what I was doing and leaned down toward her, resting my arms against the bed rail. Looking her in the eyes, really focusing on her face, I gave her a little speech:

"Dawn, no one but you will experience this labor. All we can do is try to assist you through it. Now, it's great to have a goal about how you want this labor to go. It's admirable and fine of you to want to have your baby without any medication. You've been doing well all night with the contractions you've had so far. Your control and your breathing are just great. You should absolutely go on trying, and have confidence that you can make it without pain relief. But Dawn, all the best intentions in the world won't matter if you get to a point where labor is a torture for you. You may not, but if you find it's getting rough, don't be afraid to ask for help. That's one of the reasons you're in this hospital, so that if you need the expertise, the medications, the technology, they're here for you. The true goal should be to come out of this experience with good memories. You're about to have your first child and that should not be something you think back on as a night-mare. Do what you can and use what you need so that having this baby is a positive experience. Don't let yourself get so exhausted and so wrecked by your labor that you can't enjoy your baby's birth! Okay?"

She listened intently, brown eyes watching my face. She nodded sol-emnly when I finished, and smiled good-bye as I wished her good luck and took my leave of her.

"Have a beautiful baby now and I'll try to stop by tonight to see you!"

That night I checked the delivery book to see when and how she had delivered. A cesarean in the late afternoon was reported; failure to progress— her cervix didn't dilate adequately—was listed as the reason for a surgical delivery. I didn't give it any more thought and completely forgot my promise to visit her. At 0500, the ward called for me. The nurse who took the call informed me that Dawn was feeding her baby and wanted me to come see him. I was amazed. I didn't think I had made any impression on the girl, certainly not enough to have her remember my name. Over to the ward I wandered, and slipped into her room.

She sat in her bed, her shoulders bare, lovely hair framing her face, with her newborn cradled against her right breast. She looked up at me: with quiet urgency and profound emotion trembling in her voice, she said, "Oh, Susie, just come and look at this. Look at him!"

Moving around to the side of the bed, I looked down on her son, sleeping soundly, his small face resting against the creamy, blue-veined swell of her breast. He was an exquisite newborn: unblemished skin, long dark eyelashes, a head full of feather-soft blonde hair, tiny shell ears, a cupid's-bow mouth, plump little fingers curled into a relaxed fist on his mother's chest.

"Ooh my goodness! What a magnificent baby! Oh, isn't he simply beau-tiful, Dawn!" I exclaimed as I studied his features. "I heard you had a cesarean. How was your labor? Tell me about it."

She spoke softly, briefly describing the events of her labor and delivery as she looked at her son. Her boyfriend, she reported, had been very helpful, and he'd spent hours in the nursery afterward watching this baby. She had been frustrated by her separation from the baby until now, and had spent the last hour nursing and admiring him. She asked me if I would put him back in his bed since her tummy was hurting some now.

"It would be my great pleasure. I can take him to the nursery for you if you'd like." I carefully lifted the child from her arms and held him out to admire him further. He truly was one of those lovely, lovely newborns and my heart ached with a bittersweet nostalgia for the feeling and weight of my own two babies in my arms. As I laid him in the crib and rewrapped him, Dawn announced: "He's the best thing I've ever done in my whole life!" I struggled with sudden tears, so touched was I by this young woman, so closely did I identify with the meaning of her words.

As I returned to L&D a few minutes later I found myself once again moved by what had just occurred: the unexpectedness of Dawn's request that I come see her baby, the surprise I felt that she had remembered me, that somehow the night before I had made an impression on her, that she wanted to share her pride in her son, and most of all the almost unbearable beauty of her when I first saw her in her bed. I've come to think of it as the "madonna look": a mother cradling a child in her arms, head bent down *en face*, the look of love and delight and wonder so pure in her face, that every time I see it I am knocked silly by it. To be privy to such a moment of awe and love, to such beauty, staggers me and renews all my careworn desire to be present at such beginnings. My god, Dawn and her son were lovely.

There is a particular phenomenon that I have observed that I was reminded of after my brief visit with Dawn. The first time I noticed it was the very first time I served as a coach for a laboring woman. I have seen it often since then and it always touches me. It is a shift in behavior and emotion that is quite startling. A woman will be totally engrossed in the force of her labor, struggling with pain, wrestling with these powerful sensations, frantic for relief, urgent in her need to be freed of the fetus. Sweating, pushing, hollering, crying, pleading all may occur during the final phases of her labor, and she may express absolute fury or indignation that those around her aren't responding to her great need for relief. She will look terrible: hair matted and sticky, face dripping sweat and tears, eyes bloodshot from sleeplessness and the efforts of pushing, body reeking of the effluvia of labor. She smells and looks and often acts badly, at the mercy of this inexorable activity of her body.

When the baby is born, something remarkable happens. All the pain, all the struggle, all the attention on the self and the self's vehement clamoring for rest and pain relief, all of it disappears instantly. The mother's face moves from the contortions of pain and effort to an expression of absolute love, delight, and pleasure. Her body relaxes and her entire torso leans toward the child, arms reaching out. Her voice, moments before caught in a scream or a furious grunting growl, is now soft and more high-pitched, as she croons soft words of love and yearning for the infant. If you could imagine a wild animal, a gorilla for example, caught in an act of defiance or anger, beating her breast, leaping and flailing her arms, and then suddenly imagine this gorilla stopping in mid-roar, relaxing and reaching out gently and tenderly to smooth her offspring's cheek, you might begin to visualize how abrupt, how startling this shift can be in a new mother.

There is something primal about it. It is as if the maternal instinct or drive is suddenly switched on. The focus of attention is no longer the self, but the child of the self. It is a transition of such completeness that it leaves me breathless. All the pain, the supplications, the self-pity, the exhaustion, are simply erased by the presence of this child. The unattractive, smelly, bad-tempered woman of moments before now appears lovely. Her features are softened, her voice is caressing, her body urgent only in its need to embrace the child. She has become beautiful before my eyes; I hurry to place the baby in her arms so that I may behold another madonna.

This instantaneous emergence of the maternal doesn't occur with every birth. Some women are simply too exhausted to respond to the presence of the child. Some appear distanced from their babies, as though they must have time and exposure before they are attached, or bonded, to their offspring. Some, unfortunately, even react with outspoken resentment toward the newborn, expressing their disgust with this baby that has tortured them so despicably. But when the maternal identity springs forth so dramatically and so rapidly, it is a delight to witness. One young woman, who had wept piteously during her labor, alternating between demands that we help her and apologies for her bad manners, actually squealed with glee when her daughter slid out of her body.

"Oh my baby! Oh, look at her! Oh, isn't she beautiful? I just love her so much! Hello, my darling daughter! It's okay, don't cry, your mommy's right here and I love you so!"

On and on she went, nonstop, while we tagged and wrapped and Apgared her baby, virtually singing the baby's praises, laughing with complete abandon, her face shining with pride.

One of the most disliked tasks on the antepartum ward where I first worked was taking fetal heart tones. Most of the staff just hated having to wake sleeping mothers to smear gel on their bellies, search for and then count a fetal heart rate. Though I disliked having to disturb these women, for me it was always an enjoyable duty. Interrupting their sleep at least once each night for vital signs felt so intrusive, and conflicted with what would seem to be in their best interest—a good night's sleep. Nonetheless, it had to be done; the in utero patient was my responsibility also.

What I thought was terrific was the way the mothers responded to me. Rarely did I get a complaint. Approaching the bed quietly, I'd call the mother's name. When she stirred and mumbled a response, I'd apologize for waking her, telling her I needed to listen to her baby. Invariably, each mother would turn over and pull up her gown, exposing her belly to the cold air, the gel, and the doptone—the listening device. I always asked, "Where do we usually find your baby?" The mothers usually knew exactly where to listen, pointing with their fingers or stroking the area with their palms. The willingness to be disturbed, to endure the interruption, the cold, the probing of their abdomens, simply to be reassured that their babies were alive and kicking in there touched me profoundly. I felt somehow a mystical connection with these women. *You sleep. When it is time I will come to your bedside. I will lean over you, listen and count. I will be awake and alert to any problems. Together we will guard this baby of yours. We will minimize the risk that has placed you here in the hospital.*

Those warm bellies, those sleepy faces were so poignant. On occasion, a mother and I would get the giggles about the baby. One room on the ward had some strange radio-wave phenomenon so that when we listened to the heart tones with the doptone, we also heard radio programs. This inevitably led to quiet laughter. One mother with twins just loved her babies' response to my hands and the doptone. As soon as I touched her belly, I could hear the babies move away from the instrument. She could feel it, of course. She delighted in my protests to the babies: "Come back here, you little imp! I just want to hear your heartbeat! Geez, they sure don't like me messing with their house, do they?" Many an antepartum mother would search my face in the dim light, watching me count, and then ask anxiously, "How does it sound?" or "Is it okay?" or "What's the rate tonight?"

Sometimes the little idiosyncracies of my mothers provide me with entertainment or food for thought. A strikingly handsome young woman with a virtual cloud of soft auburn hair gave birth one night with a minimum of effort. After the delivery, I offered to assist her with breast-feeding. She had three older children that she had bottlefed but she wanted to try to nurse this infant, because "everyone says how good it is for the baby." When the baby latched on to her nipple, she shrieked! "Oh, get him off! Get him off! That feels nasty!"

"Come on, now, Terri, it's not nasty!" I said, laughing. "You're just not used to the sensation."

"No, no, I mean it! Get him off!" She tugged the baby's mouth free of her nipple and thrust him at me. "Oooh, that is too nasty for me! Ugh, I don't know why any woman would want to do that! Eeeeww!" And that was that as far as nursing her baby went!

Another mother chatted away with me as I cleaned up the debris of her delivery. She talked about how easy her pregnancy had been, except for a strange desire to eat dirt. "I just craved dirt. I just had to have it!" she remarked. I had heard of this phenomenon, but hadn't previously actually met anyone who did consume dirt. I was as curious as could be: "Did it have to be any special kind of dirt?" I asked, trying to keep a straight face.

"No, in a pinch, any old dirt would do, but I really preferred red dirt."

"Red dirt? Where'd you get it? Did you buy it or what?"

"I was living with my relatives and I just dug up their backyard. I'd go out back with a spoon and just dig it up and eat it right there. There was holes all over that yard from me digging in it!"

"This is fascinating! Do you mind if I ask, uh . . . what did it taste like? I mean, wasn't it dry, or did you put water in it, or what?"

"No, like I said, I'd just dig it up and eat it dry. Didn't want no wet dirt. I guess you could say it was dry, but I liked it that way. I don't know as I can say how it tasted . . . It just tasted like dirt, I guess. It was real good, too."

Not a few young women, first-time mothers, will be absolutely mortified by the activities of their bodies during and after labor and delivery. Even if they have attended childbirth classes and have heard about membranes rupturing, bloody show, bleeding after the delivery, and so on, they appear completely surprised by the excretions of their bodies. After rupturing the membranes of one young woman, I assured her we had plenty of chucks, the absorbent pads we placed under the buttocks of laboring mothers, and that we would just keep changing them as needed. She insisted on wearing a sanitary napkin and panties in bed, and got up to change her napkin no less than four times in forty minutes, in spite of active labor contractions. She just couldn't bear being wet.

As I helped a new mother in the bathroom for the first time after her delivery, she couldn't get over how much blood was present. "Oh, my goodness! Look at all that blood! Is that normal? Are you sure I'm not losing too much blood?" she asked, concerned.

"No, no, it's okay. A lot of this is just blood that pooled in your vagina while you were lying down. But you'll have a heavy flow today and tonight, like a heavy first day of your period. Then it will ease off and turn pink and thin."

"Wow, I just can't believe I can bleed this much and not die!" She shook her head in disbelief.

Most women get pretty grungy during the hours of labor, but there have been quite a few that knocked me out with their beauty. I don't mean movie-star or magazine-cover beauty, I mean an inner loveliness that seems to glow through their skin, so that they look almost luminous. They always laugh at me when I comment on how lovely they look, but they can't see that luminous loveliness like I can. One woman was so downright majestically beautiful that I made a real fuss over her.

As she got undressed and into bed, she commented on how glad she was to be finally having this baby. She was tired of being fat and unattractive, and wanted to have her body back, and wear normal clothes. I looked at her and said, "You know, I've heard lots of women say the same things, and I understand what you mean, but don't you have any idea of how gorgeous you are?"

She laughed and said, "Sure, Susie! It's kind of you to say so, but really!"

"No, I'm perfectly serious. You could be a model in maternity magazines."

As I pulled back the sheet to put on the monitor straps, I couldn't help myself: "Louellen, I mean it, why, even your belly is beautiful! Geez, not a stretch mark anywhere. Look at this gorgeous smooth skin!" She really did have a magnificent belly, smooth milk-chocolate brown skin unmarked by any blemishes. So many pregnant bellies get scarred with stretch marks, grow more hair, and look and feel jiggly because of too little muscle tone and too much fat right under the skin.

She and her husband were laughing at me, but that didn't stop me. "You know, I was so proud of my own belly when I was pregnant that I made my husband take pictures of me, naked and nine months gone! I wanted to have a record of how my body looked." I looked at her husband. "Have you taken any pictures of Louellen during the pregnancy?" I asked.

"No, we never thought about it," he replied.

"On, no, what a shame!" I exclaimed. "Here lies one of the most beautiful pregnant bellies I've ever seen, and I've seen hundreds of them, and you don't have a picture of it? Or of this exquisite pregnant wife of yours? Shame on you! Where's your camera?" I demanded.

They both looked at me like I was nuts and then looked at each other.

"I know you think you've got a crazy person here," I spoke softly and seriously, "but I'm quite serious. This is such a special time in your life together. You've made a baby and the pregnancy is almost over. Louellen is truly beautiful in these last moments of her pregnancy. Isn't that something you'd want to have a picture of?"

Well, they quietly thought about it for a few minutes. Then her husband stood up and reached for the car keys.

"Where are you going, honey?" Louellen asked.

"Susie is right. You are gorgeous, and I'm getting the camera!" He leaned down and kissed her carefully and slowly. She smiled radiantly at him and said, "Okay, don't be away from me too long, sweetheart." When he returned with the camera, I took off the monitor straps and left the room, giving them some time to get as much of her body on film as they wanted, guarding the door so no one could interrupt this special film-taking session.

I also enjoyed teaching new mothers how to care for their babies. The constraints on my time frequently made this activity onerous and resulted in hurried, seemingly indifferent instructions from me about breast-feeding, diaper changes, cord care, and so on. But when I had the time, I really got into it and had some lovely exchanges with the women in my care. One incident in particular sits doggedly in my memory. I heard an infant screaming unceasingly from one of the postpartum rooms. Hurrying in to see what the difficulty was, I found an exquisitely beautiful young Latino woman bending over her screeching child, who lay on the bed, diaper undone, flailing her arms and legs furiously, her body beet-red, face screwed up, open-mouthed, eyes squeezed shut, caterwauling at the top of her not inconsiderable lungs. The mother was ineffectually attempting to close her diaper, whimpering with fear and frustration, terrified by her baby's awesome anger.

"My goodness! What a set of lungs! She sure makes a lot of noise for such a little thing, doesn't she?" I asked as I approached the bed. "Can I help you with this?"

The mother slumped back into the rocking chair at the bedside. "I don't know what to do. She won't stop crying. It scares me; I think she'll choke she cries so hard."

"Nah, don't worry about that. She'll get the air she needs. Let's see now, little girl. Shush, shush, it's okay, it's okay, let's get this diaper on. Now, there, wrap you up nice and tight. Hush, hush, baby, don't cry, it's okay." I wrapped her and put her up high on my shoulder, thumping her back with my hand and rocking her, speaking quietly. Within seconds she was hiccoughing the last wail away, then silent on my shoulder. As I held her with one hand, I began to clean up the detritus of her bath and diaper change, laughing about her fury. Then I looked at the mother. She was staring at me, tears streaking down her face, an expression of utter defeat on her face.

"Oh my dear. I am sorry. What is it?" I asked her gently.

"It's just, you just, I don't know. You just did that so easily. You pick her up and hold her so casually," she whispered.

What have I done, I thought. *I come in here to help and instead I've completely sabotaged this new mother's confidence in herself. Jesus, Susie!* "Goodness, I am sorry. I made that look so easy, didn't I? But you know what? I have two children of my own, and I work with babies all day, every day. It's not surprising I have some skill at this. On the other hand, you've never had your own baby before. And guess what? Knowing how to take care of a baby isn't something we all just know how to do. It's a learned skill. You should have seen me in the hospital with my first baby. She cried just like this and wouldn't stop till I just cried along with her. I felt so helpless. She vomited like a volcano after I fed her and I didn't know why. I know just how you feel, honey. I'm sorry I came in here and took over like that. I didn't think how it would look to you."

"That's okay. I don't know how to do any of this and when she cries like that, I get so scared."

"Well, of course. She's really got a temper, huh? Do you have a temper, or your husband?"

"Oh, my husband, he gets mad like you wouldn't believe!"

"Well, see there? You've just learned something here about your baby's personality. It's possible she's got her daddy's temper. You have ways of dealing with your husband's anger? You've learned how to calm him down or how to avoid situations that might set him off?"

"Yeah, I guess so."

"Well, that's what you'll have to work on with this little one. Learn how to respond to her needs so she doesn't have to lose her temper, and if she does, learn how to comfort her when she's raging. She's just a little person who you have to get to know, see?"

"I didn't think of it that way. I just thought I'd never be able to go home with this baby. She scares me so much."

We spent another half hour together, talking about basic infant care. I showed her how to hold the baby in different positions, how to thump her back to get her to burp, how to change diapers with the baby on her lap. I encouraged her to talk and sing to her baby all the time and to always think of her as a fascinating person who she, the mother, was shaping even as she learned the baby's personality and idiosyncracies. I praised her efforts thus far.

"This is your second postpartum day, right?"

"Yes."

"You've been feeling weepy and upset and inadequate today, huh?"

"Yes." The tears were flowing again.

"Well, it's okay. This is normal. A lot of what you're feeling isn't because you're not a good mother or because you think you don't know what you're doing. It's absolutely normal to feel bad the second or third day after delivery. All the hormones are shifting around inside you. You're tired from the labor and delivery. You haven't gotten any uninterrupted sleep. And all the attention you got when you were pregnant and then in labor is transferred to this beautiful new baby. All of a sudden reality hits—you're a mother! Oh my god! You're gonna have to take this kid home and take care of her! Whoa! Scarey, huh?" I grinned at her.

"God, yes!" She grinned back, wiping her tears away with the back of her hand. So we discussed baby blues, and conserving her energy, and being gentle with herself, and being sure she got people to help her so she could focus on learning how to mother this baby. When I left her she was sitting in the rocker looking down on her now sleeping infant with an expression of renewed confidence and of wonder. I learned a lot from this exchange: how important it was to encourage the mother's efforts, however fumbling, and not make her feel incompetent through my own practiced actions; how frightening it is to many women to be confronted with a newborn; how easy it can be to dispel those fears if it's done in a sensitive, nonjudgmental way. I learned as much as I taught, and over time repeated this exchange with many women.

Little Mrs. Goodwyn was a woman with whom I really connected. For three days I cared for Mrs. Goodwyn after her tiny, lovely daughter was born. Mrs. Goodwyn had married late, at age thirty-eight. Her husband had three grown children from his first marriage. For eight years the Goodwyns were childless. Mrs. Goodwyn explained that her husband hadn't wanted to start another family and that she hadn't argued.

"I had accepted the idea of childlessness long before we were married. I was comfortable with it. I didn't mind if I never had a child. My menstrual history was so bizarre that I was sure I'd never conceive. I could go a year without a period. The doctors told me it was highly unlikely and I felt relief that Clarence didn't mind. I really enjoyed his kids; we're close and I've felt like I've had children through them. So we were stunned when we discovered I was pregnant!"

"How does it feel, now that you have her?" I asked.

"Oh, Susie, you can't imagine the joy I feel. She is a miracle to me, truly a miracle! Something I never dreamed of experiencing. I touch her and look at her and can't believe that I made this baby, this beautiful baby."

We leaned over the baby together, admiring her delicacy, her true loveliness. I was filled with gladness for this woman. I put my arm around her shoulder and squeezed. She turned into my embrace, both of us crying now. "Oh Susie, how blessed I am, how lucky I am to have this baby!" she cried.

From that moment on, Mrs. Goodwyn and I were bonded. I spent as much time as possible with her, going to her bedside first thing on my rounds. She asked a multitude of questions about baby care and told me all the details of her baby's behavior while I was off-duty. I didn't mind. It was such a pleasure to watch her and Mr. Goodwyn with their daughter. They were dowdy, middle-aged, frumpy people. She had graying, permed hair and jowly cheeks. He was bald and always formally attired, in a white shirt and tie. And they were so in love with each other, with their baby, with this new life. Their elation made me high!

One day on the postpartum ward, I was orienting a new nurse. Orienting a new staff member is a demanding job: every task takes twice as long because everything you do has to be explained. A simple postpartum check can eat time faster than you can imagine. On any given day on the ward I might have to do as many as fifteen checks. Each mother was asked about her breasts, her bleeding, her bottom, her bowel movements, her urinary function. I had to touch each breast to assess engorgement, examine each nipple for cracks or bleeding, massage each abdomen and feel for the uterus and assess its tone and position, check each leg for red or hot spots and pull back on each foot while asking if it hurt to do so, and then have the mother turn over on her side and expose her genitals to my inspection. I looked for cleanliness, swelling, an intact incision, and hemorrhoids, gently pulling aside the labia as I looked and probed. All the while, I was talking, asking the mother about each item, how she felt, what she was doing with episiotomy and breast care, how the baby was feeding, teaching, explaining, informing, scolding, and praising. Then I had to write everything down.

I became proficient, of necessity, and could scoot through a bunch of checks pretty rapidly, but always felt frustrated with the lack of time to really attend to the mother's needs. Frequently, I would fall way behind because I made myself stop and spend the time to truly teach a needy mother, to respond patiently and appropriately to her concerns and questions. Whenever I was orienting a new nurse, I also had to answer her questions and explain the rationale behind what I was telling the mothers. It was fun usually, if the nurse was sharp and responsive, but terribly demanding.

Geena was an experienced nurse who had transferred to labor and delivery from a gyn-oncology ward. She was very smart and clinically skilled, only requiring the information about new mothers to be an effective obstetrical nurse. We buzzed through several checks and found ourselves delayed at the bedside of a mother who was vainly attempting to get her infant to breast-feed. Geena stood across from me, watching and listening as I encouraged the mother in her efforts.

"Okay, now turn the baby into your stomach a little, like this. Now get his head up some more in the crook of your arm. Cup your breast with your left hand, like a C, and tickle his mouth with your nipple. That's it. He's not real sure about this, is he?" I asked. The baby nuzzled and fussed around the mother's breast, mouth open at the wrong times and closed at the right ones. We worked at it for a few minutes, trying to hand-express some colostrum, the premilk substance, from her breasts. All our efforts were fruitless; the baby just wouldn't open his mouth and latch on. I was getting worried about all the other things I needed to do that weren't being done while I stood there trying to get this kid to nurse.

"Now, don't get frustrated, Mom. A lot of babies are like this. People think babies just automatically know how to breast-feed, but guess what? Many of them don't. It's just a question of patience and learning. You're finding out about his personality, what kind of feeder he is, and he's got to figure out that this thing is his food source. It can take time, but believe me, he'll catch on when he gets hungry enough. I'm going to show you a little trick I learned for pokey babies like this. Sometimes you've got to show them with a little moisture that this is the place to lick and suck."

The mother and Geena watched and listened avidly as I reached into a drawer of the baby cart and withdrew an infant bottle with formula in it. "I prefer using a bottle of sterile water for this, but there aren't any in here so we'll just use the formula," I explained as I prepared the bottle. Normally these little four-ounce bottles come packaged with a screw-on top that has to be removed. A nipple-topped lid is then screwed on so the baby can be fed. I was so totally involved with what I was saying to my audience that it didn't register that this particular bottle already had a nipple top on it. Blabbing away to the mother and Geena, I removed the top and leaned over the baby, still in his mother's arms, face against her bare breast. My intention was to sprinkle a few drops of milk on her nipple to wet it and induce the baby to suck up the moisture. What I did was pour from the uncapped bottle four ounces of formula right into this baby's upturned, open-mouthed face!

We three stared in horror at this baby's face, mouth wide open and filled with milk, eyes blinking rapidly to clear the formula from his soaked face as he gagged! Mom's breast, stomach, and gown drenched with milk! The baby was spluttering and spitting!

"Oh, my god! Oh, what did I do?" I yelped as I grabbed the baby up from his mother, turned him over and pounded his back to clear his airway. "Jesus, what an idiot! I'm sorry! I'm so sorry!" Geena and the mother both looked at me with complete disbelief. Then we began to laugh in unison, me apologizing, Geena helping the mother into a new gown, baby cheerfully licking his milky lips. I was beet-red with embarrassment and kept apologizing profusely, even as we howled with laughter at the memory of the baby's face when I poured the milk all over him.

Later, Geena laughed again as she told me she couldn't imagine what I was doing when I took the top off the bottle. The mother was delighted with the subsequent attention I paid her, in my attempts to make up for her milk bath. She loved telling her family about the nurse who tried to drown her baby. After being baptized with formula, the baby breast-fed just fine.

While the focus of my attention in my work is primarily on the mother and baby, I am also paying attention to the father, or in some cases, the "significant other"—a mother, sister, boyfriend, or friend. It's not only the behavior of the women in labor that I find fascinating, it's the way the people closest to them behave under the stress of labor and delivery. When a man cries at his child's birth, I usually find myself crying, too, beaming at his tears. I love it when a man is man enough to go ahead and show the power of his emotions. It gives me enormous pleasure to place a newborn in its father's arms: I try to make it a little ceremony by saying solemnly, "Here, Daddy, greet your beautiful daughter!"

Men's behaviors during their wives' or lovers' labors are just as varied as the behaviors of the women actually laboring. Some men are so solicitous of their wives that I try to back off and let them do their thing, without interfering with the dynamics of their relationship. They will count breaths during the contractions, wipe the women's faces with a cold cloth, spoonfeed ice chips, change mucky chucks, walk their wives to the bathroom or give them bedpans without complaint, rub their backs, soothing and encouraging the whole way. Hour after hour, they will stand at the bedside, holding up legs and counting, coaching mothers who are pushing. One young man, a sports addict, kept using sports terms in his attempt to encourage his wife. "Come on now, honey! It's the fourth down with just inches to go for a touchdown. Hunker down now and go for it! Push hard through the line and score, baby, score!" She pushed for two hours and he began to get discouraged. He leaned in close to her ear and said softly, "Okay, now with the next push I want you to give it your all, honey. You can do it, I know you can win this one! Push until your eyes pop out, okay?"

Some men are terribly embarrassed by their wives' behavior. If the woman is wailing or shouting for help, the man might remonstrate with her, telling her to stay in control, or to behave in a more socially accepted manner. I always try to reassure those men that this behavior is understandable and perfectly acceptable under the circumstances. Usually this type of father will eventually relax a bit, but not infrequently these men leave the room repeatedly to visit with family or go for a smoke, or spend the majority of their time watching TV or sleeping, while their wives continue to do the work of labor.

One such man entertained me one night. His wife, who was from the Middle East, was a large woman, voluptuous and sultry looking, with masses of black hair. He was significantly shorter than her, with pink skin, coarse, sparse hair, and a mammoth case of nerves. All he could talk about was how expensive it was to have a child. She did her thing, laboring and delivering without the need of analgesia, graceful and cheerful throughout. He stood at the door of the delivery room, clearly hesitant about even being in the room. Nothing I said could induce him to approach the delivery table and hold his wife's hand. He remained by the door until everything was finished and cleaned up, visibly trembling and talking nonstop about the cost of a college education for his new offspring.

Cultural differences make a difference in the man's behavior, of course. Another young Middle Eastern woman came in one night. It was her first baby, she was in hard labor, eight centimeters dilated and accompanied only by her husband. She spoke very little English but was screeching with each contraction. We hustled her into a room and got ready in a hurry for an imminent delivery. Her husband sat stiffly on the couch, overwhelmed, I suppose, by her screaming. I told him he could approach the bed and hold her hand, but he declined to do so. After just a few minutes, he abruptly left the room. We were too busy to worry about him; the baby crowned within ten minutes of the couple's arrival. The mother continued to scream in Arabic with each contraction, even though two nurses were talking to her softly and soothingly, gripping her hands and trying to quiet her. She kept hollering her husband's name in the most nerve-wracking wails. I felt sorry for her, sorry that she didn't have any female family members with her to share this "woman thing" with her. I knew it wasn't the norm in their country for the man to be involved with the birth process and I felt badly that she was alone with strangers when her baby was born. When I stopped by her room the next evening to say hello, she lifted her arms to me for an embrace, with a look of such gratitude and appreciation, I figured I had been a reasonable substitute for the absent women of her family.

We had an antepartum patient once who was from a Muslim country. She had four small children at home, was pregnant with twins, and was a diabetic having serious problems controlling her blood sugar levels. Because of the multiple gestation and the diabetes, she was in severe risk of losing not only the babies but also her own life. It was imperative that she be hospitalized and monitored very closely for the remainder of her pregnancy. The physicians providing her care were in an uproar because her Muslim husband refused to allow her to be hospitalized. He presented his case without qualms: they were alone in this country. They had no family or friends to assist with the other children. He could not take time off from work and they couldn't afford to pay for day care. But most important, it was her duty as his wife and mother of his children to stay home and take care of the family. If she lost the babies she was carrying or if she died, it was the will of Allah. It was that simple. He took her home and we never saw them again.

I spent several hours one night running interference with a man who disagreed with the plan of care for his wife. This woman also was diabetic. She had been having some false labor and had come to the hospital thinking it was time to deliver, even though she was only thirty-six weeks. Thirty-eight to forty weeks is a normal gestation period, but babies at thirty-six weeks usually do well. After almost twenty-four hours of intermittent contractions and no cervical dilation, the physician told her he wanted to go ahead and induce her labor with Pitocin. He explained that at thirty-six weeks, the fetus was fully developed and would do well and that it was risky to continue with the pregnancy because of her diabetes.

She was ready and willing, but her husband flatly refused permission. The doctor explained, argued, cajoled, and then got angry. The husband was fuming. As the night nursing manager, I was called into the fray as soon as I came on duty. Battle lines had been drawn. The physician refused to allow the patient to leave the hospital without signing an Against Medical Advice form, which would relieve the hospital and doctor of liability for her well-being. The husband had been insisting that the doctor couldn't be absolved of his responsibility, but that he couldn't force the woman to undergo an induction, either.

I stood at the nurses' station counter and let the doctor vent his frustration and voice his concerns, as I tried to sort out what the critical issues were. Then I went into the room, introduced myself, and told the couple that I just wanted to try to understand the nature of the conflict. The wife was pale and quiet; the husband talked nonstop for more than an hour. As he ranted, I began to understand that this was a religious issue for him. He belonged to some arcane religious sect. He had been in telephone contact with his pastor throughout the day and he believed that God did not allow inductions! He preached to me, spouting Scriptures, insisting that it was God's will that determined when a child would be born; no human interference could be tolerated.

I listened respectfully and finally assured the husband we had only his wife's best interest in mind and that we weren't going to force her to do anything. I explained the physician's concerns, the risk to the mother and baby, and the process of an induction. He listened quietly and relaxed visibly for the first time since I'd met him. "You are the only person who has listened to me," he claimed. "Everyone else here just passed judgment on me after a few minutes and got mad. I'm going to go eat and talk to my pastor. After that, we'll talk some more." Then I told him that the decision was ultimately his wife's; she was the patient and it was up to her what finally transpired. He flared up again:

"Oh, no it's not! By the will of God she is bound to obey me. She is subject to my will. I am her master. This is our belief, isn't that so?" He turned to his wife for confirmation. She hung her head and nodded silently. He puffed out his chest and grandly informed me he would return after eating and praying.

After he left the room, I sat quietly with the woman, asking her gently how she felt, if the contractions were bothering her. She described the past few days, crying softly, and told me she really wanted to be induced. She was exhausted, her belly hurt, and she wanted to get this pregnancy over with. When I explained again that it was her decision, she shook her head and sighed. "You don't understand," she said, reaching for my hand. "It's against our religion for me to have any say in this. I have to bow to his authority. I can't go against his will. What I want, to have this baby now and get on with my life, just isn't important. I have to obey him."

"If you want me to be your advocate, to argue with your husband and plead your case, I will," I responded. "I'm here for you first. I don't understand your beliefs but I respect them. I'll do what you want me to do. It's not my place to try to convince you to do something you don't believe you should do. But oh my dear, this is hard, isn't it?"

"Yes, it is. I wish he would go home to bed and then we could just go ahead and do the induction without him, you know?" She smiled wanly at me. "But I can't go against him. He's a fanatic about our beliefs and drives me crazy sometimes, but he's a good man and a good husband, so what can I do?"

We just sat then, holding hands, quiet together. I was stunned by the difference in our worlds, our perceptions about what a woman could do or not do, with her own body the battlefield in this clash of beliefs. The whole conflict was resolved without any of us winning. God or Mother Nature stepped in, and the woman's contractions picked up in the next hour. When her cervix was checked, she was five centimeters dilated, in active labor! She delivered a healthy baby in the wee hours of the morning, without benefit of Pitocin or analgesia, both forbidden by their religion.

Sometimes, the man is just shy and uncertain about appropriate behavior. Once I've invited him to be involved, he'll throw himself into it without further ado. A teenaged couple arrived on the unit one night. We hadn't even assessed the mother when the young father, all of seventeen years, asked diffidently where he should go to change into scrubs. At the nurses' station, the nurses were groaning about this boy; we were all tired and no one wanted to deal with somebody who would demand a lot of attention. I finally volunteered, dragging my feet down the hallway to the exam room. As usual, whenever I'm feeling negative about my work, I get a lesson in the pleasures of it. This boy was a delight!

Tall and gangly, he hadn't fully matured yet. His face bore the typical marks of adolescence, pimples around the nose and under the lank blond hair on his forehead. He stumbled and fumbled around the room like a colt still not used to its gangly legs. He averted his eyes when he spoke to the adults on the unit, mumbling and shrugging. But he was eager and avidly curious about everything.

During the night, he asked hundreds of questions. He wanted to know everything I could tell him. He asked so many questions about dilation, effacement, and fetal position, that I ended up almost teaching an entire Lamaze class about the stages and phases of labor, using a dusty, long-untouched plastic model of the pelvis and a plastic fetal head to illustrate how the baby moved through the pelvis. When I assured him it was okay to get in close and help his girlfriend and to ask whatever he wanted, he just took off. As the night and her labor progressed, his diffidence in my presence disappeared. The normal teenage mumbling and semi-muteness in the presence of an adult vanished. He lavished his girlfriend with praise and encouragement, stroking her face and telling her openly and softly how much he loved her. He looked up at me and said, "Isn't she the most beautiful thing you've ever laid eyes on?" My eyes filling suddenly, I smiled at him and agreed, touched by his love and lack of embarrassment. When the baby was born, he cried right along with his girlfriend, grinning and smearing tears all over his face as he devoured the baby with his shining eyes.

After the delivery, while the young mother held the baby, he ambled over to the instrument table to look at the placenta. He had more questions, of course! He not only wanted to look at it, he wanted to touch it. I gave him a pair of gloves and showed him the fetal and maternal sides of the placenta. He lifted it out of its basin, hefted it to feel its weight and then crowed with delight when I showed him how to lift up the thin tissues that comprised the amniotic membranes, pulling them up so he could see the bag his baby had occupied. He was completely absorbed. I could just imagine him the next day at school, telling his friends about this experience, gesticulating and insisting that it wasn't gross, it was awesome, man, awesome!

It's not easy to be the bystander when a woman you love is enduring a long or difficult labor. Many men have a great deal of trouble coping with their own feelings of helplessness and inadequacy. Some just withdraw and get quiet; some end up tearful with frustration and exhaustion; and some act out with anger. Cursing, demanding better care, threatening lawsuits or even physical violence are not infrequent reactions to hours of perceived pain and suffering. Usually, if it's possible to talk to the father, reassuring him and quieting his fears with explanations of the normalcy of what his wife is experiencing will ease some of his distress.

When I came on duty one night, I noticed a tall, ruggedly handsome man sitting on a chair in the hallway outside one of the labor rooms. He looked whipped, his head hanging, arms leaning forward on his thighs, hands dangling between his legs. He lifted his head, wiped sweat from his forehead, and sighed deeply, shaking his head in what looked like defeat. When I asked if he was okay, he said, "Yeah, I'm okay. It's my wife I'm worried about. Jesus, she's been pushing her heart out for three hours now. I just don't see how she can take much more. I don't know if I can, and I'm not working as hard as she is, goddammit!" I murmured some comforting, reassuring words and brought him a cup of coffee. He stood up after sipping his coffee, shook himself all over like a great hounddog, and walked back into his wife's room.

Not too much later, I helped their nurse wheel the mother into the delivery room, as the laboring woman had finally succeeded in pushing her baby down far enough for a forceps delivery. I remained in the room to do baby care and assist the primary nurse with the delivery. As I stood at the mother's side, counting with her during her pushing efforts, I noticed her husband was standing against the wall, several feet away from the table. "Come over here, Daddy, come on. You need to be here next to your wife, you can hold her hand."

"I don't want to get in your way," he answered.

"No, no, you're not in the way. This is your place, reserved just for you," I urged him forward. As he took his place by his wife, I realized his face, mostly hidden behind the surgical mask he wore, was twisted and red. "Are you okay?" I whispered quietly to him, holding his arm. "Yeah, I'm okay. This is just . . . just . . . oh, man . . ." He broke down in audible sobs. I pulled up a stool for him, plunked him down on it, and rubbed his shoulders while I laughed and teased him about his tears: "Oh you nut, you, go ahead and cry, this is a pretty good thing to cry about! I love it when the daddies cry!"

After the baby was born, I took him by the hand and walked him around all the equipment to the warmer where the nurse was tagging and printing the baby. "Go ahead and put your hand on her. This is your own terrific little girl. Isn't she lovely? She's doing great, has good color and a strong set of lungs, huh?" He leaned down from his great height, put his face right up nose-to-nose with his baby's, and talked softly to her as he stroked her belly and limbs. I just backed away for a minute and watched silently; what a marvelous moment of greeting. When I placed her, bundled in warm blankets, into his arms, he just stood there sobbing, blubbering a torrent of tears. Finally, we took the baby to her mother and I sat the daddy down on his stool at the head of the table. They kissed each other and exclaimed over the baby for a few minutes. Then, to my complete surprise, the father turned to me, wrapped both arms around my waist, put his head against my breasts, and bawled like a baby for at least three or four minutes. He was totally overwhelmed with emotion. I patted him as his wife looked on with loving amusement: "Oh, everyone in his family cries at the drop of a hat!" she informed me. After the baby went to the nursery, accompanied by her now ebullient father, he returned to our unit and hugged every single person who was working that night, thanking all of us effusively for all our help. I loved it!

Another night, another surprise pleasure with a daddy. . . . I'd been working for eight hours in the exam/triage room, assessing an unending stream of patients. It was a wild night: by three in the morning we'd delivered eight or nine babies and we were all exhausted. A woman arrived in active labor with her fourth baby. She was in good control but wanted an epidural. When I examined her, I felt a cervix dilated to about four centimeters. I was instructed by the charge nurse to take her to a room and be her delivery nurse. There wasn't a single pair of extra hands to help me pull the gurney down the hallway to the last empty room available, so I enlisted her husband's help. We got her on the bed and then I scrambled for equipment, none of which was in the room, naturally.

As I struggled to pull a fetal monitor into the room, followed by a warmer for the baby, a light, a stool, the delivery instruments table, her husband gave me a much needed hand.

I squelched a smile when he told me he was a landscape gardener, because their last name was Gardiner! And he looked like one—strong, tan, weathered face, rough hands, and a smile in his eyes.

"Man, maybe ya'll should hire some more help around here, Susie!" he said with a laugh.

"The job's yours, I'll take whatever help I can get! What a night! The babies just won't stop coming!"

After I arranged everything, took vital signs, and got the mom strapped up with the monitor belts, the anesthesiologist arrived and gave her an epidural. Once she was comfortable, I checked her cervix once again. As I felt around inside her, her husband said, "What is it exactly that you're feeling for? I mean, I know you're checking the cervix for dilation, but how do you know what you're feeling?"

"Well, when you put your fingers in there, you can almost always feel the baby's head, if he is head-down, which most are. Then you feel around for cervix. It can be thick—as much as a half-inch—and mushy feeling, with an opening in the center, or real thin like a wafer-thin unbaked pie crust, tight against the baby's head. When you think you've got your finger on it, then you stretch the other finger to the other side of it and estimate how wide open the os, or mouth, of the cervix is. If you can only put one finger in the opening, it's not very dilated, maybe one to two centimeters, but when I have to stretch my two fingers completely apart and have trouble reaching both sides at the same time, that's getting close to ten centimeters." I demonstrated with my fingers as I explained.

"Wow, I can't imagine trying to feel that. I mean I've had my fingers in there . . ." Mr. Gardiner blushed, paused, and then laughed as his wife grinned at him. "You know, I've tried to check her cervix in the past few weeks, but I couldn't tell what I was feeling at all."

"I know," I replied. "I had the devil of a time learning how to do this. It just felt like warm oatmeal for the longest time and I couldn't tell where the cervix was. But hers is easy to feel. She's about seven centimeters now." I looked back and forth at both of them. We'd been chattering away at each other. They were a very personable couple, easy with each other and with me. "If it's okay with your wife, you can check her now and I'll tell you what to feel for."

Mr. Gardiner looked at his wife questioningly, obviously wanting to do this. She laughed and said, "Hey, now that I have the epidural, you can do whatever you want! Go ahead, honey, learn something new about me!"

He put on a sterile glove very carefully under my watchful eyes, leaned over his wife and gently inserted his two fingers into her vagina. "Do you feel the head?" I asked.

"Yep, wow, it's right down there, honey. It's way farther down than the last time I felt for it."

"Now, smooth your finger over the baby's head until you feel a thin membrane over to the side from the center of his head. Feel it?"

"No, uh, wait! Yeah! There it is!"

"Now move the other finger to the other side of the head, just spread your finger out until you feel the same thing on the other side."

"Yeah, I feel it on both sides now. Oh wow! That's seven centimeters, huh? Geez, honey, I could get a job doing this, it's not so hard, now I know what I'm feeling for!" Mr. Gardiner stood up and stripped off his glove, crowing with pride in himself. His wife and I just laughed and laughed.

One night, after hours and hours of sitting in a room with one couple, watching the fetal monitor and periodically checking a very slowly dilating cervix, I grew concerned about the mother's flagging spirits. All my routine words of encouragement were falling on deaf ears. She was discouraged and finding it difficult to continue her breathing, even though she was highly motivated to have a natural childbirth. Her husband had been unwavering in his support, cajoling, praising, and encouraging her in a soft voice through hours of contractions.

As I sat at the bedside, charting her progress, the husband said, "Wait just a minute, I think I may have something that will pick up your spirits." He walked over to the table and rummaged around in several suitcases and tote bags, his back to both of us. "Ah, here we go!" he announced. He turned around to face us and we both burst out laughing! He was standing there, wearing costume Groucho Marx eyeglasses, complete with huge nose and mustache, twirling an imaginary cigar between his fingers and lifting and lowering his eyebrows! His wife giggled through several contractions as he sat on the bed beside her and I took pictures. An hour later, he pulled out another pair of glasses which had big buggy eyes that bobbled around on the ends of wire coils as he moved his head. His joking and clowning eased the atmosphere in the room considerably.

I don't know whether his props and his jokes actually sped up his wife's dilation, but she did move from six centimeters to ten during the hour of his clowning, and the laughter renewed both of us. I told her after their baby was born how envious of her I was; to have a partner who could be so playful just at the right moment was something I dreamed of.

Sometimes a family member presents a problem of another sort. Nurses become practiced in watching out for a significant other during invasive or messy procedures, but sometimes we get caught off guard. The mother of a delivering girl went through the labor and delivery with her without any problems, with no sign of squeamishness over the blood, mucus, amniotic fluid, and feces that accompanied the process. Standing at her daughter's knee in the delivery room, she watched with absorption as the baby was delivered. After the placenta plopped out into a basin, none of us noticed as the woman quietly turned to the open doors of the delivery room. I happened to turn around just as her entire body hit the cement floor, facedown, with a wallop that made me wince!

We rushed to her and turned her over, waved an ammonia capsule under her nose, and checked her face for contusions. She broke the frames of her glasses and split her lip, but her nose survived the crash. She was terribly embarrassed by all the attention, insisting that the faint had been a complete surprise to her. She hadn't felt grossed out by the placenta, she insisted, she'd just felt like she needed some air. Following hospital policy, we wrote up an incident report, put her in a wheelchair and escorted her down to the emergency room to be checked out, against her wishes. None of us could believe she had hit the deck that hard without doing more damage to herself.

Another night I was assisting with the insertion of an epidural, and stood on one side of the bed, holding the woman in a curled position, while the anesthesiologist put in the epidural. The woman's sister was standing beside the anesthesiologist, watching everything he did. As I came around the end of the bed to gather up the refuse from the epidural tray, I saw the sister lean quite gently, almost caressingly, into the anesthesiologist. He looked down at her with utter amazement, bewildered by her near embrace. As I moved forward, she just slid down his side, silently flowing onto the floor, just as graceful as can be. It took us a few seconds to realize that she had passed out because she did it so smoothly!

The birthing center where I worked was designed to promote family participation in the birth of a baby. Each room was large and well appointed, decorated with soft colors and soothing framed prints. Visiting hours were extended and rules about family participation were few, stressing positive interaction with the mother and baby. Many nurses had difficulty with the presence of more than one or two family members during a labor and delivery, but I relished it.

My one rule of thumb was that it was the laboring mother's decision how many people, and who, might be allowed in the room. Whenever I started working with a new patient, one of my first tasks was to evaluate the atmosphere in the room. I introduced myself to everyone present, asked their names and relationships, and then, as I talked to the mother in the bed, adjusted the fetal monitor and scanned the chart, I listened to the conversations going on between family members. I could almost always feel if there was tension and conflict in the room, if the presence of a particular visitor was inhibiting the mother or making her uncomfortable.

In such cases, I usually tried to clear the room completely, suggesting that visitors leave for a few minutes while I got the mother cleaned up or on the bedpan or some such ruse. When the mother and I were alone, I asked about her visitors and whether she was comfortable having them in the room. On a few occasions I did the dirty work and asked an unwanted visitor to remain in the waiting room, pleading maternal exhaustion or whatever was appropriate. Sometimes an overwhelming family member was bossy and disruptive, trying to direct the mother and father and nurse each step of the way.

Sometimes, although rarely, a husband obstructed the flow of labor by criticizing his wife, fussing about how long she was taking or about her complaints. In such a situation, I very quietly but firmly counseled the husband right there in the room: his wife was doing her best, she needed positive reinforcement from him rather than criticism, and she had the ultimate right to decide how to be cared for and how to behave. Poor behavior in a laboring woman was always excusable. I explained to many mothers and fathers that the woman was the only one who knew what she was feeling and experiencing, and if she needed to holler or cry or curse, that was her prerogative. And she shouldn't worry about how those around her would react or what they might think.

For the most part, however, I truly enjoyed having families present for the labor and/or the birth. I didn't care how many people were in the room, as long as I could get the necessary equipment in place and move freely around the patient. I have spent long nights in rooms with up to ten people sitting around on the floor and counters. I have assisted at deliveries where families lined the walls, hugging, crying, and laughing, taking pictures as a new baby joined their ranks. Family dynamics fascinate me with their variety and uniqueness.

The birthing center had no central monitoring screens at the nurses' station. The only way I could know how the baby was doing and what kind of labor pattern the mother had was to sit at the bedside and watch the monitor. This meant I spent many a twelve-hour shift in a room with the mother and any family members who were keeping her company. After just a short while, the barriers usually came down. I actively involved family members in the mother's care: "Would you help me turn her over? Her legs are real heavy from the epidural. . . . Would you mind getting some more ice chips for her? . . . There's a clean blanket in that cupboard there; would you mind grabbing that for me, please?" I explained how to read the monitor and what all the jiggles and numbers meant. That usually led to questions about the IV, the epidural, how the delivery bed worked, and so on.

We almost always had a ball. One family of eight occupied a large birthing room all night, three children sleeping on the foldout father's couch and five adults playing cards together, while the mother and I quietly went through her labor. I have seen several families headed by ministers or pastors, whose courtly manners and personalized prayers lent a special air to the room. Videotaping births is a very common occurrence these days; lord only knows how many family video libraries I'm a part of! I've gotten so used to being filmed I don't even think about it anymore, although quite a few nurses are adamant about not being filmed. Some of the reluctance is due to vanity and some of it is a fear of malpractice suits if anything goes wrong during the labor or delivery. When I think of it in those terms, I get vaguely uncomfortable, but I believe the more open, accessible, and human we are to the people we're caring for, the less chance of misunderstandings and conflicts between us. It just makes sense to me that I'm much more likely to defuse a hostile or distressing situation resulting from a mistake I've made by honestly admitting it and apologizing rather than trying to hide it or cover it up.

The pleasure I derived from sharing a birth with a family never diminished, despite years of work, and I never ceased to be amazed by the variety of families that I worked with. There was a middle-aged man who accompanied his daughter, an unwed mother whose boyfriend had deserted her, to the hospital. This man sat on the edge of the bed, cradling his twenty-year-old daughter's head and shoulders in his arms as she progressed through labor. He wiped her face with cold cloths, fed her ice chips, and encouraged her in her pushing. When the baby was born, he wept and praised his daughter, kissing her forehead and telling her how proud he was of her efforts. I carried images of the two of them, father and daughter working together to birth a baby, around in my mind for weeks, envious of the love and closeness between them.

Years later, a grandmother observing her daughter-in-law's labor affected me as greatly. I didn't know the patient or her family, having just entered the birthing room to assist with the delivery. As I set up equipment on the infant warmer, this tall, slender woman, who leaned against the wall near the head of the bed, caught my eye. She wore faded blue jeans, a plaid flannel shirt, and workmen's boots. Her gray, straight hair was cut in a utilitarian bob at her ears. She was watching the primary nurse set up the delivery bed for the birth.

When her eyes strayed to me, I smiled. "Are you going to be taking care of the baby?" she asked, stepping toward me.

"Yes, I'm Susie and I'll be doing the baby care. This is your grandchild?"

"Yep! First one, too! I'm really excited! Can I take your picture?"

"Sure, but why don't you wait till the baby's here?" I asked. Nope, she wanted my picture at the warmer, so I let her take it, feeling kind of foolish.

When the baby was delivered, this woman stood at the foot of the bed, watching closely, hands clasped behind her back, rocking back and forth on her tiptoes. After the baby was out she turned around and grinned at me, raising her fist in the air with a triumphant thrust. I laughed and repeated the gesture. The new grandmother stood beside the warmer as I cared for the baby, snapping pictures, asking questions, stroking the baby once I encouraged her to do so. Finally I wrapped the baby and placed it in her arms. Her son, the new father, photographed her with the baby. I leaned against the cool tiles of the wall, unnoticed as attention focused on the baby.

As I watched this family, this grandmother who looked like she'd just come off the ranch, this woman near my own age, holding her grandchild, I felt a surge of emotion. My face flushed and unexpected hot tears flooded my eyes. I was trembling, holding back outright sobs. I wanted to watch that family, that woman, for hours. I wanted to cry with the marvel of this event, this new person being enveloped in love and pride by its family. There were two generations to cherish and shape and share in the life of this new being. The emotions I felt were so powerful they actually frightened me: I had to leave the room and take a few minutes to still the spasms of tears that burst out of me. At the same time, I was furious. It was a busy night on the unit; I didn't have any time to stand against that wall and enjoy the beginnings of this now-enlarged family. I had to clean equipment, enter the birth data into the computer, restock the delivery cart, and the warming bed. There was no time to acknowledge what I had witnessed.

The presence of children during a delivery is another hotly argued subject among obstetrical personnel. Personal bias comes into play here; nurses and doctors who would never dream of having their own children present find it more difficult to accept a patient who wants her kids to be with her. One night I cared for a woman whose husband and three-year-old daughter were at the bedside. This woman was quiet and controlled throughout her labor. Her husband sat close beside her head, holding their adorable little redheaded, curly-haired daughter, who watched everything, her enormous eyes filled with curiosity. Her parents explained everything that was going on, answering her questions openly and in terms she could understand.

The obstetrician came in near the end of the labor and asked who was going to care for the child during the delivery.

"I am," responded the husband.

"But aren't you planning to be in here?" queried the doctor.

"Yes, and our daughter is, too," he replied.

The doctor frowned with disapproval. "Do you really think that's a good idea? She's awfully young, isn't she?"

"We've prepared her for this. We've talked about the whole thing and we want her to be with us. I don't expect she'll be any trouble at all," the father said quietly and firmly.

The doctor shrugged in acquiescence. I turned away to hide my grin. *Right on, Daddy. You want her with you, stand up for your rights! This is your family, not the doctor's! Yeah!*

That little girl was good as gold. When the baby was born, she was agog, eyes so wide they were almost bugging out of her head; mouth open in amazement. Then she smiled the biggest smile and reached for the baby.

This family stayed together for the entire thirty-six hours they were in the hospital. The baby went to the nursery only for his physical, as Daddy watched closely from the window. To sleep, big sister and father shared the small foldout cot. The little girl changed the baby's diaper, with assistance from her father and then sat in her mother's encircling arm, watching her brother breast-feed. They did it all together, a true family. I thought it was marvelous.

One night, as I set up baby-care materials on the warmer, I learned the mother in labor was having her first baby, but the father had two children from a previous marriage. The mother was pushing well when the father asked their nurse if he could bring his children in. "You want them to watch her deliver?" she asked, taken aback.

"Yes, they'll stay here at the head of the bed, so they can't see her bottom, but we want them with us when the baby's born."

"Well, whatever," the nurse shrugged with obvious disapproval.

Into the room he brought his daughter, around thirteen years old, and his son, who was six. They sat close together on the couch. The little boy was dying of curiosity and had to be pulled back to the couch several times as he ventured near the end of the bed where all the action was. His older sister fussed at him gruffly and sat tensely on the couch, twisting her plastic earrings and frowning, answering questions almost rudely, with all the mannerisms of a tough little teeny-bopper. Her father enthusiastically tried to engage her in conversation, but she rebuffed him. I recognized my own daughter at a younger age in her behavior, and wondered if she was unhappy about this baby.

When the baby was born, there was a lot of cheering: "It's a girl! It's a girl!" The older sister jabbed her brother's arm, "Hah! I won the bet! I told you it was going to be a girl!" The little boy stood by his stepmother's side, watching everything avidly. The nurse dried the baby on her mother's chest and put a little cap on her head. After a few minutes the baby was brought to the warmer for a Vitamin K shot, bracelets, and ointment in her eyes. I called both siblings to the warmer as I worked on the baby. I talked to them about how the baby looked, why her head was cone-shaped, how the cord would dry up and fall off, and so forth. I encouraged both kids to touch her. When the little boy reached out, the baby grabbed the finger he held against her palm. He grinned beatifically.

Out of the corner of my eye, I was watching the tough, prepubescent sister. She stared at the baby with utter fascination, her eyes soft with tears, chin quivering. I took her hand, stroked the baby's abdomen with it and then let go, telling her she could caress the baby all over. She did just that, crooning to the infant, "It's all right, little Nancy, I'm here, you don't have to cry, your big sister is right here." I brought the scale into the room to weigh the baby. I'd already lifted her before I realized I hadn't put a towel on the scale. I placed the naked baby into her sister's arms: "Here, hold her while I get a towel."

That young girl-woman gathered the naked, squirmy, mucky little body into her chest and arms, holding the baby tightly against herself, oblivious to the blood and mucus smearing her crisp white blouse. I had her lay the baby on the scale, read the weight, and then wrapped the baby in warm blankets and handed her back to her sister. The girl could hardly wait: she was reaching for the baby with her whole body.

I stood and watched, a catch in my throat as I flashed back to when I was ten years old and fell completely head-over-heels in love with my youngest baby brother. I remembered rushing home from school so I could tiptoe into the bedroom where he slept to sit silently watching him until he awoke and I could gather him into my arms. Tears came as I watched this girl instructing her little brother how to sit and how to hold the baby. All the surface patina of the hard little teenager was gone; there was only a young girl responding to the wonder and delight of a new baby.

All the crowding, the noise, the rough-and-tumble of a family participating in a child's birth pleases me no end. I don't care how messy the room gets. I don't care if it's hard to weave my way through a room filled with family. I love taking family portraits for them, gathering grandmothers, grandfathers, aunts and uncles, cousins and siblings all together around the mother and baby in the bed. I only wish I had copies of all those pictures, all those families welcoming a new member into their ranks! I fantasize about running an alternative birth center where I could mother all my families without so many rules and policies and technology. When I think of how women used to be shut up alone or on a ward with other laboring women, without any loved ones near for support, I'm so pleased at the changes that have come about in hospitals today, and I'm frantic for even more freedom and access for the families. I don't know if it makes a difference in the long run for the child who is born, or for the family, but I can't help but believe that being surrounded by people who love one another and this new baby has to be positive.

Chapter Ten

SAYING HELLO AND
SAYING GOOD-BYE

Everybody thinks that working on a labor and delivery unit is special. To most people, including those in health care, L&D nursing is "nicer" than any other type of nursing, except maybe pediatrics. It's "nicer" or "more fun" because "it's a happy event," "it's joyous," "exciting." I always thought that myself. The idea of being a L&D nurse was attractive because most of the time the "patients" weren't really patients. They weren't really sick. They were just in the hospital for safety's sake, in case something went wrong while they were engaged in the healthy biological task of giving birth. Everybody knows there's some suffering going on. Lots of people who've come in to have their babies have said to me, "I don't know how you do this. I couldn't stand it," *it* being the messiness of labor—urine, feces, blood, mucus, vomit—or the seemingly endless hours of watching someone in pain, or the cries of agony that sometimes fill the halls.

Nobody wants to think that the place where new babies are born is anything but a happy place. However, death is a common occurrence on L&D. It shows its face on a regular basis, and you never know if the next woman who walks through the door is going to be the patient with the fetal demise. Every time you're in the delivery room, there's the slight but very real possibility that this unknown human being about to emerge into the light may not make it, may actually, God forbid, die on you.

The death of a baby, an unborn fetus, is different somehow from other deaths. If the fetus isn't full-term or nearly so, if it's young in gestational age, the response to its loss by its parents, their families, and by the medical staff, is so varied and so unpredictable, it just can't be lumped in the same category with other deaths. For some people, passing the products of conception cannot be equated with the death of a three-year-old or a seventy-year-old. It's just tissue, just a miscarriage. But to others, the loss of that fetus is the most devastating loss imaginable. It isn't comparable to the death of a three-year-old; at least the three-year-old had three years. This little piece of nothing that fits in the palm of my hand hasn't had anything. It hasn't even gotten its eyes open yet, much less breathed or cried or wet its diapers or felt the warmth of its mother's breast, or seen the sky, or snuggled in its father's arms. It's gone before it even got started.

The worst thing is that most people who lose their babies had never even considered the possibility. Pregnancy is about new life, about beginning. It is not about death, loss, ending. If the couple wanted the baby, the loss is horrific. There is no understanding it. No explanation can remove the bewilderment. For those who were ambivalent about the pregnancy or who disliked the reality of a baby, the loss is compounded by unspeakable guilt. All of this is exacerbated by the fact that nobody knows how to deal with this loss. Hospital personnel, the parents' family and friends—everybody brings his or her own ideas about what a fetal loss is to the bedside, making the mother and father writhe with their lack of sensitivity or understanding. Heck, even the mother and father don't know how to deal with this. *The baby's dead? The hell you say! Babies don't just die. I'm pregnant. I'm going to have a baby. You're saying this baby is dead? He hasn't even been alive yet. He hasn't even been born yet. How can you tell me he's dead? I felt him move yesterday. No way, no sir. Babies don't die. They're just getting started, not quitting, not dying!*

Some women, of course, know before they're told. They'll call and say they haven't felt the baby move for several hours, or a day or two days. Those words cause shudders among the medical staff. *Oh no, not a fetal demise, God, I hope she's wrong.* These women may come in unannounced and say they just felt like something was wrong. Sometimes it's a woman who's been through a miscarriage before: she's really tuned into her body, she's sweating out each day of this pregnancy, and may drive us crazy with her frequent calls and visits—but she's always forgiven once the staff knows she's had a previous loss.

Other women have such powerful denial mechanisms that they smile at you and tell you you're wrong about the baby being dead all the way through labor, until the evidence, a dead fetus, is presented to them. Most women, however, are caught unaware when they're told their babies are dead. Suddenly all the plans, all the images of a future with this unknown little being are gone. Furthermore, the body isn't in the hospital or the morgue or the funeral home. It's still there, inside the woman, and she can't go on with her life, can't have a funeral and have the family and friends comfort her, because first she has to produce the body. She has to go through childbirth, to get a dead body.

I had been working only about five weeks when a young woman came into our exam room, saying that she felt that "something's been wrong since yesterday." In her early twenties, Mrs. Maxten was the mother of a two-year-old boy. Her body looked sturdy, not too fat or too thin, with just the beginnings of a pregnant belly. She was neatly dressed, lightly made-up, with a no-fuss cut to her clean straight hair. She answered my questions with composure, giving me the impression of a responsible, straight-forward young adult. She was twenty-seven weeks along in her pregnancy (forty weeks is term) and had no overt signs or symptoms of a possible miscarriage, just a gut feeling that something was wrong.

When I went across the hall to retrieve the doptone, to listen for the fetal heartbeat, I bumped into Tom, the chief resident. I spoke to him very briefly, warning him to go gently because I thought there might be a problem. He came into the exam room with me, asked a few questions, and listened with the doptone. After a couple of minutes, he left the room to get the ultrasound machine. When he returned, he was accompanied by two medical students and the first-and second-year residents, all males. None of these men greeted Mrs. Maxten or identified themselves. I told her quietly that they were students and residents learning about ultrasound.

They scanned her belly for at least ten minutes. Tom called his supervisor, the obstetrical chief, Dr. Dixon, into the room to look at the scan. There, in that darkened little room, the woman lay on an examining table, her protuberant belly smeared with conducting gel; the soft blue light from the scanner's screen illuminated the faces of the six men who stood around the exam table, their attention focused on the gray sworls and clouds on the screen. I stood next to her, holding her hand and watching her. She lay preternaturally still, breathing tiny, shallow breaths, foreboding wrinkling her brow, her eyes wide with concern, searching the ultrasound screen and the faces of these strange men.

Tom pushed the machine away from the exam table, switched on the overhead lights, and sat down on the stool beside the table. I was totally unprepared for his words. At that time, I wasn't experienced enough to understand what the previous ten minutes had been about. I couldn't tell one shadow from another on the ultrasound screen, and I failed to understand why the chief had been called into the room. I did know something bad was coming. With five men standing around him, Tom leaned forward and said, "Mrs. Maxten, your baby is dead." He went on, "We couldn't see a heartbeat, or any limb movement . . ." but the words, *your baby is dead, your baby is dead*, just reverberated around that room. I felt Mrs. Maxten stiffen under my hand. She turned her head toward the wall, away from all those men, away from Tom, who kept on talking professionally about inducing labor to expel the fetus.

Dr. Dixon interrupted Tom in midsentence, speaking soothingly. "This didn't happen because of anything you did or didn't do, Mrs. Maxten. I think it would be a good idea to give you some privacy for a few minutes now, and then we can talk again." The men were out of that room faster than you could blink an eye. I started to follow Dr. Dixon, but he turned and placed his hand on my shoulder. "I think you should stay with her."

"I'd like to," I fumbled. "Is it all right if I stay with you?" She nodded, her face still turned away. Then she wailed, loudly and forlornly, and reached out both arms for me. I sat on the stool holding her as she sobbed incoherently, and tried my feeble best to comfort her as the world she knew tumbled down all around her. No baby, no daughter or son to raise; no more pregnancy, no more life within to nourish and protect, only a tiny dead fetus. She had known "something was wrong."

This was my first experience with a fetal demise. My ignorance with ultrasound was short-lived; I learned very quickly to look for that little heart pumping away, to recognize limbs and watch for their movement. I was sickened by the way this woman had been told of her child's death. I fumed silently about it for days, cursing those thick-skinned males in their white coats, surrounding her with their "authority" and expertise while she faced the knowledge of the death within her body. The day before she had been fecund with life. Now she was a living tomb for a tiny corpse. After I had the unfortunate opportunity to hear Tom tell another woman "Your baby is dead" a few days later, I gathered my courage and confronted him. I asked him if I could speak to him privately, not wanting to appear critical of him in front of anyone, and said: "This not meant as a criticism, just constructive suggestion. Please, Tom, try to be less blunt about it. Tell her the evidence first. You know, like 'There's no heartbeat,' and then, 'Your baby isn't alive anymore.' Please don't blurt out 'Your baby's dead.' Break it to her gently, instead of hitting her over the head with it."

Actually a wonderfully warm young man trying his best to be a good doctor, Tom was grateful for my suggestion. He acknowledged that he never knew how to tell someone, or what words to use, and thanked me. He remembered my suggestions and was careful of his phrasing from then on.

Just three days after this conversation, a comely Hispanic girl was wheeled into L&D by ambulance attendants. She was hugely pregnant, glowing and laughing, the very picture of health and excitement. We greeted her and moved her into one of the labor rooms. She'd been transferred to our unit from an outlying clinic via ambulance after the clinic had verified that her membranes were ruptured. She was carrying twins and had made it to thirty-seven weeks without complications, a fact we all made much of, since multiple gestations automatically place a woman at risk for premature labor. As I put the monitors on her belly, she chattered away at me, laughing about having two babies, what their names were going to be, and how glad she was to have carried them so long. I found one heartbeat without difficulty, but couldn't find the other one. I called another nurse in to give it a try. No one thought anything amiss; sometimes it's difficult to find both heartbeats, depending on the babies' positions.

When I returned to the room after taking care of another patient, I found Tom, Dr. Dixon, and the ultrasound machine in the room. My heart sank as I moved to the bedside and took this beautiful young woman's hand in mine. I watched her face as they talked to her, explaining that the baby on the left was alive and well, but the one on the right was dead. She was calm, apparently stunned with disbelief. She asked several questions—why, how, what—and then began to shake. Again, the men vacated the room and I held her in my arms, reaching for tissues and murmuring softly, "I'm so sorry, oh, I'm so sorry," as she sobbed. After a while, she gathered herself together and took charge. She asked for a phone to call her husband and peppered me with questions about how we would be inducing labor. Dealing with the facts, asking about concrete details of her impending labor helped her put aside, if only briefly, the reality of the dead child within. I'll never forget how she looked when she arrived, carefree and exhilarated, totally unaware that her life was about to change radically; that death had already entered her unsuspecting world.

It doesn't take very long to learn the signs, the clues, that death has arrived. Anytime a woman says she "hasn't felt the baby moved since . . ." I cringe inwardly. Anytime it takes more than sixty to ninety seconds to find a fetal heartbeat I get nervous. Sometimes, late at night when all the patients were asleep on the ward, a devoted, diligent night LPN, Mrs. Strong and I would sit and talk about her experiences on the unit over the years. She would tell me about how horrible it always was to be the one who couldn't find a baby's heartbeat. We would walk the hall at 0500, taking vital signs together. She always preferred to have me do the fetal heart tones because she had been stung too many times.

It was almost five years before it happened to me. I knew eventually it was going to; there was no way I could avoid it during the hundreds of nights, with the hundreds of bellies I touch with gel and doptone. Even so, as I listened to other nurses tell about how it had happened to them, I counted my blessings that thus far I'd been spared.

One morning, early, about 0530 at the civilian hospital where I was night manager, one of the nurses called me into a room, telling me she couldn't find a heartbeat. I was instantly alerted to the possibility of a fetal death because this nurse had many years of L&D experience. I introduced myself to the patient and her husband: "Hi, I'm Susie, I'm just going to give a listen here. Sometimes it's hard to hear the heartbeat if the baby is turned a certain way." I listened, moving the doptone systematically over her abdomen from the navel down, from one hip to the other, down to the pubic hair. The patient, Mrs. Stubblefield, wasn't obese or even well padded. I could feel baby parts under my hands and I knew within two or three minutes that the baby was probably dead. I stopped listening, wiping the conducting gel off her belly and the doptone as I said, "Look, I know this must be nerve-wracking to you, so rather than waste any more time and make all of us even more anxious, I'm going to get the resident to run the ultrasound over your tummy, so we'll know more than I can find out with this thing."

I called the resident, waking her up. We would have to call the patient's private physician after the ultrasound scan was completed. I stood at Mrs.

Stubblefield's bedside with my hand on her shoulder and watched the screen. I knew almost immediately that the baby was dead. I watched the resident push the scanner back and forth over the abdomen, twisting it, moving it repeatedly over the same areas. I could see the head, the spinal column, and the limbs, but no heartbeat and no movement. The resident continued the scan longer than necessary. I noticed that she had turned her whole body away from the bed. She was weeping, the tears on her face shining in the blue light from the screen.

She asked me to bring in any attending physician who might be around, to verify the scan. The doctor I recruited muttered unhappily, "Oh, no, I'm not good at these things." He looked and the resident looked and then they turned off the machine. They told Mrs. Stubblefield they were not totally sure about what they were seeing, asking when she had last felt the baby move. They said they would have to wait for her doctor to verify the scan, and that they would call her doctor right away. They left the room. Mr. Stubblefield had his face down on his wife's shoulder. She looked up at me. The silence in the room was unbearably heavy.

The Stubblefields were an impossibly normal looking couple, their very ordinariness somehow an added insult to this scene. Clean, healthy, physically nondescript, they were just regular people. Despairingly I thought something this bad shouldn't be happening to such regular people. Shouldn't there be something about them that would warn us of impending doom? But looking into her face, I saw now that her demeanor was anything but "nondescript." A pallor of grief had already invaded her dark eyes. The knowledge of loss tightened the skin around her features, accentuating the bones of her previously plump-looking face. I could almost see the morbid leer of death itself in the skeleton beneath her skin, as if for one microsecond death possessed the mother's face as it had her child, to remind me of its ultimate dominion over us all.

Squelching my own dread, I looked her straight in the eye and said, "We're not going to jump to any conclusions right now, okay? We'll wait until Dr. Strickland gets here, but you know and I know, you're too smart not to know, that this isn't looking good. I'm so sorry, but let's hang onto our hope for a bit yet, okay?" She nodded and thanked me. I asked her if there was anything I could do for her while we waited, or if she needed anything? In a normal tone of voice, she said, "I really need to go to the bathroom. Is that okay?"

"Sure," I replied, and helped her get out of bed. Her silent husband walked her to the bathroom. As she moved into the lighted room, I saw her slump down in his arms, wailing cries rising, piercing the silence. I closed the door quietly, her sobs echoing in my ears.

This patient's misery was compounded by the complete disbelief of her physician. Dr. Strickland burst into the room, distraught and disheveled, shaking his head and insisting to the Stubblefields that he just couldn't believe this. He didn't do another scan. Many of the attending physicians at this hospital weren't really proficient or comfortable with ultrasound and relied on the residents and radiologists to perform them. The doctor and the Stubblefields talked briefly about the scan that had been performed four days earlier and how everything had seemed normal. The pregnancy had been without complications. There was no explanation to be offered.

Then Dr. Strickland, without explaining that labor was necessary or how it would be accomplished, performed a cervical exam and asked for a fetal scalp electrode, "to make sure." He attached the electrode and, horror of horrors, we got a heartbeat on the monitor. It was a horror because it wasn't the baby's heartbeat, it was the mother's. I palpated the pulse in Mrs. Stubblefield's wrist, and it synchronized exactly with the pulse on the monitor. The doctor was gleeful at first, his excitement filling the patient and her husband with desperate hope. I had to be the bad guy. I insisted that the pulse was the mother's. The doctor felt around inside Mrs. Stubblefield, checking the placement of the electrode, insisting it was on the baby.

I was aghast: if it was a fetal heartbeat, the baby was in trouble since the rate was in the seventies and eighties, instead of the normal 120s or higher, so why were we standing here like idiots staring at the machine? I was screaming at the doctor in my head, *Get the ultrasound, scan her, crash her, do* something *for Christ's sake, but* don't *mislead her that this baby is alive just because you've got an intermittent beat on the monitor.* When Dr. Strickland rechecked the placement of the electrode, the heartbeat more or less stopped, an errant beat bleeping now and again on the monitor. He insisted he had the electrode properly applied and that it couldn't be the mother. Certain that the electrode was picking up the maternal pulse through the baby, knowing the baby was dead, I left the room, unable to watch their faces, as the couple and the doctor vainly hoped and listened for bleeps.

Later, after my anger had dissipated, I realized yet again how difficult it is for anyone involved with a fetal demise. Dr. Strickland wasn't intentionally trying to make things worse for the parents. He naturally felt a certain amount of denial. He was responsible for this woman's care during her pregnancy. The unexpected had occurred with absolutely no forewarning, and he hated it, just as I did, and I hadn't even met Mrs. Stubblefield until an hour before. But I couldn't help but feel appalled at how awkwardly the physician had handled the situation.

Just as I finished giving the morning report to the oncoming shift, Dr. Strickland came into the report room. He told me the patient had wanted me to start her IV and had asked if I could be her nurse. I went back to her room in my street clothes to say good-bye. I held Mrs. Stubblefield's hand and cried as I told her how very sorry I was. "There isn't anything anyone can ever say to make this any easier. I'll be thinking about you all day, and my prayers are with you." She thanked me, smiling at me as she told me how much she appreciated my being there. I leaned down and kissed her cheek and we hugged each other tightly, two strangers bound together by her loss.

In the beginning of my practice, I was somehow able to care for parents who were experiencing fetal deaths with an equanimity that impressed my bosses and co-workers. I was quite effective in helping the mother and father through the hours and days of grief, holding their hands, acknowledging their loss, answering questions, helping them accept the emotions that hit them. The first time I had to see a dead fetus, my friend Nick was looking out for me, as usual. He took me aside and spoke to me about how the baby looked, then barred the door to the room where the baby lay and stood close beside me as I studied this small, cold being. It was a little girl, about thirty weeks, well-formed and newly dead. It didn't look too bad. I leaned down on my elbows, cradled the little body in my hands and said a private prayer: *Oh little girl, it just wasn't your time, was it? Go in peace, little one, back to where you came from. Come again another day, when it's the right time and you can be with us here on earth.*

Crazy, loony, maybe, but my own philosophy about life and death sheltered me from the pain of these little lost bodies for a time. I became the nurse who got assigned to fetal demises and to patients whose babies had fetal anomalies or defects. It was rewarding work; I somehow knew what to say, what to do. The responses I received from patients and their families verified my effectiveness. But gradually, it began to get harder and harder. Emotions that I thought I had in check would suddenly flood over me and tears came without warning.

A month or so into my first job, my head nurse told me she wanted me to "special" a patient whose thirty-two-week fetus had fetal ascites, an abnormal accumulation of fluid in the abdomen. The patient was having some bleeding and premature contractions. Furthermore, she was at risk for a complete previa, since the placenta was positioned over the cervix. If the doctors were unable to stop her contractions or if she continued to bleed, an emergency cesarean would be necessary. In the meantime, my boss wanted me to stay with her and watch her very closely.

For the next three hours I sat at the bedside, holding Mrs. Gently's hand. I talked her through each contraction, giving her my eyes and voice, helping her stay in control, checking her peri-pads frequently for blood. She was frightened and in pain; she knew her baby had an anomaly, with an unknown prognosis, yet she remained calm and dignified. But with undeniable urgency, she quietly asked me not to leave her bedside. "I need you to be with me," she whispered. Suddenly, she felt a gush of blood. I looked under the sheet at her pad and rang the call bell. We rushed her back to the delivery room, as blood poured from her vagina. Fourteen people—obstetricians, anesthesiologists, pediatricians, a neonatologist, nurses, med students, and scrub techs—raced furiously to get her positioned, prepped, and delivered. I sat on a stool at her head, holding her hand, assuring her repeatedly that I would not leave her side.

When the baby was delivered scant minutes after Mrs. Gently had been put under, I glimpsed the neonatologist lifting the fetus from the surgeon's hands. I saw translucent skin, tiny limbs, and a grossly enlarged abdomen which spilled over the sides of the doctor's hands. The brief glimpse made me shudder with horror; this ugly thing was the first malformed infant in my experience. I was greatly relieved that the baby was whisked into the NICU immediately because I felt my stomach heave at the sight of it.

Several days later, I spotted Mrs. Gently in the day lounge with her family. I had been off for a few days and hadn't seen her, but I knew her baby had died. I went to her, knelt before her, and hugged her close. We spoke softly, sharing tears over her tiny lost baby. I marveled at her composure and praised her strength during the hours before and after the surgery. She told me that having her baby, even for a few hours, meant everything to her, and had made letting go easier. She had such dignity, such grace; I hoped to be able to emulate her if I ever found myself in similar circumstances.

As time went by, I was exposed to many more such babies. Babies that had been dead in utero for several days, even weeks, so that they had begun to soften and rot. Babies whose color was almost black, skin peeling away, sloughing off in my hands when I touched them. Babies with deformities that horrified me, making me wonder at the bizarre nature of cells gone mad. Babies who were so small, so unformed that gender couldn't be differentiated, eyes sealed, fingers and toes just buds. One mother, an obese woman with a gentle, sweet demeanor, sat in her bed, knees propped up, hands cupping her nineteen-week baby, as she made her farewells to this fetus. She had been trying for nine years to conceive: now she was spending what little time she could with her only child. She smiled at the baby, talked to it, delicately stroked its miniscule limbs, as if even these moments were the greatest treasure.

Another mother had been in and out of the unit as an antepartum patient with premature labor. Mrs. Crocker had a disturbing effect on the nurses because she was so distant. Her face remained cold and flat; she spoke in monosyllables and never smiled. She had long, dark hair, twisted in a tight bun at the nape of her pale white neck, and a wen, making me think of a fairy-tale witch. I had no interaction with her until her final admission. She was contracting, with ruptured membranes, and was only twenty-two weeks or so. When I came on duty, she had just delivered a tiny nonviable female. The baby died not long after birth. The off-going nurse reported that Mrs. Crocker had not spoken during or since the delivery.

On the other hand, her husband had surprised everyone by comforting the medical staff. When I introduced myself to Mr. Crocker, he greeted me warmly, emphasizing how supportive everyone had been. I asked him bluntly how he felt himself. He smiled and explained that he was a minister; death was familiar, and this loss hadn't really hit him yet. I asked him how he thought his wife was bearing up; imagine my shock when he informed me that she was a forensic pathologist. She had learned how to mask her emotions, which was why we had been unable to tell what she was feeling. Her flat, blank demeanor began to make sense to me. I could only wonder how she would feel when she went back to work, while still dealing with the premature death of her daughter.

I was startled when Mr. Crocker asked me, "Would you do us a great service? We want to baptize our daughter and we would appreciate it if you would be our witness." I agreed immediately and a little later carried a tiny dead baby, wrapped in a receiving blanket, into Mrs. Crocker's room. Her husband and I uncovered the baby and gently placed it in her hands. He touched the baby's forehead with holy water, baptizing and naming her, as the mother and I watched, both weeping openly. Then the parents studied the baby, Mr. Crocker pointing out recognizable features, calling her by name. Mrs. Crocker held each miniscule hand, curling the tiny fingers around her forefinger, while I shook with grief. She cried, but never spoke a word.

It is policy everywhere I've worked to encourage parents of dead infants to see, touch, and hold their babies after delivery. Many parents are horrified initially at the suggestion that they do so, but almost all eventually opt to at least see the fetus, after we have explained that this contact facilitates the grieving process. Research has shown that parents resolve their loss more effectively if they know what the baby looked like and have had an opportunity to say good-bye. This contact makes the baby more real for them, and almost always the baby looks better, whatever its defects, than their fantasies had led them to expect. Only once have I discouraged a mother from viewing her infant.

This particular baby had been dead for at least two weeks. It was literally rotting; blackened skin covered bones that were so mushy that when I held its head, the skull bones gave way under my fingers. Black fluid oozed from its mouth and nostrils. My attempt to get footprints and fingerprints for the parents' "memory packet" failed; the feet smushed under even the slightest pressure of my fingers. I was revolted by the amount of decay; sickened by the thought of this rotting flesh inside a living woman; and I couldn't stomach the idea of her looking at this putrid mass of tissue. I knew it was wrong of me to decide for her, but I couldn't overcome my unwillingness to expose this woman to a lifetime memory of this pathetic little creature. As a compromise, I talked to her husband.

"The baby looks really bad, sir. It's been dead for a good while and has begun to decay. I am so sorry to have to say this to you, but I really feel I have to warn you. We know it's important for the parents to see their baby, but I don't know how you feel about this, since the baby does look pretty bad. I'll leave it to you to decide. If you would like to see the baby, then you could know better whether or not your wife should see it also."

He thought about it briefly, and then replied that he wanted to see for himself. I took him into the scrub room where I had left the baby, wiped as clean as possible and wrapped in a receiving blanket. I lifted away the blanket and held the man's arm as he gazed down at his son. His face twisted with the smell and tears filled his eyes, but he studied the baby for several long minutes. Then he turned to me and said, "I appreciate this. I don't want my wife to see the baby. It's too hard. Thank you for preparing me." Years later I still feel guilty that I denied that mother the right to say good-bye to her baby. But the feeling of bones giving way to my hands, the sight of that child was so horrific to me, that I couldn't help my reaction.

One of the most difficult patients I ever encountered was an obese thirty-five-year old diabetic. Mrs. Malinger had carried none of her seven previous pregnancies to term because of her diabetes.

She was completely insulin-dependent, requiring large doses of insulin around the clock to counter her steadfast refusal to comply with her dietary restrictions and to modulate her wildly fluctuating blood glucose levels. She was only five feet, four inches tall, and weighed close to three hundred pounds. She had a little girl's fat face, stringy, mousy brown hair, bad skin, and a shrew's disposition.

When I first met her, Mrs. Malinger was on the L&D unit, being treated with IV and oral medications to stop premature contractions. The medications had done little to soften her manner: when I answered her call bell, she was sitting on the bedpan, fussing loudly about how often she had to urinate. As I removed the bedpan, I saw that it was filled with bright red fluid. Upon perusing her chart for an explanation for the bleeding, I discovered that not only was she a 'brittle diabetic,' a premature laborer, and a seven-time miscarrier, but she also had a complete placenta previa.

This abnormal condition, in which the placenta implants and grows directly over the cervix, had been overlooked by the staff during her clinic appointment as they focused on the diabetic problem. Placenta previa is not uncommon in diabetic patients, adding a further serious risk to the pregnancy. Having a placenta positioned over the cervix effectively eliminates the possibility of a vaginal birth: the baby cannot pass through placental tissue. If premature labor occurs, also not unusual in diabetics, and the cervix begins to dilate, the placenta will tear. Such tears may cause massive hemorrhaging, jeopardizing the lives of mother and baby alike. Because of all these significant risks to her pregnancy, we knew this woman would be our patient for as long as we could sustain her fragile pregnancy.

Eventually, after several days on L&D, Mrs. Malinger stopped contracting and was moved to four-woman antepartum room for a long stay. The nursing staff was pushed to the limit with her. She was extremely gregarious, talking endlessly and obsessively to everyone in her vicinity. Her favorite topics of conversation were the "terrible care and total indifference of the staff to her problems," the refusal of the staff to let her eat what she wanted to eat, the filth of the hospital, and her husband's deficiencies, which in her eyes were all-encompassing. She was shrill and blatant in her assaults on the poor fellow, insulting him to his face in the presence of others and relishing his embarrassment. She engaged in intrigue with her roommates, inciting them to complain about hospital routines, meals, staff members, and treatment. She appeared to enjoy working everyone into a frenzy, then lolling back on her bed, sneering at her roommates' tears and the nurses' anger. She made illegal trips to the canteen and hoarded junk food under her bed, in the bathroom, in her suitcase, on the windowsill. She argued about her insulin doses and the necessity of our taking routine vital signs.

We held a multidisciplinary conference about Mrs. Malinger with psych nurses, social workers, and the OB residents. We coordinated our efforts to contain her damage on the ward by refusing to respond to her negative remarks, praising her whenever possible for compliance with her treatment plan, and spending extra time with her roommates to counter her effect on their morale. The physicians continued to monitor her diabetes and her fetus closely; weekly and then biweekly nonstress tests and biophysical profiles were performed to assess the well-being of the baby, while the nursing staff struggled to stay calm under her verbal attacks.

This challenging patient was with us for several weeks, until she reached her thirty-sixth week of gestation. One morning the night nurse couldn't find Mrs. Malinger's baby's heart tones. During the 0100 check, Mrs. Malinger had complained stridently about being awakened, shaking her massive belly with her hands as she exclaimed, "I wish this baby would just die so I could get a good night's sleep!" Unable to find the fetal heartbeat at 0530, the nurse was aghast. She related her feelings to us in morning report: "I went over her abdomen, all of it, four times, back and forth, up and down. She and I both poked and massaged her abdomen. She joked, 'I guess the baby's dead, huh?' I just couldn't believe it! I had heard that baby loud and clear four hours earlier. How could it have died, just like that, and after what the mother had said? Well, you know, she got real quiet after twenty minutes of me listening. Then we got the ultrasound and scanned her. Yep, the baby is dead."

What a horror. This woman, whom everyone disliked, who had created an atmosphere of tension and hostile defensiveness on the ward, who had defiantly broken every rule she could short of signing out AMA (against medical advice), had lost her baby. This is not an unusual event in diabetic women who are at great increased risk during pregnancy, but the suddenness of the death upset everyone. She had been given the best of medical care. She and her baby had been monitored closely for weeks. Nonetheless, her disease inexorably took its toll; wildly fluctuating serum glucose levels, gross obesity, flagrant nutritional insults, and maybe, a nasty personality—I know, it's wicked of me to suggest—contributed to this death. Her baby was delivered by cesarean, eleven pounds of dead infant pulled from her bloated body. What a pity. Mrs. Malinger was subdued and tearful for two days. Then, true to her nature, she launched into lengthy diatribes about her medical management, along with constant threats of a malpractice suit.

The death of this particular baby elicited some strange reactions from the staff. Because the mother had been such an unpleasant character, some people actually said that she had it coming to her, finally venting their anger at her obnoxious behavior. Other people were suddenly and ostentatiously solicitous, offering syrupy condolences and encouraging her mad monologues about her loss. I felt extremely uncomfortable: I didn't like the woman. I had despised the hostility and conflict she had brought to the unit. It was difficult to maintain my equanimity in the face of her insults, but I had managed to provide care without losing my temper or acting out against her. When her baby died, I felt pity at last. She was a pathetic human being, driven by unknown compulsions to behave badly, but nonetheless her loss was real and great. I expressed my sympathy to her once, which she accepted, amazingly enough, politely and quietly. Then I left her alone and tried to avoid the gossip about her among the staff.

Obviously, staff reactions to fetal deaths are as complicated and variable as those of family members. One first-year resident went through her own ordeal during the small hours of a night on duty. A nineteen-week fetus had been expelled after the mother had ruptured and labored prematurely. The resident delivered the baby with quiet, sympathetic dignity, interacting with the parents in a compassionate, caring way. We worked together cleaning up the mother and attending to paperwork. Unfortunately the fetus was "alive" at birth: it had a heartbeat. Eyes fused, unable to breathe on its own, cut off from its life source, its mother, its miniature heart just kept on trying. Unable to do anything for the fetus because of its gestational age, the neonatalogists had left the body with us to dispose of, after the parents had had time to say good-bye. The heartbeat was simply a neurologic reflex that eventually would cease. For all intents and purposes, the baby was dead and gone.

I remembered when my father had dissected a turtle for all the neighborhood kids, back when I was ten years old. We were fascinated by the turtle's heart, which kept on beating for four hours after being removed from the body cavity and placed in a jelly jar of salted tap water. That memory of my first gross anatomy lesson helped me distance myself from the tiny human form lying alone and cold on the scale in the delivery room. But the resident was haunted. She sat at the desk long after she finished her notes, staring into space, a frown creasing her forehead. Four times she asked me to go see if it was still beating. I comforted her as best I could, quietly reassuring her that she'd done everything possible, massaging her shoulders and trying to get her to go to bed.

"I know it's not my fault. I know there wasn't anything we could do to stop this from happening. I know the baby's not really alive. But God, Susie, all my training, all I've learned . . . It makes me feel so helpless. I'm sorry I keep asking you to go look. I should do it myself. But I just find it so hard to sit and wait like this. Why won't that darned heart stop beating?"

She kept her vigil with that baby all night, sitting at the desk, refusing to get desperately needed sleep while the heartbeat continued. I sat with her, my presence the only support I could offer as she struggled with questions about living and dying and the work we do.

As I've mentioned, the strange ability I had to work effectively with parents experiencing a fetal loss led to many such assignments. But eventually I lost my composure. The sudden tears, the unexpected grief over a stranger's loss would choke me; the dread I felt when I saw IUFD (intrauterine fetal demise) written on the census board at the beginning of my shift, all contributed to a mounting reluctance to be assigned to these patients. None of the nurses enjoyed these assignments; the work was demanding and emotionally draining. We tried to take turns, but by my seventh year of employment, I actively avoided such assignments whenever possible.

Of course, I couldn't always duck my turn without feeling really guilty about not carrying my share of the burden. I hadn't worked a demise yet at this particular hospital, and knew it was time to learn the routines and paperwork for a fetal death. I volunteered, with a queasy sensation in my belly, to take over the care of a woman whose full-term baby had expired in utero. The death was discovered at her regular prenatal visit; Mrs. Graves had then been admitted for an induction to deliver her dead baby. This poor mother had been in labor for almost forty hours, with very little cervical dilation. The obstetrics group managing her care were extremely reluctant to deliver her surgically because she had a chronic bleeding disorder. If they opened her abdomen for a cesarean, there was a risk of aggravating that disorder, resulting in further serious postoperative complications.

However, a vaginal delivery was looking less and less likely by the time my shift began, because the baby was presenting face first. This meant that the soft tissue and bones of the face were pressing against the cervix, not the firmer, rounder crown of the skull, which normally helped to dilate the cervix. As I was getting report on this patient from her off-going nurse, the physicians were attempting, for a second time, to reposition the baby, trying to move it back enough from the cervix so they could tilt the chin down and bring the crown of the head against the cervix. By the time I arrived in the patient's room, the attempt had failed. Her cervix was badly swollen from the long hours of labor and the doctors' manipulations. There was very little likelihood that the cervix could be dilated by further labor, so the doctors instructed me to prepare her for surgery.

I can't remember what that woman looked like. I can't recall *anything* about her or her husband, except his grief. But I will never forget their baby because of how it affected me. I was assisted by another nurse in the surgical prep: belly scrubbed and shaved, urinary catheter in place, jewelry and nail-polish removed, consent forms signed, lab work accounted for, documents to be filled out in hand. In a small room down the hall from the operating room, a nurse's aide set up supplies for me to use to clean up the baby's body before giving it to the parents for a farewell. I intended to bathe the baby, take hand and foot prints, and photograph it both naked and wrapped in baby blankets. The prints, its identification bracelets, a lock of hair, and the photographs would be given to the parents in a "memory packet," along with a booklet about the grieving process and a list of support groups for fetal demise parents.

Soon after the preoperative preparations were completed on this patient, my night went to hell. The labor and delivery unit was subjected to a flood of unanticipated patients just as I was ready to transport Mrs. Graves to the operating room. It was impossible for one person to move a labor bed out of the labor room, in tandem with an IV pole with two unwieldy pumps attached to it, down a long hall, and through three sets of heavy double doors. I phoned the charge nurse for help.

"There isn't anyone available from L&D," she responded. "Get some of the mother-baby nurses to help you. And Susie, get through with that case as fast as you can. We are drowning in patients and I need you ASAP!"

"Well, it's gonna be a while, you know. We're just going for surgery now, and I've got to clean up the baby and do all the paperwork, which you know I haven't done before."

"Just do it as fast as you can, okay?" She hung up. I stuck my head out of the room and saw four mother-baby nurses gathered at the nurses' station. Everyone was busy. It was the beginning of the shift, the postpartum unit was full and these nurses had a lot to do. But when I called out for assistance, everyone ignored me. *Okay*, I thought, *I'll just manage without them*. There wasn't any point in being annoyed: they all had as much to do as I did. I enlisted the aid of the patient's husband and her father. Between the three of us, we managed to maneuver the clumsy, heavy bed and the IV pole out of the room, bumping into the sides of the doors, pushing and pulling together, my face red with exertion, irritation, and embarrassment.

"I'm so sorry, Mom," I apologized to Mrs. Graves. "I know how uncomfortable it is to be hauled around like this and banged into the door, in the bargain! Can you believe this? When they built this magnificent maternity center, they didn't make the doors to these rooms wide enough to get the beds through with the railings up! Then the equipment purchasing people brought around a bunch of different bed models and asked the nurses which one they thought would be best suited for our needs. The one bed all of the nurses vetoed is, naturally, the one you're in! It's too heavy and too cumbersome for one person to manage. But the people who buy the stuff and design the rooms aren't the people who have to use them—isn't that always the way it goes?" I joked, grinning at her sheepishly as I walked backwards down the long hall, pulling on the foot of the bed with all my strength, trying to keep it from careening into the walls. I could feel the muscles in my back spasm with effort and had a silent moment of terror that I'd ruptured another disc, as sharp pain shot down my leg.

When we made it through all the double doors, I voiced my heartfelt thanks to Mr. Graves for his help and asked him to wait outside the OR until we began the surgery. In the operating room, Mrs. Graves was unable to hoist her heavy body from her bed to the table because she had had an epidural. I climbed onto her bed, and kneeling beside her, grasped the sheets under her torso. On the count of three, the OR nurses and I lifted and pulled the mother onto the operating table. My back screamed at me the whole time. Then I pushed the labor bed out of the OR, lighter now without its patient's weight, but still cumbersome. Sweating and beet-red, I slammed the bed around, taking out my frustration and worry about my back on the walls outside the operating room.

Forty-five minutes later, I had given report on the patient to the OR nurses; gotten the father into paper OR scrubs, hat, mask, and booties; escorted him to the operating room, where I seated him near his wife's head and shoulders; and wrote the required notations in the mother's chart about her vital signs, rate and dosage of medications, pre-op prep, urinary output, and transport time. Now I could stand by, waiting to receive the baby's body from the obstetrician's hands. I positioned myself right behind him, holding a sterile sheet across the front of my body. Like everyone else in the room, I was gowned, masked, bootied, and gloved in blue paper scrubs and plastic. I took several deep breaths and calmed myself.

I watched over the surgeon's shoulder as the operating team cut through and delved into the abdominal tissue—skin, fat, fascia, muscle—down to the uterus. I saw the scalpel incise the red uterine muscle. With the scalpel, the doctor nicked the amniotic sac enclosing the baby and a flood of dark, meconium-stained fluid spilled out over the operating field. The fluid reeked; a foul odor of infection and decay filled the room. The obstetrician, his surgical assistant, the circulating nurse, and I all jerked our heads back reflexively in an attempt to evade the stink. Then the doctor put his hands into the mother's uterine cavity and groped around for the baby's head. Tugging and then lifting, he was able to pull the baby's face away from the cervix and deliver the head and body into the light where we could see it.

Oh my God! Oh sweet Jesus! I recoiled, flinching at the sight of this infant. *There has to be something wrong with this baby. Some genetic defect or something. This is a deformed baby. Oh my God.* The baby's face was directly in my view. I turned to the circulating nurse, who stood next to me. Above her mask her eyes were huge, red, and flooded with tears. Hugging herself, she stood immobilized with horror, mesmerized by this travesty of a baby. The baby's face was as round as a softball—cheeks, chin, forehead, and the tissue around the eyes were all swollen and puffy, everything purpled with bruising. The nose and mouth were dwarfed by the swelling around them. But the eyes were the worst. The eyes were open, and almost extruded from their sockets. I could see three-quarters of the entire eyeballs, bulging out of that face with such hideousness that I almost vomited into my mask. I heard the surgeon and the assistant gasp simultaneously.

Before the surgery, the obstetrician and I had assured Mr. Graves that we would let him see and probably hold the baby very briefly, right after delivery. As the doctor clamped and cut the cord, he spoke over the sheeted screen that protected the surgical field from contamination and the view of the parents.

"It's a girl, Daddy. I'm going to ask Ms. Diamond to take her back to the examining room now, so I can check her out before we let you hold her."

He placed the baby in the sheet I held, signaling me with his eyes to make a fast getaway. Flipping the sheet over the baby and enfolding it quickly in my arms, I turned away from the father and headed for the doors, mumbling, "I'll get her cleaned up a little before you see her."

Walking down the hall, holding that baby against my breasts, something happened to me, something I'd never felt before. I felt something give inside, a physical sensation of something breaking down, or loose, or just quitting. *Enough! I can't do this! I just can't do this! Somebody has to help me do this. Enough already!* A torrent of emotions tore my breath away. Ripping the mask from my face, I gasped, shaking and groaning incoherently. Saliva flooded my mouth; I swallowed convulsively, trying to dislodge the glob of hot bile that had risen in my throat. This had never happened to me before. In a couple of bad cases, situations in which the mother or baby had been in real peril, I'd been afraid. After those incidents, I had to fight my fear of being involved in similar cases, but I had never felt like this. Now—holding this baby, knowing I was supposed to unwrap it, bathe it, print it, measure it, weigh it, photograph it, and hand it to its parents—some inner strength, some sense of my own capabilities, snapped within me. I simply felt inadequate to the task. *I just cannot do this. I just can't. No more. Not again.*

In the worst possible way, I wanted to put that body down, very carefully, turn around, and walk out of the hospital. Just walk away. Leave it behind. For the good of my soul. I felt like I would just wither up and die if I had to do what was expected of me with this baby. Adrenaline spurted through my veins: this was full-blown fight-or-flight syndrome and I wanted to flee! I staggered into the examining room and deposited the body on the warmer. Swamped by all the sensations and thoughts storming over me, I walked in circles for several minutes, hyperventilating, gulping back tears, wringing my hands, grimacing with revulsion at the bundled body lying before me, trying to make sense of the psychological crisis in which I suddenly found myself.

Okay, Susie, slow down. Slow down. Breathe deep. In and out. Breathe deep. Get control now. This is ridiculous. What's the matter with me? I've done this before. This isn't something new. I know how to do this. But I just can't, I just can't, it's too much, it's too much. Someone needs to help me with this. I'll call the charge nurse. No, I can't—they're all too busy. Besides I'll break down if anyone gets near me. Breathe deep. Slow down. Get control. Just do it.

Removing my gloves and eyeglasses, I rubbed my face, pushing hard against my cheeks and my eyes. At the scrub sink, I splashed some water on my face and swallowed a handful of the cold, chlorine-tainted water. I picked up a towel, dried my hands, and put on fresh latex gloves. Mechanically, I unwrapped the baby. Emotionally disengaging, with conscious effort, I cloaked myself in professional dispassion. I weighed the baby. I measured it. Futilely, I tried to bathe it, stopping when I realized the infected waters in which it had floated for two days after its death had hastened the process of decay: the skin and bones mushed under my fingers. When I smoothed the washcloth over the bloodied, mucus-smeared skin, it peeled away. I managed to get prints of the hands and feet, even though the gentlest pressure caused my fingers to sink sickeningly into them. Swallowing my gorge, I tried vainly to push the eyeballs back into their sockets, to pull the eyelids over them. *How am I going to show this baby to her parents?* I studied the body, trying to discern whether its gross features were the result of a genetic anomaly. The limbs and torso looked relatively normal, but the head seemed far too large. I wondered about hydrocephaly. I was no expert on fetal abnormalities; I couldn't say what was wrong with this baby, but it looked WRONG.

After I swaddled the baby in cheerful baby blankets, little pink and blue ducks and bunnies dancing across the fabric, and placed a knitted cap over its huge head, I stripped off my gloves and walked out where the father waited for me, sitting alone on a stool in an empty room.

"Mr. Graves, I've prepared the baby for you. I tried to bathe her but she's so delicate, I couldn't do a very good job. I'll bring her out now, but first I want to prepare you for how she looks. I don't know why, it's possible there may be some abnormality, but she isn't going to look as pretty as you might expect. She doesn't smell good—smells like there was an infection in the uterus. Her color is gray and her face is bruised and blotchy from all those hours she spent pressed against the cervix. Her eyes are really sticking out, too. I'm sorry to have to tell you this, but it's better to hear it before you see her, okay . . . ? Are you ready now?"

He nodded mutely. I went back and gathered up the baby. Returning to his side, I handed him his daughter. I squatted down beside his stool and put one arm gently around his shoulder. Together we looked quietly at the hideous little face before us. I felt him shake with silent tears and began to cry myself.

"I'm so sorry. This is so hard, I know." He nodded and reached out a forefinger to touch the baby's cheek.

"I'd like to unwrap her now and have you look at her body. It helps with the letting go if you have a chance to see and touch her everywhere. You up to that?" I asked.

"Yes," he croaked. He lowered the bundle to his knees. I unwrapped her and then, to my own great surprise, I found myself touching her, stroking her still form, holding a small, lifeless hand in mine as I talked to her father.

"See, her body looks okay, relatively speaking. I don't see anything obviously abnormal. It may just be that her face looks so wounded because of the presentation. You can see the ring around the edges of her face here, where she was pressed against the cervix. Her torso looks fine. Look at these wonderful little fingers and see, fingernails. I'm not sure of her hair color—there isn't much hair there, is there? Check out her feet, Daddy. Please, feel free to touch her, caress her. I'm going to give you some time alone with her now. You're not feeling faint, are you?"

As I touched her and talked to her father, I suddenly became aware that she wasn't hideous to me anymore. She was just a sad little form, a lost dead baby, battered and bruised after her death. I was able to see the lovely infant that might have been if she hadn't died and then been jammed against a cervix for so many hours. All my revulsion had mysteriously vanished. I stood up and searched his face, looking for distress signals. He lifted his eyes to mine, smiled so sadly at me, and said, "Thanks. I'm okay. I would appreciate a little time with her. Thank you so much."

I walked away, asking him to call me if he needed anything or felt faint. Removing my gloves, I washed my hands twice. I put on another pair of gloves and cleaned up the mess of dirty towels, bath water, measuring tape, and so on, and then washed my hands again. I could taste the rank smell from the corpse in my mouth and felt contaminated, as though my clothes and hair were permeated with the stench. I desperately wanted a shower and clean clothes. I completed the paperwork and tried to figure out what I had to do next to meet the death protocols. The parents had to sign autopsy and body-disposition papers. I had to deliver copies of all the documents related to this death to six different offices within the hospital. I had to take the body to the morgue after the parents had time with her and the obstetrician and pediatrician had examined her. Then I had to take on another patient assignment: my shift had eight and a half hours to go.

After a few minutes, Mr. Graves called me. I retrieved the baby, deposited her gently on the counter, and escorted him to the recovery room to await his wife. I hauled the labor bed back down the long hall to the labor room, called housekeeping, entered birth information into the computer, filled out more papers. The charge nurse phoned as I worked at the nurses' station. I listened numbly as she asked, "Are you finished yet?"

"No, I'm sorry. I've still got to . . ."

"Look, don't tell me what you've got to do. I don't have time to listen. I'm really sorry I couldn't help you with this and I'm sorry I've got to nag you now, but I am desperate. I need you to finish up as fast as possible and go to triage for another patient."

"But I've got to take the baby to the mother in the recovery room, and I've got to deliver all these papers and take the baby to the morgue."

"Take the baby to the mother. Everything else will have to wait. Just hurry up, please."

Wrinkled and sweaty, I trudged back to the OR where I found the obstetrician filling out his paperwork. Together, we returned to the examining room, collecting a pediatrician from the nursery on our way, and I watched as they examined the baby. It seemed more and more likely that the severe distortions and swelling of the face were just results of the presentation, but the head's enlarged size ensured an autopsy and genetic studies. I carried the baby to the mother's bedside and spoke to her for all of two minutes before I laid the infant in her arms. I asked the recovery room nurses to return the body to the examining room, where it could stay until I took it to the morgue. I returned to labor and delivery after restocking the infant warmer. In the triage room, where we evaluated all incoming patients, I recorded the birth data in a large ledger. The room was awash in patients, harried nurses trying to evaluate each mother and send her to a labor room. The charge nurse, a friend and a wonderful nurse, grabbed me by the arm.

"Susie! Thank God! Are you finished?"

"No, but the paperwork can wait till later, I guess. What have you got for me now?" I tried to smile at her, gamely pushing out of my mind everything I'd just been through. Apologizing yet again, she introduced me to a couple waiting in one of the cubicles. Autopsy and death certificate papers tucked under my arm, I started a whole new admission. The rest of the shift, I was occupied with this couple, in the early stages of their first labor. They were excited, filled with anticipation of the imminent arrival of their baby. I managed to take a break from them for fifteen minutes, which I spent delivering death papers to different offices in the hospital.

I smiled and laughed and encouraged this new mother and her husband. I took notes, assisted in the administration of an epidural, watched the monitors, emptied the bedpan, prepared the instruments and supplies for the delivery. I never said a word about what I had been doing before I met these people, but I couldn't stop the thoughts from invading my mind. *Here I am, getting ready for a new baby with these nice, friendly people, and they have no idea what I've just been doing. This is too strange. It's bizarre. I need to talk about it and there's no time. This is the pits.*

Finally, my twelve hours were finished. I gave reports to the oncoming nurse and said good-bye to my couple, wishing them a lovely birth, then called Security for an escort to the morgue. The last thing I did that morning was slide a bundle of dead baby onto a shelf in a stainless-steel refrigerator. As I drove home, I wondered about the whole experience. I wondered whether I'd finally hit the wall; whether that feeling of inadequacy and that urge to flee weren't signals of burnout. I fumed about the lack of time, the absence of help, the demands of the unit that prevented me from completing my work in a timely fashion and denied me the chance to unwind after emotional trauma. I remembered a research article describing the effects of the stress of dealing with life-threatening situations and death on emergency medical personnel. The research indicated that if such people are provided with an opportunity to ventilate, to express to co-workers their emotions and describe what they had to do immediately after such situations, the incidence of burnout and stress-related illness were greatly reduced. And here I was, going through a wrenching experience all by myself, having to take on a new patient without a chance to relax or even grab a snack afterward.

It wasn't just that I was feeling sorry for myself, although I was. I was recognizing how rotten the whole thing was: rotten for the parents of that baby, rotten for the baby, rotten for me, rotten for the charge nurse who had to hassle me instead of comforting and helping me.

The more I thought about it the more I knew I had, in fact hit the wall. I wasn't going to do this again. I didn't know how I would avoid it, but I knew it was time to give serious consideration to some other kind of work. Yet, even as I acknowledged these convictions, I found myself amazed by the emotional shift in perspective I'd experienced as the father and I caressed that small dead body. That I could somehow be lifted out of my horror and enabled to appreciate the lost potential of that baby was a remarkable, mysterious gift. I didn't know where that gift came from, but it had ameliorated the revulsion, bringing me some small portion of acceptance and calm within. I had leaned my head against that father's shoulder and whispered through honest tears, "I'm so sorry. She would have been a beautiful little girl." He had nodded, smiled at me, and whispered back, "Yes, I can see that." Then together, we stroked her little tummy and her arms and legs, her soft scalp, saying hello and saying good-bye.

Chapter Eleven

THE WAY IT CAN BE

Almost every obstetrical unit has a room set aside for the purpose of evaluating potential patients. Called the exam room, the clinic, or triage, this is the point of entry for all patients. Every woman must go through the exam room before being admitted to a labor room. The women come to the unit with their bodies full of life and they give themselves over to us, the health-care professionals. They enter the hallway, ring the bell, and wait, their hands on their bellies, their eyes speaking volumes about their fear, their hope, their pain. They look to us for advice, for help.

I'm contracting.
I'm having pains.
It's time.
I'm bleeding.
My water broke.
I've been having pains since last night.
I need something for the pain.
Am I dilated?
Is my bag of waters broken?
Is the baby okay?
I'm scared.
When will I have the baby?
When will it stop hurting?

Each one has her own story. I am only someone to deal with for these next few minutes/hours/days to get through this crisis. Then she will go on with her life, her own story, and I with mine. But right now, she is here and it's unbelievable how she gives herself to me.

This is how it happens. She rings the bell. I groan because I hate "doing the exam room." I greet her and ask her name so I can pull her chart. I give her a gown and a urine cup. I encourage her significant other to come into the room with her, so she doesn't feel alone. I talk quietly and/or cheerfully, depending on how tired I am, kidding and joshing, murmuring sympathetically, whatever is appropriate, to try to help her relax a little, to let them know it's safe here, it's a normal place with normal crazies who understand what she's feeling. She takes off her clothes, gives me the cup of urine. Neither of us even questions my right to touch her body. These are just things doctors and nurses do.

I have her lie on her left side, because if she is lying on her back, the weight of the gravid uterus presses against the major blood vessels, inhibiting circulation to the uterus and fetus. This weight can also elevate her blood pressure. If I want to get a more accurate blood pressure, she needs to be on her left. I wrap a blood pressure cuff around her arm. I listen to the pulse in her arm, while I hold her elbow in my hand, my finger pressing the stethoscope bell against her artery. I place a thermometer in her mouth as she opens it for me without question. She answers my inquiries.

How old are you?
What pregnancy is this for you?
You had an abortion—was it a miscarriage or an elective abortion?
When did your contractions start?
How long do they last?
Do you smoke?
Do you do any drugs—heroin, marijuana, cocaine?
Are you married?
Is the father of the baby involved?
Did you have the HIV test?
Are you bleeding?
Are you leaking fluid? What color is it?
Is there mucus?

She answers my questions. She will respond to the same questions repeatedly over the next few hours. Most women are eager to answer them. In fact, if given the opportunity, they'll often tell you more than you need or want to know. Then again, some women, usually young girls, will be so frightened and tongue-tied that it is a struggle to get a history from them.

Then the tummies. God, the tummies. I cover the woman's legs and pelvis with a sheet and carefully pull up her gown. "I need to listen to your baby's heartbeat." I try to remember to tell her what I'm going to do before I do it, but sometimes I forget and just touch her without thinking of the way I am violating her privacy, her modesty. She allows it: this is part of the tacit agreement between us. Because I am a nurse I can touch her. So, up goes the gown and there is a huge tummy. I palpate her belly. I can feel a baby's rump. I get my hands kicked. I touch the stretch marks. I see the linea nigra, a pregnancy-caused dark line of pigmentation down the middle of the belly. I rest my palms on her abdomen while I talk to her. I ask her where they usually hear the baby so I don't have to smear the conducting gel all over her belly. She usually knows; she shares her knowledge of herself and her baby with me. She helps me do my work, even when she's terrified, because she needs my help.

I listen with the doptone, holding my wrist up so I can watch the second hand as I count the beats. The earpieces cut off all sound except what's going on inside this woman's body. She lets me listen. She watches me while I look at my wristwatch and count silently. I am withdrawn from her, exposed to her scrutiny while I concentrate on her baby's heartbeat. The sound is reassuring. I may first just hear the swish of blood through the umbilical cord, but I keep moving the doptone until I hear the running rhythm of the fetal heart, fast, regular, and to me, just like the sound of horses galloping on a beach. I count for thirty to sixty seconds and then offer the earpieces to her and to her companion. We smile and talk about what a nice sound that is.

Then I get the doctor. When he or she enters the room, the dynamics change. No longer is it just me, the nurse, and the patient—and the rapport we have begun to establish. Now the "expert" has appeared. The doctor introduces himself and asks the same questions I've just gone through, even though I've already told him what she's said, what her "complaint" is, and he has perused her chart. She goes through it all again, and interestingly, often will be less forthcoming with him than she was with me. Sometimes even her language will change, becoming more sparse. She's more selective in her word choices. Some women will even freeze up and not be able to talk at all. If she is suddenly shy as he questions her, I will prompt her, reminding her what she has described for me.

With the doctor, there is relief—"Ah, finally the doctor"; distrust—"Is he really listening to me, does he know what he's doing, he looks awfully young"; trust—"Now it's okay, this is the doctor"; and anxiety—"Please demonstrate to me that you are going to help me, not hurt me, be kind to me." He tells her he needs to check her cervix, to examine her internally. He puts on a glove and I squeeze the lubricating gel onto his fingers, careful not to touch him with the packet to maintain the glove's sterility, since these fingers are going inside her body.

I stand at her side and tell her to bring up her knees, put her feet together and let her legs flop open. I pull the sheet up carefully so her legs remain covered and so she doesn't have to see the doctor's hands entering her. This is a particularly difficult moment. Few women are comfortable with a pelvic exam, no matter what their background. In some cases, a woman may never have had a physician examine her before her pregnancy. Even if she is not in pain with contractions, her genitals are swollen with the increased vascularization and weight of pregnancy and are more sensitive to touch and manipulation. I hold her nearer knee with my hand, gently pulling her leg to lean against my stomach. The table is so narrow that to completely relax her legs would make her feel as though she might fall off. Stirrups aren't used except for sterile speculum exams. The doctor usually tells her "you'll feel my fingers now," and I take her hand in mine, smiling at her, and tell her to "take a deep breath in, good, now blow it off, good. Breathe again. I know this is uncomfortable." I try to make eye contact with her, reassuring her with my voice and hands and female presence. The doctor's fingers slip in and probe around, reading her signs through touch only. If she is in labor, her cervix usually hurts when it's touched, and most women will stiffen and pull away automatically, trying to guard their inner self against this invasion.

Occasionally a woman will fight the exam with a ferocity that infuriates doctors—"How can I do my job if she won't cooperate?" they complain. Typically, in my experience at least, this will be a young woman. Her legs go rigid, the inner thigh muscles contract and try to clamp together like a vise. Her back arches as she pulls away; her belly thrust upwards, her hands try to push his away, her eyes squeeze tightly shut or open wide with horror, mouth open, crying or even yelling. I hold onto the one leg and tell her to squeeze my hand hard, to breathe: "Come on, don't hold your breath, breathe for me, deep breaths, it's almost over, I know it hurts, breathe."

Some women lie very still, staring at the wall or ceiling, their bravery betrayed by the silent tears that leak from the corners of their eyes and roll accusingly down their cheeks. Some apologize for their stiffness, for that initial involuntary jerk of their body as this stranger touches their labia. Some distance themselves from the procedure by talking objectively about their symptoms as though it is someone else's vagina being probed. Muslim women usually lie absolutely silent, eyes averted, a flush on their cheeks and a look of abject shame in their eyes. And of course, there are even a few women who appear to enjoy the process, seeming to take pleasure in having their genitals manipulated.

When it is over, the doctor gives his verdict as he strips off the smeared glove, looking at the secretions on his fingers, assessing them for blood, mucus, meconium, and unobtrusively smelling them for telltale signs of infection.

You're dilated three centimeters.
You're not dilated.
The baby's head is down.
The baby is breech.
I can feel a bulging bag.
Your cervix is unchanged.
We'll put you on a monitor and check out these contractions.
We'll admit you.
You can walk for an hour and come back to be rechecked.

If she is to be admitted, or just observed for a while, I gather her clothes, and assist her off the table. I wrap the sheet around her so she won't be flashing everyone as we walk to the labor room. She shuffles down the hall, while I help her hold the sheet up around her. Then we begin the dance of labor together. . . .

"There's a patient in the exam room. I don't know if she's going to be admitted or not. Will you take her, Susie?"

"Sure, no problem."

A young woman lay on the table in the exam room. She was tall, with a thick mass of auburn hair that fell to her shoulders. Her pale complexion was unblemished, but she sported two bright pink patches on her cheeks, the common butterfly flush or rash of pregnancy. She wasn't fat, but her body looked well-nourished, as we say. Under the sheet that covered her, her huge belly was strapped with external fetal and uterine monitors. Her husband stood nearby. Neatly attired in jeans and a polo shirt, he was tall also, slim and well-built, with a crewcut and a clean-shaven face. They were pleasant to look at, a regular middle-class American couple.

Both looked at me expectantly, as I entered the room and began the routine. This was the beginning of my sixth year of obstetrical nursing. After four years at the military medical center where I started, I'd spent a year as an assistant manager of a large labor and delivery unit in a civilian/private hospital. Now I was working as a staff nurse again, in another military hospital. I wasn't employed by the hospital directly; I was working as an agency nurse, contracting for shifts as needed at this hospital. The work was the same but I could plan my own schedule, which gave me the freedom to work on this book.

"Hi. I'm Susie, one of the nurses. I'll be working with you tonight, if you stay. We're waiting for Dr. Fairley to come check you. She's in the emergency room right now, but she'll be up here soon, so hang loose, okay?"

"Okay. Jeez, I really hope this is it. They've sent me home twice already. I don't think I can take much more of this."

"Yeah, I know. Well, you're really punching out some heavy-duty contractions here, aren't you? Every three minutes or so, looks like. How do they feel to you, strong or what?" I put my hand on her belly, pushing gently with my fingers, pressing the flat of my hand against her abdomen as her belly tightened with a contraction. It was strong to palpation: I couldn't push my fingertips into the rock-hard uterine muscle underlying her skin.

She breathed, pant-pant-blow, pant-pant-blow, as she focused her eyes on the wall opposite her. As the contraction waned, she turned to me. "They hurt. It's been going on for hours. I want drugs!" She grinned at me and shook her head.

"I hear you," I answered. "Not your ideal way of spending a Saturday night, huh? Let's wait and see what Dr. Fairley has to say about your cervix. If it's changing, then we'll get you admitted and go from there. I know you're tired, but you really are going to deliver eventually."

I left the room then and spent a few minutes reading her chart. Her name was Claire. She was twenty-six years old, married, and this was her first pregnancy. There had been no complications. She was almost forty-two weeks along and scheduled for an induction on the following Monday, since her baby was at increasing risk as the pregnancy continued past her due date. Normally, placental decline begins in the eighth month of gestation, and finally insufficient placental perfusion can place the fetus in serious jeopardy. She had been given a non-stress test—an NST—to determine the status of the baby. In the test, external monitors recorded the baby's heartbeat and any uterine activity for a period of thirty to sixty minutes. If the heartbeat showed accelerations with the baby's movement during that time, the non-stress test was judged positive: the accelerations indicated that the baby was receiving an adequate blood supply via the placenta and was doing well. Claire's NST the previous day had been positive, but the doctors were concerned about her passing the forty-two-week limit; after forty-two weeks, placental insufficiency and resultant fetal risk were highly probable.

When Dr. Fairley appeared, I joined her in the exam room and stood by as she checked Claire's cervix.

"Well, you're ninety percent effaced and three centimeters. So your cervix has changed from earlier today in terms of effacement: you were fifty percent earlier, but I think it's early still to admit you. How far away do you live?"

"About twenty-five minutes. I can't believe this. All these contractions and so little has happened in there. I don't think I can stand going home again."

"Well, you have the option of walking for a couple of hours if you want to."

"Then you'll check my cervix again and if it's not changed, we go home?"

"Right. We can give you something to help you sleep if you go home. Don't get too discouraged. This is the latent phase of labor you're in now, and that can take a long time. It's up to you, walk or go home until something changes."

Claire and her husband, Sam, agreed they didn't want to go home for the third time. Dr. Fairley advised them to come back to L&D after two hours, or earlier if her water broke, the contractions got more intense, or she had any bleeding. I unstrapped her belly and left her to get dressed. She was dispirited, her face a study in disappointment as she heaved herself off the table and slipped into the bathroom for her clothes.

Two hours later I saw them walking down the hall toward the nurses' station. "How are you? Still contracting?"

"Yes, and they're stronger. I want drugs!" She smiled at me, but I could see the fatigue and frustration in her face. Upon examination, her cervix was now five to six centimeters: she was in active labor.

"Yea! Come on, we'll go across the hall and get you in bed and admitted." I helped her off the table and held her arm as we moved into a labor room. The fatigue, so apparent minutes before, was gone: she was excited now.

"Thank goodness! I'll tell you, I wasn't going to go home without some drugs! I didn't think I was ever going to be admitted. I was really dreading the induction on Monday. It's going to happen now, right? How long do you think it will take?"

"Claire, every woman who comes through this unit asks me that, unless she's dropping the baby as she arrives. I've learned never to predict, 'cause soon as I do, I'm proved wrong! It's just a matter of going with the flow. Every labor is unique and happens according to its own clock. You've made excellent progress in the last two hours, so let's just assume things will continue to move forward, okay?"

We laughed and joked together as I got her into bed and plugged in the monitors again. Another nurse took Claire's history for the admission assessment form as I started an IV. True to form, I got blood all over her hand and the floor but had no difficulty slipping in the long catheter. "God, I always make such a mess! I'm sorry, I'll get you cleaned up in just a minute."

"That's okay. You don't need to worry, either," Claire solemnly reassured me, "I don't have any diseases."

Thus we began our time together. Claire was pleased to finally be in active labor. During her walk, the time between contractions had increased to about six minutes, but each contraction lasted almost two minutes. She breathed through them with excellent concentration, maintaining control without difficulty. She asked many questions. She had read extensively about childbirth and had attended childbirth classes.

"I know I'm asking a lot of questions. I'm just so excited now. Wow, I feel so much better it's amazing. It really hurts in my back, though. What happens when you rupture the membranes? Do you do it in here? That makes the contractions a lot stronger, doesn't it?"

"Listen, you ask all the questions you want to, okay? Questions are great, they tell me you care about what's happening to you, and help me know how to help you. Now, we break the bag right here. It doesn't hurt; it's just like a cervical exam. There may be a gush of water, like a flood, or it may be just a trickle. Sometimes the baby's head is so well applied to the cervix that the fluid behind it can't run out. And yes, usually the contractions come closer and are stronger after the fluid is released. That's why Dr. Fairley wants to rupture you, since your contractions are fairly far apart. She wants to keep up the momentum so your cervix will go on dilating. Sometimes things will sort of plateau out at six centimeters, and you've had a long enough latent phase as it is."

Dr. Fairley performed the amniotomy. I placed several chucks, the ubiquitous blue-backed absorbent pads, under Claire's bottom and told her how to position her legs: ankles together, knees flopped open and out. Dr. Fairley slid her gloved fingers into the vagina, holding the long plastic amnihook in position, and nicked the amniotic membranes with its tiny sharp end. I watched as fluid streamed out, a nice clear color with no meconium stain in it.

"Good, it's clear. That means the baby's okay so far. You know what meconium is?"

"Yes, it's the baby's bowel movement and if it's in the water, the baby might be distressed, right?"

"Yep. This lady knows her stuff, huh, Dr. Fairley?"

I was glad the fluid was clear. The fetal heart rate tracing was flat, without the reassuring little jagged fluctuations that indicated beat-to-beat variability. A flat line could be due to a number of factors: the baby was in a sleep cycle or resting period; the baby wasn't getting enough blood flow and therefore was inadequately oxygenated, the baby was being stressed, or the baby just had a flat line for the moment, for reasons unknown to us outside observers. That flat line could be benign, or it could be ominous. There was no real way to tell, short of taking a sample of the baby's blood for a scalp pH, but clear fluid was a reassuring sign and there were steps we could take to improve the variability before we had to resort to scalp sampling.

"Claire, let's get you onto your side. If you're hurting in your back, the first and best thing to do for back labor is to get you off your back. It also will get the weight of the uterus off your major blood vessels, so the flow to the baby will be better."

"I know." She started to turn to her left side as I lowered the head of the bed. "I tried to lie on my side earlier, but it felt so uncomfortable."

"That's it. Go all the way over. Move over toward me so you're in the middle of the bed and not banging your head on the railing there. Let the bed hold your belly, all the way over now. Get this shoulder back underneath you and put the pillow like this." I readjusted the monitors as we talked. "It's going to hurt more at first. Usually a change of position will bring on a contraction, see it's coming now. I know it hurts. Breathe with it like you have been. That's right, just like that. In and out, nice and steady, nice and steady. Keep your focus. That's the top, it's not going to get any worse. Now it's starting to come down, keep going, nice and steady. Now slow down your breathing, ease off, it's almost over. Good. The first couple of contractions when you turn to your side are always really rough, but your body will adjust to the new position and it'll get easier, trust me. You'll contract more effectively with better blood flow, so these contractions will be accomplishing more, okay?"

"Whew! That was a hard one. But you're right, it didn't hurt so much in my back. Sam, you need to press against that place in my back, okay? Not too hard, not so hard. Oh here comes another one. Heh-heh-fffoooo, heh-heh-fffooo . . ."

She panted and blew, her husband pressing his fist against the small of her back. She kept her eyes open, focusing on something across from her. She began to move her legs in small bicycling motions, a telltale sign of the intensity of her pain, and her hand moved forward to grab the bed railing. I slipped my hand into hers and said, "Put it into my hand, Claire, put the pain into my hand. Squeeze my hand and show me how strong the contraction is. Center yourself up in your face. Think about what you're doing with your eyes, your nose, your mouth, your breathing. That's it, try to stay up in your face, not down in your belly. That's happening to someone else, you're just up in your face. Keep the breathing going, nice and steady, you're at the top, it's going to start coming down now. Good! Good girl, you're making it just fine. Nice and steady, now slow down your breathing. Great, just great. Excellent breathing, excellent concentration. You're doing this so well!" I stroked her leg and then patted her hand. She released me from her fierce grip and exhaled a long deep breath, slumping back into the bed.

"It doesn't feel like I'm doing well at all. That one was really rough."

"I know, it lasted almost two minutes. But you handled it just fine. Trust me, I've watched a lot of women do this, and you're managing like a champion!"

We went through a few more contractions. She breathed and gripped my hand with all her strength, squeezing harder and harder as the contraction peaked. I squeezed back and talked her through, making her focus on my voice, trying for a hypnotic sort of chant, keeping her grounded with my hand and my soft words, encouraging, praising, singsonging her through the pain, not letting her sink into it or tense against it or flail around without control. She was wonderful. Her husband pressed her back, murmuring along with me, our voices contrapuntally cheering her on.

I left them alone for a while. It was important not to usurp Sam's role as coach and to give them a sense of being together and in control without my presence. I went downstairs for a smoke and a Coke, and relaxed for a few minutes. When I returned to the labor room, Claire told me she was ready for some medication. "What are my options? I don't know if I can handle this much longer."

"Well, you qualify easily for an epidural since you're at least six centimeters."

"I don't think I want to go that route yet. What else is available?"

"Now, Claire, you promised you'd wait fifteen minutes after you wanted pain medication before you took anything," Sam interrupted.

"I know, but I just don't know if I can do it. . . ."

"Before you decide we have to get Dr. Fairley to check you again. We can give you some Stadol if you're not too close to delivery, but if you're almost ready to push, it wouldn't be a good idea because the baby might be born with it still in his system. Your body can metabolize it for him while he's still inside, but if he comes out with it onboard, he could be depressed. So if you want me to get Dr. Fairley to check you, I will. If you want to wait fifteen minutes, that's fine too. Sam and I can't know what you're really feeling here, so it's your decision."

Another contraction came. She reached out for my hand. "Can I have your hand? It really helps." She made it through another ten minutes and then asked me to get Dr. Fairley. I went out to the desk and reported to Dr. Fairley.

"She can have some Stadol."

It had only been two hours since we had admitted her and I knew that according to labor flow charts she was probably only seven to eight centimeters, but you never could tell. I wanted to be sure she wasn't ready to push before I put any narcotics into her system.

"Would you mind checking her cervix, first, Dr. Fairley? She might be farther along than we expect."

"Sure, I'll be there in just a few minutes."

I gathered up a vial of Stadol, a synthetic narcotic, and a syringe before I returned to the room. Claire was reaching for my hand as I dropped everything on the table. A powerful contraction hit her: it peaked almost instantly and continued for more than two minutes. At the end Claire's eyes widened as she exclaimed, "Oh! Oh! I felt the baby move! It just dropped down, wham!"

The door opened and Dr. Fairley and another nurse flew into the room. I had been so focused on the contraction I hadn't noticed that during the contraction the baby's heartbeat had taken a nosedive down into the fifties. The sound on the monitor had been turned down and I hadn't heard the heartbeat drop. Silently I blessed the monitor screens out at the desk so the staff outside could see what I had missed. I lowered the head of the bed, opened the IV line to run fluids in fast and snapped an oxygen mask over Claire's face. Dr. Fairley put her fingers into the vagina and stimulated the fetal scalp with gentle scratching to raise the heartbeat. As we worked, the other nurse and I explained to Claire and Sam what we were doing. Again Claire cried out, "Oh! There! It moved again! Oh it just lurched!"

With two sudden movements, the baby had descended down the birth canal. This rapid descent was probably why the heartbeat had decelerated so suddenly. Dr. Fairley announced that Claire was completely dilated and could start pushing as soon as the baby had recovered from his fall. We went through two more contractions. Claire wanted to push.

"I have such pressure in my rectum."

"I know, but don't push yet. Pant, Claire, pant like a puppy. Like this, pant with me. Heh, heh, heh, heh, heh, keep going, keep going. Good, now slow down when you can, slow down when it eases off. Great! Hot dog, Claire! You made it through first stage! No drugs! Wow, aren't you great!"

After three contractions, the heartbeat looked better and I told Claire how to push. She was lying on her left side, oxygen mask over her nose and mouth. She grabbed Sam's hand with her left hand and reached down to pull back on her upper knee with the other hand. I sat on the end of the bed and pushed against the soles of her feet, telling her to open her legs and get her knees back as far as she could, to open the pelvis a little.

"Now, when it starts, take a deep breath and blow it off. Take another deep breath and blow that one off. Take another and hold it, tuck your chin down to your chest and push down as hard as you can, like you're having a bowel movement, right into your butt. Pull back with your hands as you push down. Hold it to the count of ten, then blow off the breath as quickly as you can, take another deep gulp of air, and push again. We'll try for three counts of ten."

She pushed, listening to my instructions and Sam's counting. I watched her perineum, uncovered and exposed in the soft light from above the bed. Her face grew dark red as she strained, her hands pulling against Sam and her knee, her knees back against her belly, feet pushed up by my hands. Her rectum bulged and her labia began to separate as she pushed the baby down. I wiped away the bit of stool she expelled, changed the chucks smeary with the ooze and slime of childbirth. She complained about the pushing.

"I thought this was supposed to feel good. That's what they said in class, that pushing would feel good. It doesn't. It hurts."

"I know. I didn't like pushing either. It felt awful and I was pissed because everyone said it would be the fun part."

"At least it doesn't feel like the dilating contractions. Those were terrible."

She worked and Sam and I helped her as best we could. After an hour, her perineum was bulging outward, a round, hard firmness that remained between the pushes. The baby's head was visible each time she bore down, slipping back only slightly when she relaxed the pressure against it. I called Dr. Fairley in to gown and prepare for the delivery. A nurses' aide had opened up the supplies for the delivery and turned on the warmer for the baby. Sam had changed to scrubs and we were ready to deliver this baby.

"Okay, Claire, your final moment is at hand! Turn over onto your back. Sam, will you hold that leg up so we can take the bottom of the bed away? Here, put your feet on these foot rests in between the contractions."

"Is the baby crowning?" she asked as she slid down to the edge of the birthing bed.

"Yes, he's crowning! Has been for the past few pushes. You're about to be a mother, honey!"

"Can I have him on my belly right after he's born? Do I still grab my knees and pull back or do I have to keep my feet on these things?"

"Go ahead and grab your knees just like you were on your side. Sam and I will help hold your legs up."

She pushed through another contraction. The baby's head emerged centimeter by centimeter, wet and gray, wisps of blondish hair smeared with blood and mucus. Dr. Fairley ran her fingers around the stretched vaginal opening, feeling the space and the elasticity of the tissue.

"I think we're going to have to do an episiotomy. You're stretched real thin and don't have much space left here."

"That's okay. I don't care about an episiotomy. Let's just get this baby out."

Another push, more of the head emerging, then a rest, Sam and I holding her legs up and back toward her chest during the rest interval, rather than placing her feet on the stirrups since she said it felt better to have them up and back.

"Okay, this one will do it, Claire," Dr. Fairley announced. "Push now."

"Open your eyes, Claire, and watch your baby come out," I told her. The head came forth: crown, temples, forehead, ears, eyes, nose, and mouth all free now.

"Now pant, Claire, don't push for a second, while I suction the goop out of his nose and mouth. Okay, now a little push for the shoulders. Get her legs way back, this is a big baby, and I don't want to have his shoulders get stuck," the doctor instructed. Claire pushed. Dr. Fairley pulled downward on the baby's head to free the anterior, upper shoulder and then lifted the baby toward the ceiling for the posterior, lower shoulder and *shwoosh!*—the body slid out, deftly held in Dr. Fairley hands.

"A boy! Claire, a boy!" I yelled.

"Oh, Sam, look at him. We have a son!"

"Here, Daddy, you want to cut him free?" Dr. Fairley handed a pair of scissors to Sam and showed him where to cut the cord.

"Thank you Claire, thank you. I love you!" Sam cried as he kissed her.

"Here's your kid, Mom!" Dr. Fairley laid the wet, screaming infant on Claire's bare abdomen. I grabbed towels and began to dry him off. The aide handed me a warm blanket from the isolette as I rubbed the baby all over. We needed to get him dry and keep him warm. His mother and father cradled him with their hands, stroking his fresh, new little body, talking to him and each other as I filled out his I.D. bracelets and put them on his wrist and ankle. I smeared his feet with ink and printed him. I clamped the cord with the plastic clamp and cut off the excess cord. It was messy: Claire and I had blood, mucus and footprint ink all over us, but I didn't want to take the baby away from her. I listened to his heartbeat, checked his muscle tone, his color, listened to his loud cries and then softer hiccoughing breaths as he calmed against his mother's breast, her familiar heartbeat under his ear now, instead of above him as it had been in utero. The aide handed me more dry, warm blankets while Dr. Fairley delivered the placenta. I filled out all the damned paperwork, in between taking the baby's temperature and making sure he was well covered on his mother. As Dr. Fairley began to repair the episiotomy, Claire found it hard not to cry out from the stinging pain of the needle.

I thought to distract her. "Are you going to breast-feed, Claire?"

"Yes. Ouch! That really hurts!"

"Let's see if this little guy will take your nipple. He's kinda rooting around there, isn't he? Bring him up a little in your arms, get his head firmly in the crook of your elbow there. Turn his tummy to yours. That's right! Now cup your breast—make a C-shape with your hand—and tickle his mouth with your nipple. Wow, look at him latch on! What a natural, like he's been doing this all his life!" I laughed as the baby took the nipple after two exploratory licks, and sucked away. The parents and I watched with pleasure as he nursed, quietly reviewing the labor, the birth, commenting on how it had gone, how well Claire had done.

"Where's your camera?" I asked.

"We left it in the car."

"Well, if you want pictures of the baby in here, run down and get it, because I have to take him to the nursery before he's an hour old."

Sam left for the camera and I helped Claire switch the baby to her other breast. He protested loudly when I lifted him from his mother's warmth but latched onto her proffered nipple with renewed interest. I cleaned up the debris of the birth—instruments, bloodied towels, papers, gloves, garbage— as Claire nursed her infant, rocking him gently in her arms, talking softly to him. Sam returned with a video camera and filmed the baby, Claire, and me as I took him from her arms. I lifted him and gave the camera a front and a rear view of his naked, pink, lovely little form and then wrapped him tightly in two warm blankets. Dr. Fairley had returned to the room. She filmed the family as I placed the baby in Sam's hesitant arms.

"I've never held a baby before. This might not be a good idea right now."

"Oh crap, he's your son, no better time than the present! Just get his head secure in your arm there. Now turn to the camera and show us this beautiful baby!"

He was beautiful! No caput, or swelling under the scalp, no cone-head, eyes wide open, checking out the world, warm and secure in his father's strong arms, pursing his lips in endearing little moues. The first forty-five minutes of his life he had spent on his mother's belly, held in her arms, suckling at her breast. Now his father cradled him. It was a perfect beginning.

I sent him off to the nursery in the infant transport, a rolling isolette pushed by the aide, to whom I had given instructions to report to the nursery staff that the baby had breast-fed very successfully on both sides for forty minutes! Sam accompanied the baby to get his weight. Claire and I talked as I began her recovery routine: vital signs, fundal massage, ice packs on her perineum, lochia checks.

"That was amazing, Susie. I'm so glad I didn't take anything. I wanted to, but it went fast enough, huh?"

"Claire, you were terrific. I want you to keep this thought with you for the rest of your life. You did an outstanding job! You stayed in control and did exactly what you needed to do and you should be very proud of yourself always. You passed the woman's big test with flying colors."

"I am proud," she said softly. "I couldn't have done it without you. You helped me so much, I can never thank you enough."

"You don't have to thank me. It was my pleasure. Really. Sharing a birth like this one, with a woman who does so well is why I do this job, why I love it. It was a privilege for me to be here with you. You made a beautiful child."

I have been told that before: "I couldn't have done it without you." I always appreciated hearing it, having my efforts recognized. But I also knew she *could* have done it without me. I wasn't indispensable; she would have delivered probably just as well without me. But I did know that this birth experience had been enhanced by my presence and my willingness to buck routine, to bend the rules, to individualize her care. My hands, my voice, and my instructions helped her through two hours of hard labor. Without my willingness to stay in the room and give her my help, she probably would have resorted to medication. And without question my presence made it possible for that baby to lie on his mother's belly, to breast-feed immediately, to be comforted by his parents for the first hour of his life.

I knew there are nurses out there who encourage immediate bonding and breast-feeding, but I had had precious little personal experience of them. Invariably, unless I intervened, the aide or LPN or nurse would have removed the baby to the warmer for Apgars and drying and tagging. They might have allowed the father to hold the baby briefly. Sometimes they might let the mother hold the baby, but then it's off to the nursery, parents and child separated for the first four hours, within minutes of the baby's delivery. I hated that separation from my own babies and I hated it for my patients. There wasn't any medical reason to hurry the baby away, as long as he was pink, breathing well, warm and dry. The babies were moved because it was easier for the staff. That was the simple reason: get the baby to the nursery so we don't have to be responsible for him; so we can get on with the mother's recovery; so we can get her moved off the unit to the postpartum ward; so we can be finished with our paperwork, our clean-up, our patient.

It's so easy to lose sight of the reality of this event. It's a new baby, a birth, a life-changing event for the mother and father, not just another delivery. It's the beginning of a lifelong relationship fraught with love and worry and danger and joy. The days and nights of meeting an infant's needs, of listening to his cries, of responding to his hunger and pain and fear, of watching him learn the world; the years of growth and development, the all-encompassing responsibility, the demands of this helpless human being, the joy of getting to know his personality, the changes in his size, shape, and abilities, all begin here. It demands a little time. It requires a little grace period. It necessitates a few moments of simple pleasure in the fact of his being.

Giving that time is one of the most important responsibilities I have as an L&D nurse. I make time available for the parents whenever it is possible and I do it vehemently, angry that I must be assertive and inflexible in order to achieve those few minutes of bonding for my patients. It galls me that I must fight and coerce other staff members to do this. It angers me to know that the nursery will be upset if the baby isn't in their hands within one hour. It enrages me that the staff gets pissed if the patient's recovery period is longer than an hour because I haven't been checking her blood pressure and massaging her belly while she's nursing her baby. It infuriates me that the next shift is ticked off because the mother is still on the unit two hours after her delivery and they have to move her to the ward.

Everyone's priorities are askew here. Everyone wants to accomplish the delivery and move the patient out as expeditiously as possible. All the routines are designed to meet the needs of the staff and the unit, not the needs of the mother and father and baby. Of course there are times when the routines and rules are meant to be followed. A large baby needs to have his glucose level checked to be sure he doesn't become hypoglycemic. A baby with respiratory problems like grunting or nasal flaring needs to go to the nursery right away for careful assessment. A baby with goopy sounds in his chest needs to be properly suctioned in the nursery. A cesarean mother probably can't relate to her infant very effectively right after surgery, and the nurses need to be able to attend to her recovery closely. But a normal labor and the birth of a normal, healthy baby should allow for some quiet time for parents and infant to spend together. Without me, Claire and Sam would never have had that first hour with their son. I went home proud of my guardianship and angry about the complaints of the day shift over why the patient was still on the unit. A pox on them all! I made that family a gift that morning, a gift of time together, and I would do it again, no matter what!

A couple of years after this birth, I took a job in the family birthing center that I mentioned earlier. I can't begin to describe my delight when I found myself expected, even required, whenever possible, to keep the baby in the mother's arms immediately after birth. An infant warmer/resuscitator was kept in the birthing room, but in the first few minutes after birth we did our baby care at the bedside. While the mother held the baby, we dried it and wrapped it in warm blankets. We put on its I.D. bracelets. We suctioned its mouth and nose and did the Apgar scoring. We listened to its respirations and counted its heartbeats. I was vastly amused when I heard of a physician who complained that some of the nurses weren't leaving the baby in the mother's arms long enough! Oh, how times change! Twenty years earlier, my Rebecca was whisked away from my body to an infant cart across the room where I couldn't even see her. I had to beg to have Michael placed on my abdomen for two minutes after his birth. The first five years I worked, the babies were automatically handed to me as soon as the cord was cut; I carried them away from their mothers to the warmer where I performed various tasks before handing them to their parents. After those five years, I had to argue with co-workers and insist that I be allowed to do initial baby care while the mother held the baby. Now, finally, in some hospitals at least, it is actually policy to encourage and facilitate immediate and prolonged physical contact between infant and mother. I love it!

Chapter Twelve

THE QUESTION OF PRIVACY

When I decided to pursue nursing as my work, I was unaware of how I would be required to become involved and actually interfere with other people's lives. Well educated and well read, I had considerable exposure to and awareness of the critical issues of society at large. But my knowledge of these issues was purely intellectual. As the child of a small-town physician, I had glimpses of a great variety of people who were served by my father's general practice, but our family enjoyed an elite status that sheltered us from much of the economic and social hardships experienced by many of Dad's patients. My mother has been an active do-gooder all her adult life, devoting her considerable energies to decades of volunteer work. As a result of her many interactions with the needy in our town, Mom became the person to call when no other solution could be found for individuals in immediate need of shelter, medical care, and/or food. Because Mom has trouble saying no, there were more than a few occasions during my adolescence when strangers were taken in, sheltered, and fed under our roof. But in spite of these inter-actions, by virtue of our middle-class status we were somehow still removed from the harsh reality many other people faced. Indeed, my mother's good works and my father's prestige imbued us kids with an unconscious snobbery. We were raised with the belief that we were among the fortunate few: blessed with good health, better-than-average intelligence, advanced educations, and a comfortable home; we were obligated to help others less blessed. Even as we embraced this philosophy—becoming doctors, a nurse, and teachers—by virtue of our privileged lives we were insulated from and largely ignorant about other, less advantaged people.

The safety and isolation of my adult upper-middle-class home perpet-uated my ignorance. As a nurse, I knew that I would be working with all manner of people; I was eager for the exposure to this great variety. For fifteen years, my circle of friends and acquaintances had been limited to academics, graduate students, and professors and their spouses. Eventually, though I loved my friends, I became bored with the sameness of my social group. I longed for the stimulation of the unknown. I knew I would find it in nursing.

However, I never gave any serious thought to how invasive my work would be. Embarrassingly naïve, I thought I would just be helping women go through childbirth. It didn't occur to me that I would be expected to evaluate the way my patients cared for their own children; that my scrutiny of their actions and behaviors could lead to public interventions in their families. By entering the hospital and placing themselves in my care, patients effectively relinquished their rights to privacy, in spite of legislation designed to protect that privacy.

My nursing education and training provided me with the wherewithal to perform my nursing tasks. However, in assuming the role of nurse, I automatically accepted a larger role—that of both judge and jury—with the power to pass judgment on whether my patients were capable of caring adequately and appropriately for their children. Over the years, I have intervened on any number of occasions when I have recognized symptoms of dysfunction in my patients and their families. It is my legal and ethical responsibility to do so if there is evidence of serious marital discord, wife or child abuse, substance abuse, or dire financial need.

Even as I intervene, I remain discomfited by this responsibility. Deep within, I continue to be amazed by both the complete absence of privacy for hospitalized people and the unquestioning way health-care providers are expected to act because of that absence.

Of course, I recognize that I can be accused of disingenuousness as I blithely recount in these pages stories of my patients' most intimate experiences. But in telling these stories, I am attempting to reveal my own inner turmoil over the paradoxes and conflicts inherent in my work as an obstetrical nurse.

I'm sure nurses and doctors, indeed everyone who works with patients, would be unhappy to called voyeurs, but we all are avidly curious about our patients. We are no different from all the people who slow down on the highway to gawk at victims of car wrecks. Actually, we work in an environment where the equivalents of car wrecks happen every day. People come in and bleed and scream and do all sorts of "unusual" things right in front of us and we have a legitimate right, by virtue of our work, to witness what happens to them and how they handle it. In our professional roles, we don't spend a lot of energy thinking about the exposure of our patients and their families to our scrutiny, but beneath our professional identities lurk the very same human characteristics that make rubberneckers out of people on the highway—morbid curiosity, titillation, concern, empathy, and even compassion.

So, voyeuristically, we watch our patients and their families. And we talk about them. Many a night, idle nurses sit around the nurses' station, gossiping about the people we have cared for. Most of us try to protect our patients' privacy by avoiding conversing about them in public places like elevators or hospital dining rooms. We rarely discuss one patient with another, even though patients themselves press us for details about other patients.

The patient's medical chart contains the most personal information: her history and physical describe her body systems, her allergies, her medical care, her previous surgeries and diseases, her drug and alcohol use, her family's medical history, her mental, marital, and parental status. While she is an inpatient, her chart is passed from hand to hand, shift to shift. It will be perused not only by doctors, but by nurses, medical students, social workers, physical therapists, respiratory therapists, lab techs, secretaries, medical records personnel, utilization review, quality assurance personnel, etc. The chart is not only referred to for legitimate medical reasons, but also to satisfy our insatiable curiosity.

More than any other, an obstetrical unit is privy to the most intimate information about the patient. Her presence on the unit is a direct result, after all, of sexual activity. That activity and its consequences, not just pregnancy but all sorts of reproductive diseases and complications, are the focus of an obstetrical unit. It isn't surprising then, that closely held secrets become common knowledge in spite of the best efforts of the patient to guard those secrets.

Medical personnel are legally obligated to guard the confidentiality of a patient. From the first days of nursing school, the importance of the right to privacy is stressed. We are instructed not to discuss our patients, never to identify them by name to outsiders, never to reveal information about them to any person who doesn't have a need to know. In the military system, telephone calls about a patient's status were strictly limited: we were not permitted to give out any information about the patient except that she was in fact a patient. In the civilian hospitals I've worked for, information is released more casually, even though the laws are the same. Many a time I've been yelled at over the phone by an irate grandparent or sibling who insist they be told whether the baby has been delivered yet, or if the mother is still in labor. "But I'm her mother, her husband, her brother, her best friend!" they cry. Answering them truthfully about the mother is always dicey.

On some occasions, I have met the caller in the hospital previously. If I recognize the voice, I relay information over the phone, in spite of the rule not to do so. Other times I have been puzzled by the loopholes in the rule, when I have been expected to give information about a patient to a caller who identifies himself as her commanding officer, or the nurse who transferred her to our unit, or a doctor who cared for her previously. How do I verify this person's identity? What about the nursing supervisor who calls asking for information to put in her report? How do I know she is who she says she is, and why does she need to know all these details?

The most common privacy issue in obstetrics is the number of pregnancies. It is significant in the patient's care to know for certain how many pregnancies she has had, how many infants she has carried to term, how many she has miscarried, how many she has electively aborted, how many she has lost prematurely, how many still live. The first question a woman is asked, after her name and age, is "How many times have you been pregnant?" Most women answer this question truthfully, recognizing that previous pregnancies have an impact on the course of this labor. For example, a mother of three living children will probably labor and deliver more rapidly, since her uterus and vaginal canal are experienced. Anticipating a rapid delivery is important in terms of maintaining control over the delivery and being prepared with equipment and supplies. A woman who has had two or three or ten abortions but who has never delivered a term infant will probably experience as lengthy a labor, particularly the pushing stage, as a first-time mother. Likewise, a woman who is a chronic miscarrier is a patient who requires extra vigilance, since this fetus is so hard-won.

But occasionally, women will answer the question with a lie. They will say that this is their first baby, because they don't want to reveal the fact or number of abortions they have had, or that they gave a baby up for adoption. The lies usually occur because the woman's significant other, her current husband or boyfriend, or sometimes her mother, is present during the history-taking. One such woman was hospitalized for severe diabetes and hyperemesis gravidarum—excessive nausea and vomiting—during her pregnancy. Not only were there problems stabilizing her blood glucose levels, but she vomited almost everything she ingested, so her nutritional status was in serious jeopardy, as was her fetus. Everyone on the ward knew she had been pregnant four times, but the previous three pregnancies had been terminated via elective abortion.

Her obstetrician requested that a gastroenterologist review her chart and consult on her vomiting, since she was unresponsive to various routine treatments for nausea and vomiting. This physician paid her a visit one morning. In the presence of her mother, he began to question the patient about her previous pregnancies, casually mentioning her three abortions. The patient denied the pregnancies, insisting he was mistaking her for another patient. The slow-witted doctor produced her chart and argued over the data therein until she threw him out of her room. Her mother, not surprisingly, was outraged by the information: a loud family argument ensued, complete with tears, shouting, and recriminations. The end result was a lawsuit against the doctor and the hospital for invasion of privacy.

When I was an assistant nurse manager, I had the unfortunate chore of counseling a nurse who had argued with a patient, in front of her boyfriend, about the number of her pregnancies. The boyfriend hadn't known about the two previous abortions and was furious with his girlfriend. The nurse tried to exonerate herself by saying that the chart listed two previous pregnancies: if the information was supposed to be suppressed, she felt the doctor should have marked it thus in the chart, "in red ink so we notice it." I remonstrated with her, reminding her of the right to privacy, the risk of lawsuit, and the necessity of accepting a blatant lie when the patient was attended by other people. "You can always verify the information with the patient when you are alone with her, but you must be very careful in your questioning if other people are present."

One of the most blatant abuses of patient privacy I ever witnessed occurred when a lab technician used his access to the hospital computer system to learn when one of our patients was admitted. This woman was estranged from her boyfriend, the baby's father, and had refused to allow him to visit her in the hospital. The lab tech found her name and room number in the computer and called the boyfriend. The boyfriend phoned the woman, right during her labor, yelling about his rights to see his child. A great furor erupted. The woman was enraged about the breach of privacy. The obstetrician was angry because the woman was out of control, hampering our efforts to get her delivered. The lab tech blithely explained to the furious obstetrician and hospital administrators that he didn't think it was right for the woman to deny the baby's father access to his child.

Nurses and doctors are hampered in L&D units because of the almost universal acceptance of a coach. Information previously readily divulged by the patient to the nurse is now often withheld because of the presence of significant others. One young woman arrived on the unit with her mother, grandmother, and mother-in-law. Before any questions had been asked, the patient's mother drew aside the nurse assigned to her daughter. Whispering urgently, the mother explained that the patient didn't want her mother-in-law or grandmother to know she had genital herpes. While every attempt is usually made by the staff to guard such secrets at the patient's request, this patient had active herpetic lesions that necessitated a cesarean section. Her membranes had ruptured, which meant that we needed to deliver her infant expeditiously to reduce the risk of herpetic infection, a life-threatening possibility for the fetus. The baby could not be allowed to pass through the vaginal canal where the virus lurked, shed from the lesions on her cervix.

The women accompanying her couldn't understand why the patient was being prepped for surgery when she hadn't even begun to labor. The patient's mother was upset when we explained that it would be difficult to avoid answering their questions about the surgery. If she didn't want them to know her daughter had genital herpes, why had she allowed them to accompany the patient to the hospital? We were placed in an awkward position. While we wanted to protect the patient's privacy, we weren't required to lie to her relatives to protect their sensitivities. In the face of our uncomfortable silence as we prepped the patient, the women forced the mother to explain. Sobs and raised voices emanated from the room, while the poor patient lay on her bed trapped by her IV, monitors, and urine catheter as the older women castigated her stupidity in contracting the virus.

On several occasions, I was made aware of how some women will attempt to bury a secret so deeply that they hide it from themselves. Denial is an unbelievably strong coping mechanism. Judy was brought to L&D in a wheelchair from the emergency room, hollering with pain, in full-blown active labor. She was twenty-three years old and unmarried. When I went into her room to admit her, she yelled at me to "get it out, take it out." I told her we would help her with her labor but she needed to calm down so I could put the monitor on her baby. "It's not a baby! It's my appendix! It's not a baby, goddammit! It's a tumor!" she cried.

"Listen, Judy, it's a baby in there. Absolutely for sure, you're real close to giving birth."

"No, no! I can't have a baby! It's not a baby. Oh, oh, it hurts! It's killing me! Take it out, take it out!"

"Now look, Judy. I know it hurts. I know you're scared. But work with me, okay? Listen to me and I'll help you handle this."

"Oh, give me something for this pain. I can't stand this pain. Put me to sleep and take this tumor out of me. Give me something, give me something!"

"Judy, we can't give you anything now: you're eight centimeters dilated. Your cervix is almost completely open. If we give you something now it would be bad for the baby, the baby would be depressed and couldn't suck or breathe like it needs to."

"I don't care about a baby. It's not a baby, anyway. There's no baby there. It's a tumor. I don't care about a baby."

"Listen to me, young lady. You don't have to care about this baby. You don't have to see it or touch it or keep it. But you do have to deliver it. I will help you all I can, but you are going to have to cooperate with me. I cannot give you something for your pain if it will put this baby at risk. I'm responsible for the baby as well as you. Now pay attention to me. Stop fighting me. Do what I tell you and we will get through this together."

My firm, schoolmarm voice stopped her in her tracks. She hiccoughed and nodded at me, wiping her tears away with her forearm. She brushed back her mop of unruly blond hair and straightened the sheet over her firm young body. As a new contraction began, her face filled with panic, but I could see her push it away. Her green eyes held mine, pleading for my promised help. We breathed together, eyes locked, her hands gripping mine fiercely.

Just as we reached a state of calmness a woman entered. Dressed in a stiff black suit, hair glazed to helmet-strength with hairspray, with lacquered nails and expertly, if heavily applied makeup, she clutched a shiny black purse tightly with both hands. I couldn't immediately recall when I had seen anyone as uptight as this woman. She was Judy's mother. Visibly nervous, she fidgeted at the bedside, her shrill voice nattering away about her own labors.

"You do what the nurse says now, honey. Remember the nanny we had? She was with me in labor and she made me concentrate just like this."

"Where's Daddy?" Judy asked.

"He's downstairs in the lobby, waiting," replied her mother.

"What does he think, Mom?"

"Well I told him it was your appendix like you wanted, but he knows, honey, he knows. We've both known you were pregnant. How could we not?"

I was stunned. How could these parents have stood by for months, knowing their daughter was pregnant, and doing nothing, literally nothing about it? What did they think would happen to the baby? Why hadn't they talked to their daughter? An entire family had engaged in massive denial, pretending nothing was different, as the daughter grew a new life. I wanted to slap the mother, scream at her, berate her: *How* could *you? What kind of mother are you? How could you ignore this? How could you let her go all these months without bringing it up? How could you? What did you think would happen when she went into labor? Did you imagine the baby would just disappear?* I was so appalled, so furious that I had to abruptly leave the room to collect myself. As I tried to control my anger, I told myself that I was there only as the nurse, only to assist with this birth. It wasn't my place to pass judgment on the dynamics of this family. But I was angry, nonetheless.

Judy moved rapidly into second stage and needed to push. I talked her through a contraction, explaining how to hold her breath, when to breathe again and how to push down and out. The urge to bear down was savage in her. Her eyes would widen with alarm as she took a cleansing breath and curled up her body. Positioned on her side, she grabbed onto her knee with one hand and wrapped her other arm around my waist. She tucked her chin down to her chest and pushed her head into my stomach as she strained with all her energy. I counted aloud against her head, curled around her, holding her other knee, both of us laboring mightily to bring this baby down. "That's it, push with all you've got, four, five, six, push, Judy, push! Ten, breathe! Quickly, and again, two, three, four, down and out, six, seven . . ."

No more denials, no more requests for medication or anesthesia, no more tears. Just a ferocious, completely focused intent to push the baby out. Committing herself totally to the urgent messages of her body and my voice, she worked like a Trojan, almost frightening me with the intensity of her effort. Her mother, thank goodness, had left the room, so we were able to concentrate on this task. We moved to the delivery room after an hour of tremendous exertion. The baby was delivered, a large girl. Another nurse assessed her at the warmer as I attended to Judy. Knowing nothing about the patient's denial of her pregnancy, the other nurse spoke brightly, "What a beautiful big girl you are! Wouldn't you like to see your baby, Judy? You want to see your mother, don't you, little girl?"

From the moment of delivery Judy hadn't taken her eyes off the baby. "Do you want to hold her?" I asked her quietly. She looked up at me, eyes wide and brimming with tears, an impossible green. She nodded and held her arms out for her daughter.

"She's so big, isn't she? I was worried about her size, if I was eating right. But I guess I did everything okay, huh? 'Cause look at her, she's really big and healthy, huh?"

She's a beautiful baby, Judy," I responded. I knew she had tried to hide her pregnancy: her belly was elongated and squashed-looking; I suspected she had bound her belly for months. At that moment her mother slipped into the delivery room. I watched, with not a little righteous satisfaction, as she took in the scene of her daughter holding this swaddled infant. Her haggard face distorted with dismay and outrage.

"What are you doing?" she cried. "Just what in God's name are you doing? Why are you holding that baby? You shouldn't even see it. You can't have that baby! You can't keep it! Why are you doing this? You can't keep it, Judy, you know you can't!" She looked apoplectic. I tried to calm her.

"She wanted to hold her. Holding her doesn't mean she's going to keep her. If she's giving her up for adoption, seeing her and holding her will make it easier for her in the long run." As I spoke, I couldn't help feeling vindicated, however meanly, in my earlier anger at this woman: Now *you make a scene? Now you walk in here and try to tell your daughter what she can and cannot do with this baby? It's a little late for that. This is the reality, lady, that you so blithely ignored for months. You chose to ignore it, but you can't anymore! You've got a grandchild. Here she is, whether you like it or not. What did you think your silence would accomplish? Did you just assume we would know the baby wasn't wanted, that we would just automatically whisk her away and you wouldn't have to have anything to do with her? Christ, are you really that stupid?*

"Look, Mom, isn't she something? She's big! I made a big baby, Mom," Judy interjected, oblivious to her mother's anger. The mother stepped close, uselessly berating her daughter, but studying the baby intently. Judy completely ignored her, talking right past her about how handsome the baby was. Shortly after, the mother departed "to tell your father." The baby was taken to the nursery and as her episiotomy was repaired, Judy finally talked about her circumstances, probably for the first time. I began the conversation by quietly remarking to her, "You have a lot to talk about and work through with your parents, don't you?"

"Yes. See, I broke up with the baby's father right after I got pregnant. I didn't even know then. He was real bad for me, and I knew it was over with him. I'd just gotten a good job that I was doing real well with, and five months ago I met a great guy. I'm really crazy about him, but I didn't know how to tell him about the baby. So I just didn't. I just kept quiet. Things were finally working out for .ne with the job and this guy and I just, you know, didn't want to lose it all. . . . What am I gonna do?"

"Well, you're going to have to do some serious thinking and talking, with your folks and your boyfriend. We'll get you together with the social services people today. They can help you a lot with information about resources available for single mothers, adoption if that's how you decide, and so forth. You don't have to make any decisions right now. Just take your time over the next three or four days, and talk with your folks openly now, about what you want, what you need, okay?"

"Okay. She's really a beautiful baby, isn't she?"

She kept the baby. My back hurt for a week afterward and I'm still angry at her parents.

Judy's pregnancy wasn't truly a secret; it was an unacknowledged reality within her family. A couple of years after I worked with Judy, another woman on our unit gave birth "unexpectedly." She was forty-four years old and had been married for twenty years. In report we were told that she had been sent up from the emergency room completely dilated and gave birth within thirty minutes of her arrival. She had insisted she had no idea she was pregnant. Her periods were always erratic; she gained and lost weight over time without deliberate changes in her diet. She explained the fetal movement she'd felt as "just gas, something I've always been subject to." The nurses who assisted with her delivery commented on her composure: "She didn't seem at all surprised when we told her she wasn't having a stomachache—she was having a baby! She didn't even blink at the news. She just said she thought maybe it was appendicitis and then went on and had the baby as calmly as you please! It was something else!"

It was a busy time on the ward. We were inundated with patients and no one had time to speculate further about this woman's equanimity in the face of an unanticipated baby. She wasn't my patient, but I answered her call bell the day after she delivered. When I delivered the diapers she had requested, I spoke to her briefly, checking on her recovery status. She was holding her baby against her shoulder, patting his back and swaying gently from side to side, murmuring endearments to him. I asked her how it felt to become a mother so unexpectedly.

"Oh, it's absolutely wonderful! My husband and I gave up trying years ago. We always wanted children, but it just didn't work out. I'm thrilled about it!"

She gave no evidence of shock or surprise to find herself a parent so suddenly. She smiled at me, a defiantly smug grin on her face, as if to say, "Yes, no question, this is exactly what I've always wanted!" I wondered about her complete acceptance of this dramatic, surprise birth. She worked with the baby as if she had given lots of thought about how to care for an infant. There was an air of confident self-satisfaction about her. The blatant smugness of her smile puzzled me.

As we talked, I studied her. She was dark haired and tall, with a body thickened by age and pregnancy. She moved with such deliberate carefulness, changing the baby's diaper, wrapping him in his blanket. I scanned the room, noting an open suitcase, jam-packed with baby clothes, receiving blankets, baby powder and shampoo, diaper-rash ointment. She had delivered this un-anticipated baby only the day before, but here was a suitcase loaded with baby supplies. As I watched this woman handle her baby with obvious plea-sure and without any hesitancy, something clicked in my head. *I bet this wasn't a surprise. I bet she got pregnant on purpose, with someone else. No way was this a surprise! She looks and acts like it was all planned. . . . Oh well, more power to her, I guess she's gotten what she wanted.* I was too busy to ask about her husband's reaction to the baby, but I didn't doubt for a second her ability to handle whatever dismay he might feel about becoming a father in his late forties.

I was charge nurse one night when the emergency room called to announce the impending arrival of a sixteen-year-old who had delivered precipitously at home. In due course, lying on a gurney pushed by paramedics, Susan arrived on the unit. The baby had been taken by one of the ambulance par-amedics to the nursery. We were to evaluate the new mother for lacerations before sending her to the postpartum ward. As the admitting nurse took her history, I listened to her story, studying her physical appearance. She looked healthy: smooth, unblemished skin, clear blue eyes, shiny blond, permed hair. She wore no makeup, her face white but for flushed cheeks that somehow emphasized her pale complexion. Although she spoke softly, dipping her chin with embarrassment, her voice betrayed her agitation, trembling and spilling words in a staccato manner. She was scared.

"I was on the phone with my mom and I got this terrible pain. I hollered and told her I was sick—that I had to go into the bathroom. I told her that and I just dropped the phone! She called the paramedics. I guess. I didn't call them, so she must have. I was on the toilet when the baby came out and fell in the water! I heard him gurgling under the water, so I fished him out. He was still attached to me, you know. By the cord. So I held him between my legs and walked to the hall closet. I knew we had some new scissors in there. So I got them and cut the cord."

"You must have been really frightened," I remarked. *Good God in heaven—gurgling in the toilet?*

"Well, I was. I knew I should've told my mother before now. I knew it! I wanted to, but I just couldn't. I tried to get up my courage, you know and tell her, but I didn't, all the time I was pregnant. I just kept on going to school. She said I was getting fat, but that's all. She would've understood, I know, because she had me when she was only fifteen. But I was scared."

"You live with your mother?"

"Yes. She was out when it happened. We were just talking on the phone."

I quizzed the paramedics out in the hallway. Did they find the placenta? What had they seen? The girl wasn't able to recall the placenta. I was wondering why she hadn't hemorrhaged if she hadn't tied off both sides of the cord before cutting it.

"We just got a call saying there was a medical emergency at this address. We didn't have any idea it was a baby. We figured a heart attack or something. Boy, were we surprised to go in the bathroom and see this baby lying on the floor! She wouldn't answer the door at first, she was afraid to let us in. Don't know whether there was a placenta or not, there was a good amount of blood and fluid on the floor of the bathroom. We were just focused on the baby, drying it off and clamping the cord."

The mystery of the placenta was solved in the delivery room when Susan expelled it. The paramedics had clamped both sides of the cord after she had cut it. Evidently they had arrived in the nick of time, just as she was cutting the cord, otherwise the baby and she might have bled to death. The medics were so shaken by the event they had forgotten one end of the cord they'd clamped in Susan's bathroom was hanging from her vagina, still attached to the placenta inside. I had to spend some time calming them down. They were worried about the baby's well-being, repeatedly insisting that they would have handled it better if they had known before their arrival.

"You did fine, just fine. You clamped the cord and wrapped the baby, maintained its temperature," I reassured them. "You were great!"

About thirty minutes later I was standing alone at the nurses' station, watching a young woman—surely no more than thirty—walk up the hall toward me. She was a looker, meticulously dressed in tight jeans, a frilly red blouse that fell off one shoulder, and shiny fire-engine red high heels. Gold chains draped her neck, dripped from her earlobes, and rattled around her wrists. Heavily sprayed blond hair was teased high on her head, falling around her shoulders in the windswept style so favored among what I called "mall-crawlers." Like her body, her face was fashionably thin and lovely, in spite of the complicated makeup, which had to have been applied with great care. I was impressed by several shades of eye shadow, heavy mascara, foundation creme, blush, and (what else?) fire-engine red lip gloss that duplicated the color of the perfectly manicured long nails on her heavily ringed fingers. *Wow, check out this vision!* I muttered to myself, wondering who she was and what she was doing clicking up the hall in four-inch spike heels at 2:30 in the morning.

Approaching the desk, she asked me with extreme hesitancy, "Is my daughter here?"

"What's her name, ma'am?"

"Susan Hansom. What . . . what . . . why is she here?"

"Yes, she's here, she's in the delivery room, being checked for lacerations, any tears, you know."

At that moment the phone rang. Since I was alone at the nurses' station, I apologized to the woman and answered it. It was the admitting clerk downstairs.

"Listen, Ms. Diamond, I just sent that girl's mother up to L&D and I wanted to catch you before she gets there. See, I realized . . . uh . . . I don't think the mother knows her daughter was pregnant. I didn't want to be the one to tell her she was a grandmother so I told her we send all women to L&D at night. Ha, ha!"

"Your phone call's a little too late." I answered dryly. *Oh Christ. I thought she knew from the phone conversation. I know the girl said she hadn't told her mother, but I thought she meant during the pregnancy. I assumed she told her over the phone. Lord, what have I done?* The woman was watching me with a horror-stricken look on her face. I hung up the phone, inwardly fuming at the damned admissions lady. "Mrs. Hansom, I'm so sorry. I thought your daughter told you. I assumed you knew. Jesus, I'm so sorry to have to break it like this to you, so bluntly. Your daughter had a little boy in the bathroom, right after she was talking to you."

"Jesus God. Jesus." She paled, clutching at the counter. I hurried around and stood beside her. Placing a hand on her arm, I guided her into an empty labor room and seated her in the chair. She was dumbfounded. Her mouth opened and closed, opened and closed. She looked at me as though she thought I was lying to her, then looked away. She trembled and fumbled with her purse.

"I'm so sorry. I know this is a terrible shock to you. Your daughter is okay. She was a real trooper through the whole thing. She took care of the baby and cut the cord, even though she must have been really frightened. The baby is in the nursery now, and as far as I know he's okay."

"I just can't believe this. What am I going to do?"

"Well, let's go downstairs together and get a cup of coffee. Do you smoke? Let's go have a cigarette and talk, give you some time to get your thoughts in order before you see your daughter."

I could tell she was a smoker; she'd been fumbling in her purse, moving her hands around like she didn't know what to do with them. As we started down the hall, her boyfriend appeared. She introduced him to me and then looked at him with such astonishment and fearfulness, she was completely at a loss for words.

"Do you want me to tell him?"

"Yeah."

I explained as we went down to the cafeteria. The boyfriend, as meticulously costumed and groomed as Mrs. Hansom, was courteous with me, a perfect gentleman, as he lighted our cigarettes and asked appropriate questions about the new mother and baby. With careful, stilted words, he expressed his gratitude for our help and his pleasure in hearing that Susan was okay. Mrs. Hansom sat very still, sucking on the cigarette as though it was life-giving oxygen, her head down, eyes averted. I assured them that social services would be of assistance over the next couple of days in providing information about adoption, and so forth. I cautioned them not to make any major decisions about the baby during the next few hours. "You've had a big shock. You need time to assimilate this news, to adjust to it, before you make any decisions. And you need to remember that Susan handled herself very well in the emergency. She's going to need a lot of support from you."

"Yes, of course she has our support," the boyfriend told me. I left them and went to the delivery room to see how Susan was doing. I explained that her mother had arrived and that I had told her about the baby.

"Is he with her?" She fired the question at me, with what sounded like terror in her voice.

"Who?" I put my hand on her arm, trying to calm her with a warm touch.

"Kurt. Her boyfriend."

"Yes, he's here also."

"Oh God! Oh God! Is he angry? Is he mad at me?"

"Why no, Susan. He didn't seem angry at all. He's been a real help to your mom. She's a bit shocked, you know, honey. She didn't realize what was happening when you were on the phone together. You can see her as soon as the doctor's done in here."

"I want to see her alone, okay? Please?" Her eyes filled with tears as she waited for me to agree. I stroked her arm for a minute, encouraged her to relax, and reassured her that she could see her mother alone. Then I left the delivery room, as other duties required my attention.

The nurse who had been with Susan in the delivery room told me later that the girl had been obsessing about her mother's boyfriend, what he would do, what he would say. We wondered why she was so afraid of him. I worried about whether he had beaten her or her mother. I wondered if maybe he was the baby's father. Her fear of his response was so extraordinary there must have been some underlying reason. She was a beautiful girl, living at home with her attractive, youthful mother. The mother's boyfriend looked younger than the mother. It wasn't impossible that a triangle existed there. The eventual disposition of the baby and the dynamics of this trio took place on the postpartum ward. Susan's L&D nurse passed on our request for a social-service consult, which resulted in a visit from the social worker and interventions as appropriate, to the postpartum nurses, but we never followed up with the case after Susan left L&D.

Long afterwards, I'd find myself wondering about this family. I also recognized that my speculations about them had absolutely no foundation in fact: Susan didn't come out and say anything suspicious about her mother's boyfriend. I just watched and drew my own conclusions, however wildly off-base they might have been. She wasn't my patient and she was on my unit for less than two hours, so I wasn't in a position to act on any vague suspicions, other than suggesting the social-service consult. All I did was feed the avid interest I had in other people's lives.

Another sensitive subject on L&D is the issue of drug use. Although not readily, most women will admit to the use of illegal drugs. Over time, I have learned it isn't enough to simply ask, "Do you take any drugs?" I actually list them: "Do you use marijuana, cocaine, crack, valium, speed, any narcotics?" I preface this question by explaining to the mother, "I'm not asking this to pry or just because I'm curious. I'm asking because it's important to know in order to care for you and the baby appropriately." Those women who do admit drug use usually insist that they haven't done any drugs since the beginning of their pregnancy. Occasionally, a drug user will reveal defiantly that she does abuse drugs and has throughout the pregnancy.

Any patient with such a history and any woman who has not received prenatal care or who is a walk-in—an unexpected patient with no prenatal chart—will have toxicology labs done. Urine and sometimes blood are sent to the lab to determine if any drugs are in the mother's system. This is critical information, since the presence of narcotics or other drugs in the mother's system will directly affect the baby's initial response to extra-uterine life and is a significant behavioral indicator in the first hours and days of the baby's life, potentially affecting its ability to breathe, suck, move, and respond to stimuli.

I was working in a civilian hospital when a woman arrived one night complaining that she felt "something in her vagina." Quickly we stripped off her clothes, got her into a gown, and into a bed. When we drew back the sheets to check her cervix, we were horrified. A tiny foot protruded from her vagina, moving ever so delicately back and forth. The man who had brought her to the hospital stopped me as I left the room. Grabbing my arm, he asked nervously if I would get the car keys from the patient because he was in a hurry and had to leave. He refused to enter the room, so I retrieved the keys from the patient. Visibly nervous and agitated, he grabbed the keys from my hand and took off, running for the exit.

We had no prenatal chart for this woman, no information about her medical history or this pregnancy. Every question we asked of the patient was met with vagueness: "I don't know. . . . I'm not sure. . . . I don't remember." All we could ascertain from her was that she had another child and that her waters broke two days earlier. She spoke cogently but didn't convey any sense of urgency or distress over the fact that her baby's foot was hanging out of her vagina. She said only that she'd felt "something in there" for the last day or so. Uncertain about the date of her last menstrual period, we estimated the woman to be twenty-four to twenty-nine weeks along. Upon looking at the fetal foot, the neonatalogist felt it was probably closer to twenty-nine weeks, which gave the fetus a better chance at survival. A decision was swiftly reached to perform an emergency cesarean to try to save the fetus.

We hustled around the patient—starting an IV, compiling a history, monitoring the fetus, putting a urine collection catheter into her bladder, shaving her abdomen. I wondered at her. The only way to describe the patient was laid back. Her face was flat and totally devoid of expression. She appeared oblivious to all the activity around her. Completely disengaged, she blandly watched us scurrying around and doing things to her body. She didn't even seem concerned when she was told that we would be operating to deliver her baby. As she was being prepped in the operating room, I told the obstetrician that I was going to send a urine sample from the collection bag for a tox screen.

After her delivery of a tiny fetus, twenty-nine weeks but growth retarded, the doctor approached me at the nurses' station, and complimented me.

"Really good pick up, Susie. Her urine was flooded with cocaine. I just can't believe it."

"Shit," I exclaimed. "We crashed her, put her to sleep, and she was snowed with cocaine? God, we could've killed her."

"I just don't understand it. I asked her three times if she used drugs and she denied it," the doctor said.

"Of course she denied it! She's a junkie, for chrissakes. She was obviously stoned, Doc. God, she didn't bat an eye when we told her she was going for surgery."

"But I *asked* her about drugs. How could she jeopardize her baby like that?" This young physician's naïveté astounded me.

"Doc, get real! This lady comes in and tells you her membranes ruptured two days ago! It's not her first baby, she knows what it means when you rupture. She doesn't react to all the haste, all our urgency, even though she's got her baby's foot hanging out of her vagina, for god's sake! She's a drug abuser. If she took drugs during the pregnancy, do you think she really cares about her baby? Maybe she was afraid we'd call the cops or something. The man with her split as fast as he could. Hell, she might be holding some coke in her purse right now. She doesn't care about that baby, she can't. All she cares about is her fix. The only reason she came in was because she had to, with the kid already coming out of her."

The baby was transferred to a tertiary care facility, intubated, and "wired for sound." He would require hours of intensive, minute-to-minute high-tech care at exorbitant cost with an uncertain outcome. His survival was hardly guaranteed. If he did live, the quality of life he would experience was far from good. So much against him, before he could even start: prematurity, all the attendant possible long-term effects of his care, and a mother at best indifferent to his well-being, wanting only to protect her secret, illegal drug use.

Another drug abuser displayed similar complete disinterest in her baby. A crack addict, she delivered the baby at home and didn't call anyone for help. Her boyfriend came home to discover the baby, unwrapped and un-washed, still attached to the placenta. He called paramedics, who rushed the mother and baby to the hospital. I couldn't get the mother to tell me anything about the birth or to hold or look at her baby. She couldn't even tell us with any certainty when the baby was born. The following day, the grandmother of the baby begged the nurses not to let the mother take the baby home, insisting she was so addicted to drugs that she wouldn't and couldn't care for her infant. Social workers and people from the child welfare agencies entered the case at our request. Later, I learned that the baby was placed in a foster home and did not go home with his mother.

Most obstetrical units place a heavy emphasis on patient teaching. In order to maintain accreditation, every unit is required to provide instruction to new mothers on postpartum care of their bodies and on infant care. Videos are available on every conceivable topic: episiotomy care, breast-feeding, infant bathing and feeding, resumption of sexual relations, sibling rivalry, signs and symptoms of infant illness, postpartum blues, cesarean incision care, to name but a few. Classes are given on many of these topics, with bath and diapering demonstrations, lectures on hygiene, and the use and preparation of infant formulas. Postpartum and nursery nurses fill out pages of documentation testifying to this patient instruction. Before a mother can be discharged with her baby, we review every item to verify that she's at least been exposed to the material, and we try to be sure she understands what we're talking about. She has to sign a paper indicating that she's received the instructions and understands them.

If we think a mother isn't confident of her parenting skills, if she exhibits any negative bonding behaviors, or if we suspect substance abuse and/or a dysfunctional family, we are required to take further action. In the military hospital, this meant the mother would not be discharged until we felt she could handle her baby without our help. We were required to request a social-service consult for single mothers, teenage mothers, and any mother who appeared to have physical or emotional difficulty with her baby. We watched for and documented indicators of poor bonding and/or potential child abuse. These included negative comments about the baby's gender or appearance or features, reluctance or refusal to hold the baby close and in the proper position, annoyance with the baby's cry or messy diapers or hunger, negligence in meeting the infant's needs, and so forth.

When I hear a mother repeat more than a couple of times her disappointment in the baby's gender, I am alerted to a potential problem. If I see a mother holding her new baby loosely sprawled over her knees, or watch her leave the baby crying alone and unsafe on her bed, rather than in its crib, I pay attention to the other ways in which she interacts with the baby. I also alert the other nurses providing her care. Is the baby fed on demand? Does she keep its diapers changed? Is the crib close to her bed and within her reach, or halfway across the room? Does she maintain the baby supplies she needs? Is she always calling the desk to ask for someone to do the baby care? Does she look the baby in the face, talk to it, call it by name? Has she even named the baby? When she touches the baby, does she do it gently or roughly? Does she leave the baby in the nursery all the time? Is she trying to breast-feed? How does she respond to congratulations and best wishes from the staff and her family? What is her demeanor like? How messy is her room? How involved is she with her baby? And so on and so forth . . .

There's no privacy here. Willingly or not, the mother, her baby, and her family fall under the scrutiny of many people. Complete strangers, those people observe, assess, evaluate, and make judgments about the patient's ability to parent her baby. We are trained to make these judgments and legally obligated to act on our impressions. I don't hesitate to call social services if I think a mother may be having trouble accepting her baby. I'm supposed to provide her with the resources available to help her take care of her baby: an infant car seat, bottles of formula, scrips for nutritional supplements, counseling for adoption, or marital problems, or dysfunctional family situations. I've never had a problem with any patient or family refusing such services. No one's ever accused me of crying wolf about possible child abuse, and I haven't heard of any other nurse I've worked with being so accused. In most cases, like the crack addict above, the evidence of potential neglect or abuse is obvious and the system makes what paltry efforts it can to intervene. Social workers, counselors, and psychiatric nurses carry on with each case, after they've been notified by the primary nurse responsible for the patient.

We do what we can, trying to make a difference in the sorry lives that sometimes reveal themselves to us. Most of us take it personally, worrying and losing sleep over a baby we just hate to see go home to possible neglect. On several occasions, I've watched with pride and respect as fellow nurses gave far more of themselves to patients than they were legally required to do. These nurses were women who had been victims of abuse themselves, beaten and battered by husbands or boyfriends. When they recognized a battered woman, they confronted her without hesitation. They exposed their own pain, their own shame to the woman. They spent extra time with her, telling her of their experiences, offering advice on how to escape the abuse and regain control over her life and her children's lives. They would cry with the woman, but they would also refuse to allow her to avoid the reality of her situation.

Situations like these place a heavy burden on hospital personnel. Ultimately, we are more than gossipy, curious, vicarious thrill-seekers. We are involved in the private lives of complete strangers; we have to ask questions about their most guarded secrets, watch their every movement, and intervene for the welfare of the baby and/or mother when necessary. When dysfunctional families come into the hospital, we're supposed to guard their privacy even as we invade it, for the sake of the patient, and talk about it among ourselves. Legal and medical rules dictate many of our actions and put us in the position of having to pass judgment on patients under our care. Confidentiality and privacy fly out of the window.

As time passes, even though my interest about my patients continues unabated, I have grown increasingly tormented by this unsolicited burden of judgment. Even as I have developed into a seasoned professional, my compunctions about my work grow stronger. I remember the younger, naïve nursing student who felt so claustrophobic in the locked psychiatric ward. Just as I wondered then how it can be that psychiatrists are granted the power to decide other people's fates, now I find myself wondering about my right to interfere with someone else's life.

Just as I could then easily imagine the possibility that I could find myself a psychiatric patient, I could now just as easily be the patient in the bed instead of the nurse at the desk. The benefit of this discomfiture is that it has made me far more sensitive to the issues of privacy and confidentiality. I try to keep a rein on my curiosity. I try to avoid gossiping about my patients. And I try very hard to refrain from intervening with patients without solid evidence of the need for intervention. Before calling in social services or expressing concern to my co-workers, I try to analyze whether the patient's behavior is truly dysfunctional or if it just seems strange because of my own values and expectations.

For instance, there wasn't any question in my mind about the necessity to intervene on behalf of the baby of the crack addict. Any woman so lost in her drug addiction that she is unable to seek appropriate help with having her baby obviously has serious problems. Her abnormal maternal behavior, which I observed myself, along with her mother's urgent warnings about her inability to care for her baby, were further indications for public intervention. But in many cases, we nurses jump to conclusions about our patients that are not based on obvious solid evidence of problems. I've heard nurses voice vehement objections to a patient's parenting skills simply because the patient is dirty, poor, uneducated, or of another culture. Is it right for me to decide a mother hasn't exhibited appropriate bonding behaviors because I never hear her speak lovingly to her infant or see her holding her baby the way I think she should be holding it? There may be any number of reasons why this mother behaves as she does that have nothing to do with inappropriate parenting. If a mother expresses disappointment in the gender of her baby does that automatically mean she isn't going to love the baby just as much anyway? Do I actually have any right to draw conclusions about a family's interactions without blatant evidence of dysfunction or damage within that family?

My obligation to be ever vigilant in assessments of patients' psychosocial behaviors and needs, and at the same time to recognize the difference between my own expectations and beliefs and the patients', complicates and increases the uneasiness I feel about the issues of privacy, confidentiality, and self-determination. While I acknowledge that being a labor and delivery nurse is not about just helping laboring mothers—as I so naïvely believed years ago—but is also about meddling in patients' lives when necessary, I am increasingly uncomfortable with that responsibility. The power to affect someone's life, outside the hospital and after the birth of a baby, is not a power I bargained for when I became a nurse, and it is a power I feel less and less inclined to wield. It has become yet another aspect of my work that calls into question whether I am really suited to do this job.

Chapter Thirteen

GERMANS AND OTHER
FRIENDS

Few women expect their pregnancies to be a time of serious trouble. When complications occur, the pregnant woman and her family are usually caught completely off guard, dismayed by the sometimes extreme procedures and the frightening equipment that are medicine's efforts to sustain the pregnancy and safeguard the mother and unborn child. Unfortunately such complications do arise: bleeding episodes caused by a placenta improperly implanted over the mouth of the uterus or a placenta that separates prematurely from the uterine wall; preterm contractions that might expel an immature fetus; blood incompatibilities between the mother and baby; nausea and vomiting so severe the mother's ability to provide sustenance for her fetus is compromised; fetal anomalies that jeopardize the baby's life outside the womb; complications from diabetes or other diseases; and multiple gestations that threaten to deliver before the babies are viable.

Any of these complications can result in lengthy hospitalizations, along with innumerable medical tests and a compendium of pharmaceutical agents. When a pregnancy is so jeopardized, the life of the mother ceases to be her own. She will be guarded and probed, examined and invaded for days, weeks, and sometimes months, in the effort to maintain the pregnancy and protect both her and the baby. Children and husband, home and job are relinquished. Her daily activities, diet, sleep, and recreation are circumscribed by her treatment plan. She has no privacy, no time alone. In all probability, she will find herself sharing a room with another such prisoner of pregnancy, someone she has never met before, whose personal habits and illness may intrude even further on her own daily routines. Nurses, doctors, and other hospital personnel can enter her room at will, at any time. They may be caring, indifferent, hostile, or rude; she has little recourse if certain personnel irritate or annoy her. Her hours become hospital ones, artificially divided into shifts and hourly segments of time: time for medications, for vital signs, for doctors' rounds, for ultrasounds, for fetal heart tones, for meals, for bedmaking, or for bathing.

Aside from the physical disruption of her daily life, the emotional impact can be devastating. Worry about her unborn child, concerns about children left at home, conflicts with her spouse or family members who may not understand her hospitalization, can all contribute to her distress. The effects of her treatment may debilitate her even further, so that maintaining any sort of emotional composure can be difficult at best. One woman I cared for was in the hospital for severe hyperemesis gravidarum, an illness of pregnancy marked by long-term vomiting, fluid and electrolyte imbalance, and weight loss. Mrs. Sadler's condition was so severe she had been transferred from out of state to our high-risk obstetrical unit. Her husband could not obtain leave from his job to be with her during her hospitalization, and was able to visit only every other weekend. She came from an unusually large family, but they lived across the continent, and she knew not a soul in this area. Except for hospital personnel, she was truly alone in this alien world.

Mrs. Sadler vomited anything that passed through her mouth. We couldn't stop her vomiting, so our task was to somehow maintain her nutrition and hydration until her fetus matured. We kept her hydrated with IVs. We inserted a feeding tube to her stomach to provide needed nutrients. Unfortunately, she actually vomited up the tube several times, until we were forced to insert a catheter into her cardiovascular system to infuse nutrients directly into her bloodstream.

I ached for this woman. She was frail and skeleton thin, with dark circles around her eyes. She had a private room because she was so ill, but the privacy may have contributed to her profound depression. Rarely speaking, she passed through her long days lying listlessly in bed, too weak and dispirited to move, other than to make trips to the bathroom. Submitting silently to dressing changes, ultrasounds, and frequent vital sign and IV checks, she wept piteously whenever we had to change her IV. Because of the risk of infection, every seventy-two hours we had to stop the IV and restart it in another vein. Each IV change was torture to her. Taking off the tape pulled out the hair on her forearms. Because of her weight loss, her paper-thin veins collapsed easily and finding a new vein usually necessitated several sticks. She would start crying as soon as we touched the tape, not ceasing until the new IV was secured.

I worried about her. I was new in the job, unsure of what could be done to ease her suffering. She had been on the unit so long that the rest of the staff had become accustomed to her plight. She was treated with gentle compassion; everyone felt badly for her. But everyone just accepted that she had to endure her condition, even if it made her wretchedly miserable.

Since this was my first exposure to hyperemesis gravidarum, I didn't recognize the subtle prejudice held by many obstetrical caregivers toward these patients. Nausea and vomiting are acceptable, tolerated symptoms of early pregnancy, but someone who doesn't stop vomiting after the first trimester becomes suspect in the eyes of others. It's not considered normal, and even though Mrs. Sadler's condition was and is a recognized, legitimate malady, something about it makes people suspicious. Over time, I was to hear doctors, nurses, and nurses' aides speculate, often unfairly, about the under-lying cause of the vomiting.

> *I think she's just doing it for attention. She only vomits when her family is here.*
> *She says she can't hold anything down, but I saw her eat a cracker.*
> *She must have some serious psychological problems. There's just no reason for this behavior. Let's get a psych consult on her.*
> *I don't think she's happy with this pregnancy and that's why she's puking so much.*
> *I think she's faking.*
> *She just spits all the time—it's disgusting.*
> *It's just a way to get out of work.*

This prejudice may arise out of the sheer unpleasantness of the condition. Nobody anywhere is unaffected by the sounds and smells of someone heaving. We all have to fight the reflexive nausea that hits us when we see another person vomiting. Flushing countless reeking emesis basins full with the sour contents of someone's belly, changing befouled linens and gowns, washing down splattered furniture, and mopping stinking floors are routine tasks with these patients. But no matter how many times you do these things, no matter how accustomed you become to the odor and the sight, it is never an agreeable task. After a while, if you're tired, overworked, and underpaid, and the same woman keeps making messes you have to clean up, it's all too easy to begin to condemn her for something she has no control over. I was no less subject to this bias than my co-workers and had to consciously remind myself that it wasn't the patient's fault.

By the time I was assigned as Mrs. Sadler's nurse, she wasn't vomiting anymore. She hadn't actually eaten a morsel of solid food or swallowed a sip of fluid for a month. All her nutritional requirements were being infused into her veins. But I was afraid of her silence, her refusal to respond to routine questions, her hours of inactivity and sleep, her depression. Hesitant, inex-perienced, with little confidence in myself, I wrestled with these fears and my reluctance to invade her desolate isolation. I felt such an intruder when I had to perform routine duties with her. I had to fight my own inclination to ignore her loneliness, to just do what was required for her clinical care without acknowledging her emotional state. For a couple of weeks I fumbled ineptly and uncomfortably with her care. I tried, unsuccessfully, to convince myself that I was learning how to maintain professional distance. Still, her lonely despondency gnawed at my conscience; I began to feel ashamed of myself.

The right to privacy, both physical and psychological, was a conviction deeply ingrained in me. Because my father's medical practice often resulted in my being inadvertently exposed to his patients, from early childhood on I had been trained not to look, not to question or wonder why people behaved as they did. When Dad took me on hospital rounds, he admonished me, sometimes harshly, when I tried to peek into patients' rooms as we paraded down the halls. Even in nursing school, I found myself discomfited and tense every time I had to invade a patient's space. Although I understood intellectually that normal rules of etiquette did not strictly apply to health-care providers, that my work necessitated the broaching of patients' personal boundaries, relinquishing a lifelong pattern of deference to others was a formidable task. In this first year of work, with Mrs. Sadler and other long-term patients, I was forced to confront my lack of self-confidence. If I cared about my patients, and I did, I had to learn to be assertive. The patients' needs could not be slighted because of my own diffidence and discomfort.

I had to do something for Mrs. Sadler. I brought her some coffee-table books, replete with colorful photographs and illustrations, shyly offering them as possible distractions. After consulting with the head nurse, I wrote an order in her chart requiring her IVs to be changed only by experienced personnel. This order protected her from the custom of allowing medical students to practice on her. On several occasions I conspired to get Nick to do her IVs since his skill was exceptional and his manner with her so gentle and solicitous.

She remained quiet and for the most part unresponsive until I volunteered to wash her hair. The nursing staff had left this task for her husband to perform during his biweekly visits. As I discovered, dirty hair was a particular source of distress for her and contributed to her sense of helplessness. Her IV and feeding lines made it very difficult for her to manage a thorough shampoo and rinse. Together we worked to thoroughly wash her luxuriant, long, golden-red hair. I spent an hour with her, standing behind her seated form as I gently brushed and combed her hair, working out the tangles, complimenting her on this beautiful hair. I grew nostalgic, remembering the elderly woman whose hair I had shampooed back in nursing school. As I brushed Mrs. Sadler's mane, I recounted the story to her, telling her about being hugged by that sweet old lady.

From then on, whenever I entered her room, Mrs. Sadler greeted me with a smile. I made special stops at her room before and after my shift to say hello and see how she was doing. We shared our opinions about the books I'd loaned her. Her animated responses to some of the photographs filled me with delight. We talked about her marriage and her feelings about the baby. I expressed my concern about how she might feel about the baby after suffering so much during its development. She began to come out of herself a little, actually walking in the hall for a few minutes each day. We talked about labor and delivery; I taught her some breathing techniques and tried to answer her questions about the process.

On my birthday, Mrs. Sadler gave birth to a healthy baby girl after a brief labor. I came to work just after she delivered and went flying into the recovery room to see her. She held the baby up for me to admire and gave me the best possible thank-you gift imaginable. "I was determined to have this baby on your birthday, Susie, and I did! Now I'll always remember you when we celebrate her birthday."

During my first days on the job, I didn't have much time to interact with long-term patients in any way other than superficially. I was following my preceptor around, learning the ropes, with little capacity for giving serious consideration to any one patient's individual needs. Eventually I realized that in addition to Mrs. Sadler, we had another long-term patient who was a problem. She had been in one of the few private rooms for more than two months. Staff members talked about her in a sort of shorthand that I at first found difficult to penetrate. Gradually I began to learn something about this patient.

Patricia Rockham was thirty-two years old, an African-American military dependent. Her husband was an active-duty soldier, which entitled her to military medical care. She was pregnant for the sixth time. Her first five pregnancies had terminated in miscarriages. She was a class-R diabetic. That meant that she had been diabetic since her childhood; she needed insulin to survive; and the disease had affected multiple organs in her body. Pregnancy was a profound insult to her metabolism, and it threatened her ability to survive. She was subject to bouts of preterm labor and wildly fluctuating blood glucose levels with the attendant risk of ketoacidosis, an abnormal buildup of acid and ketones in the blood, which could lead to possible loss of consciousness, even coma. She had chronic hypertension and would eventually develop preeclampsia, a serious disease of pregnancy. She was also grossly obese. In other words, she was definitely high risk.

I was terrified of her. I felt like I didn't know anything about diabetes. I was completely lost when it came to understanding the mysteries of unstable blood sugar levels and the possible consequences of brittle diabetes. In addition, I was unnerved by the sight of medical students who entered her room to take blood samples, fleeing the scene, ashen faced and quivering with fear after the tongue lashings she gave them. The regular staff took her demanding, rude behavior in stride, either avoiding contact with her or laughing about her tyranny in the tiny room she inhabited. Unsuspecting med students and interns were "initiated" on the ward by being sent in to deal with Mrs. Rockham.

Eventually, of course, I couldn't avoid dealing with her. The first few times I entered her room, I trembled as I talked to her, struggling to present a cool professionalism that I did not feel in the slightest. She lay in bed, sullen and withdrawn, a fat and unattractive woman. Her body was swollen with retained fluid, skin stretched parchment-thin over great stumps of legs. She had no neck, no wrists or ankles, thunderingly large thighs, massive breasts. She was so big all over, obese and swollen with illness, that her pregnant belly wasn't recognizable as such. She didn't like to talk. She answered my questions with indifferent grunts. If something pissed her off, she let everyone know in a fast minute. "Her breakfast tray wasn't right. . . . Someone left the light on in the bathroom. . . . The medical student asked stupid questions and hadn't read her chart. . . . We were too noisy at the desk. . . ." And so forth.

Her life was one long nightmare. Every day she had to stick her finger every four hours for a little blood, to check her glucose levels. Every other day, blood had to be drawn for lab checks. Every ounce of her urine was measured and dipped and tested. Every bite of food that went into her mouth was measured and calculated and timed. Every day she received several injections of insulin. Every four hours her vital signs were taken. Every night her sleep was interrupted for vital signs, fetal heart tones, finger sticks. Every week she had ultrasounds. Every week she made trips to the opthalmology clinic for eye exams. Every week she was visited by the respiratory therapist, the occupational therapist, and the physical therapist. Is it any wonder that this woman was a raging harridan half the time, lost in a state of depressed withdrawal the other half?

In little ways, I began to overcome my fear of her. When I needed a finger-stick result, I asked her to show me how to do it. I clowned with her, telling her I was a new nurse and didn't know anything. I focused on her knowledge about her illness, asking her questions about her treatment, her insulin dosages, her meals. Probably the most significant thing I did with her was to openly acknowledge how rotten her daily existence was, while extravagantly praising her ability to withstand all the insults to her physical person and her privacy.

"This must really be a bitch, having to stick your fingers so often. Are they as sore as they look? You are really amazing, Mrs. Ruckham. I'd be a raging lunatic if I had to put up with all this stuff. Show me how to do this, please?" She began to respond, particularly after I told her that she scared me to death and to please be gentle with me because I wanted to make life as tolerable as possible for her, but didn't really know how, so she'd have to help me. She chuckled when I told her about watching the med students leave her room quivering, and then explained to me how mad it made her to have people practice drawing blood on her. Just as I'd done with Mrs. Sadler, I managed to end the initiation of med students by writing nursing orders that her blood was to be drawn by experienced personnel only.

One day Nick and another LPN told me they were going to play a practical joke on Patricia. As they walked into the room, I followed closely behind, uncertain about the appropriateness of this play. The LPN, who had often drawn blood from Patricia, announced, "Mrs. Rockham, you've been giving everyone a hard time about getting blood from you. Now this has got to stop! We're going to take care of this today, you hear? And no more trouble from you!"

From behind his back he whipped out a 60 cc syringe—the grandfather of all syringes, it looks like a turkey baster—with a five-inch-long spinal needle attached. He waved the syringe and needle in her startled face. She jumped and scooted back on her bed faster than I'd ever seen her move. "Get that thing away from me! Get it away! Are you crazy?"

We all hollered with laughter, Mrs. Rockham the most tickled of all. I realized there was a playful little girl hiding in all that mass of misery and that she loved being teased, if she could tease back. We began to get real smart with each other. I'd accuse her of tyrannizing the med students. She'd accused me of being a know-nothing clumsy fool. I'd clown and she'd clown back. We had a ball together, laughing and joking about the craziness of my work and her treatment.

In between the jokes and clowning, Patricia allowed herself to talk a little about how she felt, how hard it was dealing with all the interruptions and the invasions of her body; how confused her marriage was right now and how it had suffered because of her illnesses and miscarriages; how afraid she was of losing the baby. I began to enjoy her. I found I liked her. I felt protective toward her. I looked forward to whatever time I had with her and worked on little details to try to ease her daily routines.

I spent four hours one shift frantically trying to cope with an episode of hypoglycemia. Her breakfast tray had been late and her blood sugar had dropped so low that Patricia had passed out. I found her, clammy with sweat, unresponsive, sprawled back in her bed, fork in hand. Doctors were mobilized. A new IV was started and glucose pushed rapidly into her bloodstream. I assisted, terribly frightened by how little I knew and how rapidly she had deteriorated. The OB chief managed the crisis, quietly instructing me every step of the way, explaining what we were doing and why.

After we had stabilized her, as I cleaned up the debris of our work, I realized how important the event had been for me. I had learned a lot about diabetes and about Mrs. Rockham. I wasn't afraid of her anymore. There was a bond between us now, one that she acknowledged, holding my hand as she quietly thanked me for finding her and getting help.

"You scared the devil out of me, Patricia. We're not going to let this happen again, no way! I'm going to haunt this room. You'll be so sick of me by the time you have this baby, you won't believe it. Okay?"

"Yep. You just better keep your eye on me! And you make sure they bring me my damned food, you hear? That's your job, you know, watching out for me!"

Patricia was with us for five months. At the end she was moved to the labor and delivery unit for one-to-one monitoring and nursing care. She was preeclamptic and having preterm labor again. She was so sick we had an arterial line inserted, so that blood samples could be obtained hourly without sticking her. Her body was so edematous that it was impossible to find her veins anyway. I took care of her for several days. She talked me through the A-line routines, literally teaching me how to obtain the samples and keep the line flushed and clear. She loved being my teacher, giggling over my ineptness, fussing at me when I made mistakes, and complimenting me gruffly when I performed well. "See, you're not so bad, after all. You just need me to teach you!" she announced with pride.

Somehow Patricia rallied and stabilized enough to have the A-line removed. We kept her on the labor deck for close observation. One morning, as I was preparing to give her a bed bath, her husband sauntered into her room, dressed in a shiny suit, collar open, tie loose around his neck. He was a large man with a loud voice and exaggerated gestures, whose casual attitude toward Patricia I found infuriating. He chattered away about the all-night party he'd just left, as Patricia watched him through squinting, hard eyes, her body rigid with anger. As I bathed her after he departed, I could feel her distress.

She sat on the edge of the bed, pillows propped behind her to hold her up: she was so weak and ungainly she couldn't sit upright without help. I soaped, rinsed, and dried her legs and feet, amazed at their swollen size and the brittleness of her skin. "Oh, man, Patricia. Your legs are so swollen. Do they hurt?"

"Everything hurts, Susie. They sure are ugly, aren't they?" She peered down at her legs, great water-filled logs.

"Well, they aren't pretty, for sure, but that's because of all the fluid inside. I wish I could siphon off some of this water you've got in here, Patricia. Since I can't do that, I guess you'll have to settle for some lotion. Maybe that'll help with this tight, dry skin, huh?" I smoothed on the lotion, handling her legs and feet as gently as I could, remembering the little old man in nursing school whose foot was blackened from gangrene as a result of diabetes. Patricia's feet didn't look much healthier than his had. Oh, do I hate diabetes. As I worked, bent over her legs, she started muttering.

"He's got a nerve, don't he? Coming in here, dressed like that. Waltzing in here, fancy as you please. All duded up, wasn't he? Having himself a high time at a party. While I'm lying here. Umphh!"

"Yeah, pretty inconsiderate, I'd say," I murmured. "Okay, I'm done, and you're tired out from sitting up like this too long. Let's ease you back down now on these clean sheets." We strained together, she hefting her weight back onto her pillows as I lifted her heavy legs and positioned them for her. Breathless with the exertion, she panted for a few minutes as I tucked her in. Finally, she was settled, resting on her back, looking like a great black Buddha that had been toppled from its pedestal.

"Oh, Susie. It's just not fair. I know I look like a damned monster, lying here, all fat and swollen and sick. But it's his baby, too, that he says he wants so much. Wouldn't you think he'd care a little about coming in here like that? Why's he have to make me feel so bad?"

"Jeez, Patricia. I don't know. It made me mad, too. You just don't pay him any mind now. You pay attention to yourself. If he's that insensitive, you need to put him out of your mind and focus on yourself and getting through this in one piece. And you're not a monster! Swollen up like a balloon, yeah! Monster, no!" I grinned at her, stroking her fat cheek, ignoring the bristles of hair on her chin and upper lip, looking for the laughter in her eyes that could turn her homely face warm in an instant. She smiled wanly at me, shook her head, and turned her face to the wall.

Upset and near tears I headed for the wardmaster's office, now occupied by Nick as a result of a recent promotion. The wardmaster was the noncommissioned officer in charge of the enlisted soldiers assigned to the unit. As wardmaster, Nick was essentially second in command after the head nurse. Closing the door behind me, I spewed out my disgust for Patricia's husband, my fear for her emotional state, my pity for her suffering and loss of dignity. He listened quietly and sympathetically, letting me rant, until I had myself under control again and could go back to work.

Later that afternoon, Patricia's mother visited. I was standing just inside the room, talking quietly with Patricia and her mother, listening to them fuss about her husband. The door swung open to reveal Nick, standing with his hands on his hips, a cocky look in his eye.

"Looks pretty glum in this room. A bunch of long faces, for sure. I think ya'll need a little entertainment." Patricia, her mother, and I all stared at him, startled by his sudden appearance. He grinned, twitched his hips, and pulled the drawstring tie on his scrub pants suggestively. I laughed and looked over at Patricia as I said, "Sure, Nick, you're always threatening us like that. All talk and no action!" Patricia was watching him closely, a small grin on her face.

"Oh, yeah?" he challenged me. "No action, huh?" And swoosh! With one quick motion his pants were down around his ankles! We all three screamed simultaneously, Patricia almost coming off the bed! Then we realized he wasn't naked or even standing there in his shorts. The man had a second pair of scrubs on under the ones that now lay around his feet! We hollered and hooted and cursed him in an uproar of hilarity. Nick stood there, grinning like the Cheshire cat, absolutely smug with glee. It took an hour to settle down the unit, with everyone wanting to know what had happened. But the head nurse's half-hearted lecture about keeping the noise down and our unprofessional behavior did nothing to dampen my gladness. Patricia's somber mood, and her distress over her husband, had been lifted neatly and effectively by Nick's prank. What a marvelous therapist he was.

After five months, Patricia was finally delivered by cesarean. The water trapped in her swollen body flooded the operating table, spilling onto the floor in great washes and puddles. Her kidneys shut down briefly, necessitating dialysis. She was on the intensive-care unit for ten days, asking for pictures of her baby and visits from Nick and me when she was lucid. She let me kiss her and stroke her face, listening avidly to my descriptions of her tiny new son, so hard-won, who was thriving in the nursery.

I'll never forget what a joy it was to watch her walk down the hall toward me a month after her delivery. I'd never seen her fully upright, much less ambulatory. She was thinner. Her skin looked almost normal. Her body had a recognizable feminine shape. And her face was aglow as she talked to me about her baby. She was breast-feeding him, getting up in the middle of the night to pump or nurse. She was bursting with pride over him, and so happy to finally have a baby in her arms. I was in awe of her strength and her resilience, her stubborn determination to bear this child, at whatever cost to herself. She taught me more than she will ever know. I loved her.

One night late in May a couple of years later, I began to care for another unusual patient. As a tertiary care facility, this military hospital was equipped and staffed to handle the most complex, high-risk patients in its branch of the armed services. It was not unusual to receive patients from other parts of the world, flown in by helicopter or plane from military bases. Their care was complicated since they were cut off from their usual support systems, often alone, in a strange hospital with only minimal personal belongings; faced with serious complications in their pregnancies, and/or grave threats to the babies they harbored. But this woman was not a typical air-evac patient.

She was a beautiful twenty-four-year old from Germany. Her husband, Peter, who accompanied her to the hospital, was a lieutenant in the German air force. He had been stationed on the West Coast where, I learned, our air force was teaching the Germans how to fly "top gun" fighter planes. This young man had been involved in a nine-month training course in flight navigation. Because he was a participant in this cooperative military program, he and his dependents were entitled to military medical care while in the States. His wife Annelise, who had joined him in the United States, became pregnant with twins. Early in her pregnancy she was quite ill with pyelonephritis, a kidney infection. After a two-week hospitalization, she had recovered and her pregnancy had continued without further problems. Until now.

Having completed the training program, Peter and Annelise were on their way home to Germany, traveling in a military transport plane. As they crossed the continent, Annelise began to experience recurrent symptoms of pyelonephritis, along with premature labor contractions. She was six months pregnant, threatening to miscarry, and she spoke no English. Her husband communicated quite effectively, after his nine months working with American pilots. He was able to convey how sick she felt to the flight crew. Calls were made to the ground, to doctors at the nearest airbase and at our hospital. Before making the transoceanic leg of the trip, the pilot and crew turned the young couple over to military medical personnel at the airbase. An ambulance brought them to our obstetrical unit.

When I assumed her nursing care, Annelise had been on magnesium sulfate (MgSo4) therapy for most of the day. She had been given other, milder tocolytics—medications that suppress premature labor—in an unsuccessful attempt to stop her contractions. She was still having regular contractions every twenty minutes or so, with three grams of MgSo4 running in her IV. Mag sulfate is a heavy-duty medication given to premature laborers because it relaxes the smooth muscles of the body, including the uterus. It can be very effective as a tocolytic, but the recipient must be watched very closely for adverse effects. While many women receive "mag" without untoward consequences, the potential side effects can be unpleasant at best, and life-threatening at worst. Severe flushing or a sensation of warmth, nausea and vomiting, loss of appetite, slurred speech, depression or absence of reflexes, confusion, lethargy, pulmonary edema, decreased urinary output, respiratory impairment, and muscle weakness are possible when doses exceed two grams per hour. Annelise was getting three grams an hour and at times during the week I cared for her, she was receiving four grams.

The young woman in the bed was one sick cookie. I could tell by looking at her when I entered the room that the mag was taking a toll. She was lovely: wavy dark hair; golden tan skin from the beaches of the Pacific; a body that was lithe and athletic, firm and well-toned, without an ounce of fat. But she was sick. She lay unmoving in the bed, deep in the drugged-out sleep of a mag patient. IV tubing and monitor wires snaked from her body. Since she was unable to urinate on her own, a plastic catheter trailed from her bladder to a urine collection bag hanging on her bed. Her husband sat in a recliner at the bedside. We spoke briefly; I complimented him on his English. He was distracted, obviously concerned about his wife. I explained that the medicine she was receiving was responsible for her weakness, but that we were watching her carefully. He looked exhausted. He hadn't left her side except to snatch quick meals in the cafeteria.

The rest of the night he dozed in the chair, rousing briefly when I entered the room to take vital signs, check the monitor, empty the urine bag. Annelise opened her eyes when I touched her and shook her head when I asked if I could get anything for her, but it wasn't clear that she was really aware of my presence, much less if she could understand me. The next night the situation was the same. Peter had a room in the hotel the hospital owned for out-of-town family members. He used the room only for showers, spending all his time at his wife's bedside in the tiny labor room, cluttered beyond its capacity with an extra monitor for the second baby, IV poles and pumps, chair, table, and suitcases.

That second night I gave Annelise a bed bath, which had not been done in the three days since she'd been admitted. Together, Peter and I sponged her body and massaged moisturizing cream all over her. I marveled at her beauty and healthy look—so many women just let their bodies go in pregnancy and are physically unattractive because of stretch marks, skin disorders, and generally poor personal hygiene.

It was difficult handling Annelise's body because it was so limp in my hands. Here was this healthy young woman rendered totally helpless by the complications of her pregnancy and the treatment she was being given. The mag had wiped her out. She was unable to lift an arm, turn over in the bed, or eat, much less stand on her own. Peter and I changed her bed linens together, Peter following my instructions with an alacrity that was touching. He wanted so obviously to be of some use and touched and caressed his wife with great tenderness. He was quite businesslike in his interactions with the staff, asking appropriate questions about her care repeatedly until he felt he understood what was being done. Since she spoke no English, he was extremely reluctant to leave her alone and politely refused any suggestions that he go to his room to sleep.

The third night, I felt mounting concern about both of them. Annelise was not eating anything. She would vomit what little she managed to swallow and she was visibly losing weight. Peter looked seriously tired. He was a good-looking young man, blond as could be, with a grin that knocked me over the few times I saw it. But the strain, lack of sleep, separation from their families and country, and worry about his wife and two unborn kids were wearing him down. I was impressed by his calm manner, his ability to laugh and talk easily with the staff and Annelise—when she was conscious. I kept thinking how ungodly alone he must be feeling, even though he had been able to call Germany over military lines, to talk to his family and to his commanding officer about extending his leave.

I began to mother him, along with his wife. I asked about his meals, making him tell me what he'd been eating, and sending him for breakfast whether he wanted to go or not. I pleaded with him to give me his laundry, but he refused, explaining with a grin that there wasn't much of it and it gave him something to do to wash his socks and underwear in the sink. He did succumb to my bossiness on the fifth night. I made up the bed in an empty labor room and insisted he shower and sleep there. I promised to wake him if Annelise needed him, and guarded the door. He slept for six undisturbed hours, the longest rest he'd had thus far, and looked the better for it. I felt better, also, my maternal instincts having been satisfied, if only briefly.

I was charmed by him and worried sick about his wife. After six days of tocolysis, she was still contracting and still not eating. She was really sick from the mag. When she was awake, she wept silently and steadily over her condition and the hopelessness of it. The two babies were the only positive aspect of the whole situation: their little heartbeats just kept right on, with good variability and regular rhythms. I'd bathe her with Peter's help, taking off the monitors to give her belly a break, worrying about skin breakdown from the constant friction of the straps and monitors. I put two foam egg crate pads on her bed and fussed mightily at the other shifts if they didn't keep her body and bed linens clean. Finally I talked with the third-year resident in charge of her treatment.

"How long can we keep her on this stuff," I wanted to know, "if it's making her so weak? Did you know that she has eaten virtually nothing for more than five days now? I'm really worried about her; she's so weak she can't lift her head or arms from the bed, and I know she's losing weight."

The resident listened to me quietly. She was a tiny woman with a brusque manner that disguised her sensitivity. To my surprise, she picked up the phone and called her attending staff supervisor. She repeated my concerns about Annelise, saying that she felt we were doing Annelise more harm than good at this point. When she completed the phone call, she informed me that we were going to stop the tocolysis and let come what may, as soon as she alerted the NICU staff.

"The mag isn't stopping the contractions and we're starving this lady to death. I just can't justify the treatment any longer," she explained. I went off duty soon after our conversation, wondering if Annelise would deliver or if the paradoxical effect I'd seen with MgSo4 would occur: occasionally, patients who continued to contract through heavy doses of mag would stop when the medicine was discontinued. I hoped for that, giving Annelise's body time to incubate the babies a few days longer, since every day in utero gave them more of a chance at survival.

Annelise held onto those kids another day and night. We continued with round-the-clock tocolytic injections, which made her feel jumpy and irritable, but she was smiling and eating a bit here and there the next night. She was able to move around in the bed, and looked so much better, her vitality restored simply by removing the mag from her system. When I came to work the following night, her room was empty. "What happened? What happened?" I asked.

"They just finished the cesarean, Susie," the evening nurse told me. "She started contracting like crazy and dilated to six centimeters. They were going to try a vaginal delivery, but one of the babies' heart rate decelled, so they went ahead and cut her. The babies are okay, in the NICU, holding their own."

I went to see the babies. They were tiny, weighing in at just barely four pounds each, but were actually good-sized neonates for only thirty weeks and multiple gestation. Annelise had done a good job growing these kids, in spite of her difficult pregnancy. Every ounce they could claim would be important over the next days and weeks as they struggled to survive.

Peter returned to the labor deck a little while after I had arrived. He was grinning from ear to ear, wonderfully excited and relieved. He hugged me, talking about his boys and how glad he was that Annelise didn't have to suffer any longer. He moved around the room, collecting belongings, asking questions about her recovery, relating what the neonatologists had told him about the boys' status. His relief and his pride in his sons was great to see, even as I worried silently about their chances. They were both on ventilators. No one could say whether they would survive or not, and if they did, whether or not they would have permanent disabilities related to their prematurity. Even in the best of all worlds, they wouldn't be able to go home to Germany for a long time. I wondered about the logistics of all this: How would Peter be able to stay here? What happened when Annelise was ready for discharge? Was the German air force paying for all this? The cost of keeping those two little boys alive would be enormous; Peter was only a lieutenant. Would his leave be extended yet again? Would he and Annelise have to leave the States without their babies?

I said nary a word of this to him. Right now he needed to rejoice in the birth of his sons. He needed to get a good night's sleep. We talked about Annelise's recovery and what to expect each day as we moved her things to a postpartum room. He finally went off to the hotel to sleep, ebullient with happiness.

The next couple of days were uneventful. Annelise was recovering well, getting up to use the bathroom, ambulating to the nursery with Peter to see and touch her babies. She was quiet, shy because of the language barrier and uncomfortable with the lack of privacy in the four-woman room she shared with other cesarean patients. Peter hovered near her all through the long days, helping her in every way, unhappy when he was forced to leave her at night. He slept on a couch in the visitors' lounge, refusing to go to his hotel room because she might need him to translate during the night. I wanted to give them a private room so he could stay with her at night, but the ward was full and she was no longer a high-risk patient; I couldn't justify moving someone out of either of the two private rooms for her.

Peter and I chatted whenever we could. I was busy on L&D and had little time to visit, but I kept track of Annelise's progress. Unfortunately, she had a complication: when the catheter was removed from her bladder, she was unable to urinate. She had to be re-cathed, much to her distress, and the doctors were unable to tell her how long it might be before she would be free of the catheter. The resident speculated with me as to the cause: it might have been from having the catheter in for so long before she delivered or there might have been some surgical trauma to the nerves in the area. She would be wearing a urine bag on her leg and remain catheterized for at least ten days, to allow the nerves and muscles time to recover. The babies were doing well, monitored closely in the NICU, with frequent, long visits with their doting parents.

Peter visited the German consulate and spent a good bit of time negotiating with his command about his leave. Discussions were beginning with the neonatologists here and in Germany about the eventual air-evacuation of the twins. Peter was handling all the details easily. He maintained his cheerful attitude, to my amazement, as he struggled with a foreign language, city, transportation, and several bureaucracies. I had been thinking about what he and Annelise would do when she was ready for discharge. I planned to ask my sister Katy if she would mind me inviting them to stay at the town house we shared. Since my son was living with his father that year, only Rebecca was home with me, but she was leaving for summer camp within a few days. We also had another guest for the summer, David, a young Ugandan man. One of my brothers was involved with missionary work in Uganda. He had arranged for David to come to the United States several years earlier for an American education. Living with my brother and his wife, David had become a member of our family. Now he was spending the summer with Katy and me while he worked for the university where Katy was a professor. We were a little crowded, but when Rebecca left for camp, her room would be available for Peter and Annelise.

Just before change of shift in the morning of Annelise's fifth or sixth post-op day, Peter approached the desk where I was searching for someone's chart. He was dishevelled, sleep wrinkles on his face, hair askew, clothes rumpled. *Another night on the couch*, I thought. *Damn, this boy needs a better place to sleep. There are people in and out of that room all night, talking, smoking, and watching TV. This is just not right.* Worse yet, he was obviously upset, close to losing it. In spite of all he had been through, I hadn't yet seen him in such obvious distress.

"Someone took my kit," he said, voice trembling.

"What?"

"Someone took my kit. I was sleeping in there. On the couch. It was right by my head. When I wakened up, it was not there."

"You mean your suitcase was stolen?"

"No, not suitcase, my kit. How do you say it, my shaving kit. What can I do? Do I call the police?"

"Well, we can report it to the MPs, but damn, Peter, things are stolen around here all the time. Are you sure it's gone, did you look under the couch?"

Together we searched the room. His kit was gone, stolen while he slept. I was sick for him. Near tears, he stumbled down the hall to his wife's room. All that he had dealt with over the last two and a half weeks, all the strain and worry and fear and loneliness were etched in his posture, his face, his brimming eyes. I couldn't stand it. I called my sister immediately and asked her, without preface, if I could offer our home to him. Not surprisingly, she agreed. I went to Annelise's room and stepped behind the curtain enclosing her bed to find Peter with his head in his hands, Annelise watching him with confusion and concern in her eyes.

"Listen, I have an invitation for you. I doubt very seriously that you'll ever see your kit again, Peter, but I just hate to see you spend another night in that room. What I would like to do is to have you come home with me. I live with my sister and my daughter; we have plenty of room. I could drive you to the hospital in the morning after I get off work and bring you home in the evening before I have to be here again. In a few days, when Annelise is well enough to leave the hospital, she could come home with you to my house and you could both still spend the day here with the boys. I really would like to do this. It's not right for you to go on like this, with no privacy and no place to sleep. You need some good food and a decent bed. Will you tell Annelise what I've said?"

He stared at me, stunned, I think, by the invitation. Then he talked to his wife. She looked at him, at me, and back at him as he talked. Before he could say anything to me, I said, "I'll give you some time to discuss it. We would love to have you both, and I'll be glad to do whatever I can to see that you can be here as much as possible."

I left them, feeling good about making the offer. I just couldn't stop imagining what it would feel like to be in another country, going through these life-changing and life-threatening events without anyone to help me. How frightened and alone I would feel. He had been managing so well, but enough was enough. The babies weren't anywhere near stable enough to transport; their parents needed a place to stay, a refuge. How could I not offer?

When I returned to the room, Peter thanked me and accepted my invitation. Annelise held his hand, stroking it lovingly and smiled her thanks to me. We talked again about the logistics of the arrangement, reassuring her that he would be there for her all day. She said she wasn't afraid to be alone at night, she didn't need much help now, and she wanted him to be comfortable.

That night I picked him up and took him home. Katy, Rebecca, and David welcomed him casually, making him feel at home, and he settled in without difficulty. I demonstrated how to use the washer and dryer and pointed out the grocery store and post office down the block. I told him he was welcome to buy whatever food he liked, but that when we cooked, which wasn't on a regular basis, he would be expected to share our meals. He offered to pay rent, but I refused, explaining that he was a guest in my home, not a boarder. We agreed that he would be responsible for long-distance phone calls and gas for the car, but nothing more. I laughed as I told him I'd always believed that Americans were supposed to be famous for their hospitality and that this was a chance for me to prove it. His gratitude was nice, but knowing he was sleeping and eating well was the real reward.

Five days later, Annelise came home with us. I had been lending Peter my car, since I slept during the day. He was reliable about meeting my schedules, drove well, and fit into our weird family as if he belonged there. I couldn't help but giggle with my sister Katy about the neighbors' bewilderment over who actually lived in our town house. Two single women, a teenage girl, a handsome blond young man, and a very black, stunningly good-looking African. Then Annelise showed up. Shortly after that, the resident who had been caring for her spent three days with us before leaving town, after completing her residency! It was wild and so much fun. Peter and David teased and joked with each other, playing with the English language and its inconsistencies as only two bright, non-English minds could. Our dinners were long and hilarious and everyone fell in love with Peter's clowning. He could make faces that made our sides split and was unmerciful in his teasing of Annelise. She would laugh and hit him, fussing at him in German. She understood a great deal of our speech, but was reluctant to talk, shyly insisting she didn't have the words.

They spent long hours with their babies. I visited with them on my days off and was touched by their interaction with the boys. Peter was incredibly gentle and loving with them, not at all intimidated by their smallness or the wires and tubes attached to them. They were progressing beautifully, off the ventilators within a few days, and into the intermediate nursery for "feed and grow" time within a week. Annelise would hold each of them, singing to them while caressing their faces and bodies. Peter took many pictures and followed their treatments and weight gain closely.

When they weren't in the nursery, Peter and Annelise went sightseeing. They drove all over the city, saw all the tourist attractions and looked for baby stores, delighted with U.S. prices compared to Germany's. Katy took them on a hike up a local "mountain," to my absolute horror walking Annelise all the way to the top. She had forgotten that Annelise was a cesarean mother, only two weeks post-op! I was frantic that the exertion might have hurt her, but her youth and exuberant good health served her well and she had no ill effects from the climb. The catheter was removed a week after she was discharged and she was able to pee, so we were all happy!

As I had anticipated, the gossip at work was rampant. I ignored it, largely, responding to nasty remarks with elaborate accounts of wild orgies, assuring the gossips that we even had animals involved, which I knew they would appreciate. That shut them up, at least around me. One of the LPNs, my friend Mrs. Strong, asked me how I could take a German military man into my home. "We fought those people in the War. He could be your enemy if we have another war. You don't know anything about him. He could steal you blind. Why would you want to do this?"

"Look, Mrs. Strong, our own government is teaching him how to navigate fighter planes. His country is one of our country's allies. Besides, I'm not having him stay with me because he's German. I don't care if he's an Eskimo. He's in a foreign country. His babies were born prematurely and are at risk; his wife has been gravely ill. He's been alone, without help, for long enough. It's the right thing to do. My mother would say it's the Christian thing to do. It makes me feel good to help them. It's a way for me to show that Americans are good people, at least some of us . . . Why is this so hard to understand? Yeah, he could steal me blind. I have to trust my instincts about him, though. My mother was always taking in people who needed help. Sometimes it cost her, but most of the time it ended up being truly fulfilling. I'm just doing what I've been taught, is all. Besides, Peter is really funny and great to be with. He entertains us all, and we're really enjoying having them." The payback for me was large: I have friends in Germany now. I had touched two strangers and been given a brief look at what their lives were like. That was enough. My mother's example had served me well.

I was sharing a special time with Peter and Annelise. He was standing in my kitchen when he was told, long-distance, that he had been promoted. He jumped to attention and saluted me, grinning wildly, jabbering away in German. Annelise's mother told me, through Peter, that their home would always be open to me; that I was a very special person to take them in; that people in Germany would never be so kind and generous; and that she was very grateful to me for taking care of her daughter.

The three of us went shopping together on their last day in America and I bought baby clothes for the boys. Annelise and I tried on jeans, laughing and gesticulating about our butts and how the jeans looked on us. We had coffee together at a café in a mall, and shared our personal stories. They told me about how they met, how in love they were, and about their plans for the future. Watching them with their boys was always an emotional experience. These tiny new babies with their lovely parents: How would they grow? What would they be? Would I ever see them again? I knew I would miss Annelise and Peter and was sorry once again that after sharing the beginning I would not be able to follow this family, except long-distance, as they grew together.

    After much planning and scrambling for passports and documents of all sorts, my Germans finally left the States. I dropped them, loaded down with tons of newly purchased items, luggage, and souvenirs, in front of the hospital so they could catch the bus to the airport with their boys for the overseas flight. Two nurses and two neonatologists accompanied them; the flight was long and uneventful. I heard from Peter twice, ecstatic reports about the boys after an initial difficult period. Several undiagnosed problems surfaced in Germany and they were in the hospital for another month. He sent me money for the phone bill and praised Annelise's mothering. He was filled with joy in his "two dwarfs," as he called his sons. All in all, this was an unqualified success story; I was enriched by it more than I could have imagined.

Chapter Fourteen

FRUSTRATION

My first four years as a L&D nurse were a time of learning. In that time, I became quite proficient in my work. I could perform a plethora of technical nursing tasks with competent efficiency. I knew what I was doing and how to do it. However, the more confident I became in my abilities and skills, the more questions and nagging doubts disturbed me. This is a paradox experienced by most working people: first you learn how to do your job; only then can you begin to question why you're supposed to do it the way it's always been done. Recognizing this phenomenon wasn't difficult, but actually doing something about my questions and resolving my doubts has been an arduous, largely unsuccessful exercise.

In the early years, I didn't actively question many of the policies, procedures, and treatments that shaped the manner in which we obstetrical workers cared for our patients. To be sure, I wasn't thrilled with the high-tech, pathological approach we took with patients. I had been, after all, a natural childbirth mother and a prepared childbirth instructor. My personal philosophy was one of nonintervention in the birth process. But I was a nurse working in a high-risk obstetrical unit. I was expected to care for women with multiple perinatal complications, so I willingly suspended my personal inclinations in order to provide high-tech care.

Gradually, of course, I began to grow uncomfortable with my voluntary participation in this care. Everywhere I looked there were examples of the problems inherent in hospital obstetrical care. There were three main areas of concern, to my mind. First is that most basic of conflicts, which infects virtually all organizational providers of human services. This is the conflict between meeting the needs of the people, in this case, the patients, for whom the organization—the hospital—works and meeting the needs of the people who work for the organization, in this case, the obstetrical staff. Job satisfaction versus job mission.

The second problem arises from the two contradictory approaches to the actual management of childbirth, that is, the pathological/technological model versus the natural/noninterventional model. The third problem is a spin-off of the second: the very nature of current obstetrical care, with its ever-increasing technological advances, creates a seemingly impenetrable barrier between the technologically adept caregiver and the technologically ignorant care receiver. Clumsily stated here, evidence of these problems has echoed throughout this book. But it took years of exposure to these problems for me to reach the levels of frustration and disenchantment that demoralize me so today.

Ideally, the aim of obstetrical care is to serve the patient. All the skills, technology, and experience we bring to the bedside should be directed, first and foremost, at causing no harm. The next goal should be to meet the patient's needs in an appropriately caring and careful manner that will result in improvement in the patient's status. Unfortunately, many of the obstetrical routines and procedures are not designed with that goal in mind. They are used because "it's easier" and/or "just in case."

For instance: We want to alleviate the mother's labor pain; we have marvelous medications and epidurals to accomplish just that. But the mother doesn't usually know ahead of time that getting an epidural will mean that she won't be able to urinate by herself; that she will have a blood pressure cuff on her arm, EKG leads on her body, and a pulse oximeter, which measures her oxygenation levels, on her finger or toe. She will have little or no muscular control of her legs; her ability to push may be reduced; her baby runs an increased risk of a forceps, vacuum, or cesarean delivery; and she may wind up with an oxytocin-augmented labor. It's "easier" for everyone involved, mother and medical staff, to give the epidural. I'm not even going to mention how much more expensive it is.

But I have to ask, what if women understood these things long before they began labor? What if nurses were trained to truly coach a woman successfully through her labor, reducing the need for epidurals? What if nurses were not required to care for more than one laboring mother at a time, so they could actually concentrate on alleviating much of the pain of labor without resorting automatically to technology and medication? So much of what we do in caring for a laboring woman in the hospital is for *our* convenience, or "just in case."

For instance: There is much controversy in the obstetrical world about the efficacy of electronic fetal monitoring. It is not definitively clear that monitoring actually improves maternal/neonatal morbidity and mortality—that it results in fewer complications for the mother and baby, up to and including death. It has been known for years that monitoring has contributed to the rapid rise in cesarean rates. These issues continue to be studied and argued over, but practitioners on obstetrical units routinely use monitoring on all patients, whether it's warranted or not, because it's easier to follow the course of the labor if you can watch the continual printout of contractions and the fetal heartbeat instead of listening intermittently with a stethoscope. It's also done just in case a lawsuit is filed sometime in the next twenty years.

For instance: Most normally laboring women do not require an IV during their labor. It's "just in case" we need to give some medicine rapidly, "just in case" the mother gets dehydrated, "just in case" we need to do an emergency cesarean. These are all perfectly valid reasons for an IV, but why does that mean that every woman must have an IV? I've spent some highly frustrating times fighting to get an IV into a woman's arm while she thrashes around the bed, her baby crowning as I jab for a vein. There is absolutely no reason for an IV in such a case. The rationale is that the patient needs an IV for a dose of Pitocin after delivery to keep her uterus firmly contracted so she won't bleed. But Pitocin can be given intramuscularly, if necessary. If the uterus is massaged gently and breast-feeding is initiated right after delivery, Pitocin isn't usually even needed. Stimulation of the nipples with suckling results in uterine contractions, the body's built-in physiological mechanism for releasing oxytocic hormones to contract the uterus. But "it's easier" for the nurses to squirt some artificial oxytocin into an IV bag. And the question of speedy access to the vein is almost always moot: when an IV is needed in a hurry, it gets done in a hurry, believe me! Adrenaline is a powerful aid in doing what has to be done stat!

I had a fight with an anesthesiologist one night over an IV. We had the patient on the delivery table. The baby was crowning. An anesthesiologist was present because the mother had received an epidural: policy dictated his presence at every epidural-treated delivery. While pushing, the mother had popped out her IV. This woman was in some pain and moved her arms around a good bit during her pushing. She needed to pull against her husband's hand or the table grips in order to push effectively. The anesthesiologist kept asking her to hold her arm out straight so he could start a new IV. He missed the vein three times and was getting increasingly irritated with the woman because she couldn't hold still. Standing on the other side of the table, I got pissed when I saw him actually wrenching at her arm, yelling at her to hold still, while the obstetrician and the other nurse were yelling at her to push. This anesthesiologist had actually shoved the husband away from the table so he could get at this woman's arm.

"Why don't you wait until she delivers?" I asked.

"No, dammit! She needs an IV now!" he snarled at me.

"But the baby's already almost out!" I insisted. "What does she need an IV for now?"

"If she needs suturing, I can't give her any more anesthesia without an IV, that's why!" he shouted at me. I shut up, refusing to be drawn into a full-blown battle in front of the patient. But he could have waited, dammit! If she needed suturing after delivery and a local anesthetic didn't suffice, then an IV could be inserted, quietly and calmly, instead of assaulting her during these harried moments of intense effort. *Her* comfort, *her* efforts, *her* needs were not paramount to this anesthesiologist. He wanted an IV and he wanted it now!

For instance: Eating during labor is a hospital "no-no." There are legitimate reasons for this rule, but I still have questions about it. Supposedly, a woman shouldn't eat because digestive processes slow down during labor and anything in her stomach is likely to be vomited up. Vomiting while you're in labor is no fun, of course, but neither is being starved for twelve to thirty-six hours. The two big hamburgers I scarfed down a couple of hours before I went into active labor with Rebecca never even threatened to reappear. I've cared for women who have eaten just before entering the hospital but never once vomited during their subsequent labors and I've cared for women who vomited through their entire labors, even though they'd had nothing to eat for hours. I just clean up the mess and go on from there.

Anesthesiologist have laid down the law against eating "just in case." If a cesarean is necessary and the patient vomits during surgery, she might breathe in some of the vomitus, which can be dangerous. This is an understandable concern, but in eight years of attending cesareans, I have seen many women vomit, whether they've eaten prior to surgery or not, and in each case, the attending anesthesiologist adeptly and efficiently suctioned away the vomitus. That's one of the reasons the anesthesiologist stands at the woman's head during the surgery, monitoring her every move and vital sign. That's why we have suction equipment lying beside her cheek throughout the operation. The risk of aspiration does exist, but it is minimal because of all the built-in safeguards. So maybe this rule could be relaxed a little, huh? For the mother's comfort during her labor? A little juice, maybe? Or some soup and crackers? Do we have to make her weak and sick from hunger for the convenience of the anesthesiologist and for a "just-in-case" scenario?

It's not only just-in-case scenarios that increase my frustration levels. It's not just the reluctance of medical personnel to attend properly to the patient when such attention might mean the nurse or doctor has to skip meal or a break. It's the combination of these problems that drive me crazy. And the worst aspect of our work is the way the technology and science of medicine actually separate us, physically and psychologically, from our patients. The case of Mrs. Plummer is a perfect example of all of this.

Mrs. Plummer was to be induced because of severe preeclampsia. A twenty-four-hour collection of her urine had revealed five grams of protein per liter, an ominous sign since the normal amount is less than a gram. Her blood pressure was borderline, with only two elevated pressures, and she had minimal edema, or swelling caused by fluid retention, but the large amount of protein couldn't be ignored. This was her first pregnancy, after ten years of infertility. Proteinuria, edema, and elevated blood pressures, along with primiparity (first pregnancy), are all indicators of possible preeclampsia. In current obstetrical practice, any one sign or a combination of the three calls for treatment of the mother with magnesium sulfate and the delivery of the fetus, particularly if gestational age is great enough to ensure a reasonably healthy fetus. Mrs. Plummer was only thirty-five weeks along, but the doctors were fearful of her proteinuria, thus the decision to induce.

The problem with inducing labor early is that the cervix hasn't been hormonally primed. It is still thick, long, and closed, a barred doorway to the interior. Before it can dilate, it must be softened artificially, via prostaglandin suppositories or gel. This can be a long and unpleasant process. The prostaglandins cause contractions, along with possible fever, nausea, vomiting, and diarrhea. So Mrs. Plummer probably had an ordeal ahead of her.

When I arrived for work at eleven that night, in my fifth year of nursing, Mrs. Plummer had been in bed since noon. She had an IV with mag sulfate piggybacked into the "maintenance" fluid of 5 percent dextrose and Lactated Ringers, the only sustenance she would receive during her induction. The dextrose provided her with glucose for energy; the Lactated Ringers hydrated her with fluids and electrolytes. She had a catheter inserted into her bladder. Fetal and uterine monitor belts wrapped her belly. She was expected to remain on her left side as much as possible, to lower her blood pressure and provide better circulation to the uterus and fetus. The prostaglandin suppositories were being inserted into her vagina every four hours.

Mrs. Plummer had been contracting all day and had received several doses of a narcotic to help her with the pain. Her nursing care for the night involved taking hourly vital signs, emptying urine from the collection bag, dipsticking her urine to monitor protein levels, and giving narcotics to manage her pain. Another nurse was assigned to her for the shift, so I had little interaction with her; I only heard the nurse's comments about her need for pain medication. The nurse-anesthetist convinced the obstetrical residents to allow him to insert an epidural catheter so "when she gets active, or you start Pitocin, we can just inject it without any fuss." No one could predict how long it would take for the prostaglandins to sufficiently soften her cervix so that Pitocin could be started for active labor. It could be a few hours, or two or more days.

The following night when I listened to report, I was distressed to hear that Mrs. Plummer was still receiving the prostaglandin suppositories. Her cervix had changed very little over the past thirty hours. The cervix had finally dilated, to a scant two centimeters, and Pitocin had just been started. She was described by the staff as being "weird" and "wimpy," crying and fighting the cervical exams, showing little stoicism. I listened to the criticism silently, not having any personal experience with this lady. Who knew? Maybe she was one of those difficult patients, or maybe she was behaving appropriately, given what she had been through during the past day and night.

I was assigned to Mrs. Plummer for this shift. When her nurse gave me a more detailed report, she expressed concern about this woman's treatment course.

"Her blood pressure has been completely within normal limits. She only has a trace of protein in her urine. Maybe she isn't preeclamptic. Maybe we should leave her alone. She's exhausted and has been in a lot of pain all day."

"She still has the epidural catheter in, right? Why haven't we gotten it injected?"

"The resident on tonight says she not dilated enough yet."

"Well, so what? We're inducing her, anyway. If we're 'pitting' her, why the hell not? She's going to have contractions anyway, so it's not like we're going to shut down her labor if we get her relief with the epidural."

"Yeah, I know. Maybe you should ask the doctors about this."

I conferred with the intern and the third-year resident. "Can you tell me why we're treating her so aggressively? Are we sure she's preeclamptic?"

The resident, a courteous, gentle man, reviewed her labs and history with me, explaining that the proteinuria simply could not be ignored, along with other suspicious changes in her liver function tests, further indication of probable severe preeclampsia. I appreciated his polite justification of the necessity for induction; I had no desire or reason to challenge his diagnosis. I just needed a reasonable explanation of her treatment before I attempted to interact with her. I asked him about getting her pain relief through the epidural. Without realizing that the second-year resident had already refused to call the anesthesiologist until her cervix was dilated four centimeters, he agreed readily to an epidural dose. "Sure, get her dosed, there's no reason for her to be uncomfortable as long as the Pitocin is stimulating regular contractions."

Aha! A major improvement, I thought as I went in to start my shift with Mrs. Plummer. After introducing myself, I explained that we were calling the anesthesiologist to inject the epidural. "Once we get you comfortable, I'd like to give you a bed bath and put an egg crate on your bed with fresh linens, okay? An egg crate is a foam pad that will make this awful bed at least a little bit more comfortable."

We talked briefly as I emptied her urine collection bag, dipsticked the urine for protein, checked her IVs, and the monitor strip, making notes on my scrub pants of her intake and output, and her vital signs. A big woman, tall and heavy with pregnancy, she looked exhausted, her gray-blond hair sweaty and matted on her neck and forehead, face shiny with perspiration, dark circles under her pale gray eyes. Her husband didn't look much better. Wrinkled clothes hung loosely on his large frame. His curly, gray-streaked hair was rumpled and his face sported a two-day stubble of silver whiskers. He'd been vigilant at her side the entire time and was wrecked from no sleep and concern over her pain. "Have you eaten today?" I asked him. "Would you like to shower? I can get you some scrubs; they're really more comfortable than jeans."

Over the next two hours we accomplished a lot. Mr. Plummer was dispatched to the doctors' locker room with towels, soap, a disposable razor, and fresh scrubs. He reappeared, much refreshed, after a long hot shower. Mrs. Plummer's epidural was dosed and a continuous infusion started by the anesthesiologist, to keep her pain-free for several hours. I gathered fresh linens, basins, soap, hand lotion, and an egg crate. Together, her husband and I gave Mrs. Plummer a complete bed bath and then changed her bed, rolling her back and forth to get the foam padding and sheet beneath her, smoothed and tucked in tidily, with proper hospital corners. Her husband rubbed lotion all over her arms, legs, and tummy as I cleaned up the bath debris.

"Where have you been the past thirty-some hours, Susie? Oh, I feel like a human being again. You are an angel!"

"No," I explained. "It's just that most patients on this unit aren't here for very long, so bed baths and clean linens aren't routine. I'm sorry you've gone so long without getting refreshed, but the staff usually focuses on the labor progress and sometimes we forget to do the simple comfort measures that make this whole process a little more bearable. I'm just glad the epidural has worked and you're not in pain. Now your job is to sleep. Nothing else. I want you to settle in and try hard to really sleep. Before you know it, you'll be completely dilated and have to push and I want you to have some energy for that, okay? I'll be in every hour tonight to do my little busy work, and I'll watch you and the baby on the monitor, but please try to ignore me if you can."

I got a pillow and blanket for her husband, did the hourly check, adjusted the monitors, and turned off the lights. As I did my charting at the nurses' station, I felt an undeniable sense of accomplishment. All I had done was provide simple basic nursing care. I had attended to Mrs. Plummer's physical comfort through pain relief, a bath, a foam pad, and clean sheets. That was all; just the basics. But to the Plummers I was an angel of mercy, the first person in thirty hours to do more than push narcotics into her IV or bring her ice chips. The neglect was not intentional. No one could have predicted that it would take so long for her cervix to ripen and begin dilating. The nurses on previous shifts might very well have considered a bath but decided against "disturbing" Mrs. Plummer. But it was so gratifying to go into that room and effect such a change in her physical and emotional state with a few simple actions. I felt rewarded: this was one of those times when being a nurse was fulfilling.

For the next five and half hours I guarded my patient. With the ultrasound, I chased the baby all over her belly several times, to keep it on the monitor, but she slept soundly most of the night, even when I fumbled with monitor straps and took her blood pressure. Her husband snored softly in the recliner at her bedside. All my mothering instincts were satisfied: my "family" in the cramped little labor room rested quietly while I stood watch over them during the wee hours of the night.

At 0545, the second-year resident wanted to check Mrs. Plummer's progress. The cervical exam revealed that she had dilated only one more centimeter, to three, during her hours of sleep. The doctor explained that she could now rupture the membranes: she wanted to attach a fetal scalp electrode to the baby to get a more reliable tracing of the baby's heartbeat. The artificial rupture of membranes was duly performed, scalp electrode attached, and the doctor left the room. Within minutes Mrs. Plummer was crying in pain from contractions. Even though the continuous epidural was still delivering anesthesia to the epidural space, she was really feeling the contractions now. I suspected the epidural catheter had been dislodged during the many hours it had been in place and might not be functioning efficiently enough to counter the stronger contractions she was experiencing. When I asked for the on-call anesthesiologist I was informed that he was in a delivery and thus unavailable for Mrs. Plummer.

For thirty minutes, Mrs. Plummer sobbed through contractions that came every two minutes. I held her hand, made her breathe with me as much as she could, and kept asking for the anesthesiologist. He was required to stay in the delivery room until that patient's care was complete. The baby had been delivered but a medical student was repairing the episiotomy under the resident's instruction, so a normally brief procedure stretched into a lengthy teaching session. Meanwhile Mrs. Plummer became increasingly distraught, wailing inarticulately about not being able to take it any longer. Her husband and I struggled ineffectively to comfort her.

As I leaned out of the doorway into the hall, asking about the anesthesiologist for the third or fourth time, I spied an unknown man in scrubs standing at the anesthesia cart, filling a syringe and checking supplies. The nurse at the desk told me to ask this person if he could help: he was the nurse anesthetist on duty for the day shift. I approached him, asking, "Can you give me a hand with this patient? The anesthesiologist is in the DR and she needs to have her epidural reinjected."

"I'm not on yet," was his terse reply. Stung by his abruptness and feeling defeated by my inability to comfort Mrs. Plummer, I turned back into the labor room to struggle through another contraction and more sobs. A few minutes later, the nurse anesthetist, evidently having changed his mind, reinjected the epidural. Another fifteen minutes of uncontrolled, sobbing contractions passed as we waited for the anesthetic to take effect. The nurse anesthetist tried to determine the level of anesthesia by pricking Mrs. Plummer with a needle, asking her which leg was more numb. Mrs. Plummer was unable to reply coherently: "I don't know. The left is sharper than the right, no, I can't feel the left."

The nurse anesthetist rolled his eyes at me and said sharply, "Well, look, you've got three options. You either wait for this dose to take effect; we take out this catheter and put in a new one; or you do without."

"Doing without is not an option," I stated flatly.

Mrs. Plummer simply cried. The nurse anesthetist stormed out of the room. I followed him into the hall, where he gestured to me to come closer as he walked away from the labor room door. To my astonishment, he suddenly whirled around, pointed his finger at me and, in a harsh whisper snarled at me, "I'm *not* fucking with her today!"

"Now look," I replied, holding up my hands in a peace-making gesture.

"No, goddammit! She doesn't know what she wants or feels. She can't even answer a simple question about her pain level for me, she's so out of control."

"You wait just one minute!" I interjected firmly. "This lady has been in that bed for close to forty hours now, contracting the entire time. She's had nothing to eat, precious little sleep, and more than enough pain. . . ."

As I spoke, I could feel my face getting red. The nurse-anesthetist realized I was working up to a towering rage: he began to backtrack. "Well, look, see," he hemmed and hawed. "I just don't think the catheter is any good and if she's gonna get cut . . . she hasn't made much progress . . . then we probably should just redo the epidural."

"That may be the case, I don't know, but she can't take much more. She doesn't have any reserves left." I walked away, furious.

It was 0700, time for report, the end of my shift. The anesthesiologist was still in the delivery room. As I gave report to the oncoming shift, I emphasized strongly my concern for Mrs. Plummer's ability to endure much more. Then I sought out the resident assuming charge of the labor deck for the day. I outlined my concerns to him, stressing the need for pain relief for this patient. He listened attentively and assured me that the day team would be certain to take care of her needs. It was now 0730 and Mrs. Plummer was still sobbing and writhing with each contraction, her husband futilely, frantically trying to soothe her. My relief, the day-shift nurse, came into the room to assume Mrs. Plummer's care. I made my good-byes to her husband and gave Mrs. Plummer a few final supportive words, stroking her legs and encouraging her to hang in just a little bit longer.

I left at 0745, feeling such outrage that I don't remember driving home. What were we doing, in the name of obstetrical care, to this woman? Forty hours of lying on a hot plastic mattress; catheters in her arm, urethra, and back; no food; constant interruptions by strangers who unceremoniously handled her body, told her in what position to lie, poked and prodded her belly, thrust their fingers into her vaginal canal, gave her medicines that only increased her pain—all in the effort to deliver her baby. This baby, this ultimate outcome, that she had tried to conceive for ten years, was now supposedly in jeopardy because of preeclampsia and was being forced to emerge five weeks early, with all the attendant risks of prematurity lying in wait.

Despite all our good intentions to deliver her baby safely, we had been engaged in a systematic torture of the mother. Rotating medical personnel, indifference to her discomfort, false expectations about how swiftly her cervix would change, differences in treatment philosophies of the various doctors in charge of her care, and simple neglect had all contributed to a nightmare of physical and psychic discomfort and startling, unremitting pain.

The five to six hours of intermittent sleep following her bath were the only relief she had been afforded by her obstetrical team. To be hurled back into the agony of active labor after those hours of pain-free rest was simply more than she could tolerate. My rage grew out of my knowledge of what she had been coping with, my frustration with the system that made "continuity of care" so difficult to achieve with a patient whose labor extended over several shifts and my fear that she would be forced to go on for hours more of this hard labor. If she was only three centimeters at 0545, and it took so many hours to get that far, she might have many more hours to endure, or even a cesarean to crown this horror.

But my real fury was focused on the nurse-anesthetist and his outrageous refusal to "fuck with" this patient. This nurse was just beginning his shift. He was just coming on, after a good night's sleep. His sole task for the day was to provide pain relief for laboring mothers. That's all. Just be there to give epidurals to women in labor and attend their deliveries. That was his job, his mission for the day, goddammit! And his very first interaction with a patient resulted in him losing his temper because the patient wasn't cooperative. Oh, I was angry! Oh, I am still angry! There is absolutely no excuse for this kind of behavior, for this kind of expectation of the patient. There is no excuse for the mind-set that thinks the patient should be cooperative and make our job easier, and if she doesn't, she's a bad patient that we have to "fuck with."

It's our job. We work with people all day, all night, who are in pain, who are belligerent, uncooperative, out of control, mean, nasty, dirty, smelly, etc. We get tired, we get frustrated. We try to do a good job, and the patient can make that so difficult sometimes. But the bottom line is that we are there to provide care for the patient. To *care* for the patient: to attend to her needs and her safety and her comfort. We are *not* there to care for ourselves, to ignore the patient's pain or fear or unpleasantness because it's too much trouble or too messy or too tiring. That nurse-anesthetist's attitude enraged me and my anger generalized to blanket all of the staff and myself with culpability in the horror of this patient's treatment. All my efforts to make her comfortable the night before were for naught, because here she was back in agony again, and the people who were supposed to help her were unavailable or indifferent to her because they hadn't been with her all night or the day before.

I was just as guilty because I left. I went home. I talked to the people who would be working with her, did my best to impress upon them how great her need for help really was, and then gave up and went home. I couldn't do anything else for her. I couldn't physically pull the anesthesiologist out of the delivery room to come to her room. I couldn't redose her epidural myself or give her any medication without the doctor's orders. I couldn't stand at the nurses' station and scream at everyone to *"Do something! For God's sake, do something!"* I could only hope that the resident would hear my concern and take action. So I went home, raging and crying and wanting never to be a nurse again. I felt so helpless, after feeling so good about the comfort I had given her earlier in the night.

I didn't sleep well, waking with Mrs. Plummer's image in my mind repeatedly during the day, tossing and turning with my frustration and anger. When I returned to work that night I learned that she had delivered a baby girl at 0910. She had progressed from three centimeters at 0545 to delivery in a little over three hours. The agony she was experiencing with her contractions as I left that morning was not surprising for active, rapid labor. Nurses' notes stated that she had obtained relief via the epidural at 0845. I went in to congratulate her and listened to her glowing reports about her beautiful little girl, both of us happy that her ordeal had finally come to an end. I said nothing to her about her labor, just agreeing with her that she had progressed far more rapidly than we had expected. She thanked me again for my help, telling me that my name was certainly appropriate, because I was truly a jewel. We hugged and laughed and I admired pictures of her baby. She endured twenty-four more hours of mag sulfate therapy, a postpartum hemorrhage, and continued complications from the preeclampsia that kept her on IVs and in the hospital for five more days.

I had no further contact with her, but she remains in my mind as a vivid example of all that is inherently frustrating and difficult about high-tech obstetrical care in our hospitals today. She suffered greatly at our hands. She got her baby, that longed-for infant, but she paid an enormous price, and we, her caretakers, made her pay it. While it is true that she or the baby might have died without our expertise, she should not have had to suffer so much.

I know there are many times in the practice of medicine in which pain is inflicted necessarily in the name of treatment, but this case was not one of those times. Her pain, exhaustion, and stress was nosocomial, or hospital-caused. We could and should have accomplished her inducement without torturing her and without blaming her when she cried out for pain relief.

Sometimes events unfold in such a manner that it isn't until the case is completed that I find myself seriously questioning the care we have given a patient. One night at this same hospital, I assumed responsibility for a second-time mother who was near the end of the first stage of labor. Working as an agency nurse at the time, I was relatively new to this hospital. Although I had five years of experience, I was not well known to the residents running the L&D unit, which meant that I was less likely to question or challenge their decisions.

My patient, Melody, was young, just twenty-three years old. When I met her in the darkened, windowless labor room, I saw a plump, placid-faced girl. Because she had a continuous epidural, she was comfortable and calm, smiling benignly up at me from her bed. She reclined on her side under smooth sheets, the monitors, the IV and epidural pumps ticking away. My overall impression of the room and its inhabitants—patient, husband, grandparents—was one of tidy tranquility. Melody's wavy black hair was unmussed and her face looked as if it had just been washed. Her husband and parents were trim, attractive, neatly attired folks. The room didn't even smell bad: the usual malodorous air of a long-occupied labor room was absent. Hours of controlled breathing usually created a cloud of god-awful bad breath, from the patient and her coach. The stench of human feces, blood, urine, mucus, and amniotic fluid, along with the medicinal odors of spilled antibiotics, IV fluids, and plastic sterile wrappings combined with halitosis and inadequate ventilation to produce an odiferous environment to which I was long accustomed. But there was no cloud of vapors here. Melody's nurse had kept her room in good order, promptly removing trash and bedpans and goopy linens, and Melody's labor had been a relatively short and peaceful one, thanks to her early epidural.

According to the intern who examined her, Melody's cervix was almost completely dilated. The off-going nurse grinned at me as she said, "You're going to have a delivery soon." She knew I enjoyed the birth process. I expected an hour or two of pushing and then a baby. Little did I know that I would spend the entire shift with this one patient.

The intern's cervical exam was incorrect. The first-year resident pronounced the patient to be only eight centimeters dilated. Two hours later, with Pitocin augmentation, Melody was finally ready to push. Her epidural had just been redosed; Melody assured me that she was pain-free but could feel the tightening of the contractions. Before we started pushing, her bladder needed to be emptied since she hadn't voided or been cathed for several hours.

A full bladder can impede the baby's progress through the birth canal. I tried three times to empty her bladder. On the first two tries, the catheter wouldn't advance past the baby's head into the bladder. The third attempt yielded only 200 cc of urine, a small amount considering Melody had received almost 3,000 cc of IV fluid. Her urethral meatus, the opening to the urethra, was swollen and traumatized by the catheterizing.

Melody pushed for almost two hours. Even though she could feel the contractions, she was unable to coordinate her muscles in such a fashion as to be successful. The baby's head sat stuck at a plus-2 station (a measurement of position in the pelvis: the baby crowns at plus-3), not budging when she bore down. The residents opted for a surgical delivery, convinced that after no progress for almost two hours she wasn't going to be able to deliver vaginally.

When I inserted the indwelling urinary catheter that would remain in place for twenty-four hours after surgery, there was bleeding from the previously traumatized urethra. We took Melody back to the OR and prepped her for surgery. The first-year resident did the surgery, his first cesarean, under the guidance and assistance of the second-year. It took him fifteen minutes to get down to the uterus. Under skilled surgical hands, this requires five minutes or so. The third-year resident was standing by, observing. She was obviously unhappy about the length of time required to get into the uterus. As the resident carefully knifed an incision across the lower segment of the uterus, I put on a sterile glove. It was probable that after two hours of pushing, the baby's head would be jammed fast into the pelvis, requiring my hand to push against it from the vagina, as the resident lifted from the inside of the uterus.

Both of the residents performing the surgery tried to lift the baby out, unsuccessfully, so I stooped down, wriggled my way under all the sterile drapes, squeezed my hand between her strapped legs and found the vaginal opening. Inserting my fingers, I felt the resident's fingers through a thin membrane that I realized was the wall between the vagina and the rectum. I wasn't in her vagina: I was in her rectum. Without thinking I slid my fingers out and up into the vagina, pushing against the baby's head. It was wedged in hard, the pushing efforts having created a sort of suction that we had to break in order to get the baby out. My contaminated hand joined the resident's as we worked to release the head. The baby was delivered.

Now we had a new problem. In the efforts to lift out the baby, the uterus had been torn upward from the end of one side of the incision. A ragged tear branched up a good five or six centimeters. As the residents began the repair, the third-year resident started barking out orders. She explained that the right ureter to the kidney might have been injured because of its proximity to the uterine tear. It would be necessary to open the bladder, inject dye into the IV, and watch the two uretal openings inside the bladder to be sure that both ureters were secreting dyed urine from the kidneys into the bladder. This was accomplished: bladder lifted up into the surgical opening in the woman's abdomen, cut and pried open, ureteral openings visualized, dye injected, blue urine observed flowing from the kidneys through both ureters into the bladder. Both were open and undamaged. The bladder was then sutured closed, the repair finished on the uterus, the abdomen closed, and the stapled incision covered with a dressing.

After three hours in the operating room (a routine cesarean takes about an hour, tops), we trundled Melody to the recovery room where I watched over her for the next two hours. I spent some time explaining the surgery on her bladder to her and her family. I told them she would be staying in the hospital for a few extra days with the urinary catheter in place, until the bladder healed. Her mother kept repeating her thanks for the wonderful way in which we had cared for her daughter. I was upset to learn that her parents wouldn't be able to stay to help her after her discharge from the hospital, and wondered how she would manage an older child and a new baby, and be able to recuperate from the physical trauma of this delivery.

Melody would have a significant recovery period. Not only did she have a uterine incision, but her bladder was also involved. In addition, my hand, contaminated by bacteria in the rectum, had probably insured an infection, necessitating IV antibiotics. Her urethra was going to be very sore, particularly after having been traumatized initially and then having an indwelling catheter for at least five days. Her rectum would probably hurt, too.

This case really bothered me. It's not unusual, in a residency program, to have inconsistency in the decision-making process. Sometimes a team of residents will let a woman push for three, four or even five hours, under the premise that her epidural kept her from pushing effectively. The guidelines for the second, pushing, stage of labor call for no more than two hours of effort. After that time, the labor is considered a failure because of "arrest of descent"; that is, the fetal head cannot pass through the pelvic bone perimeters. In Melody's case, the decision for surgical delivery was probably a sound one, given how firmly wedged the baby was in the pelvis, but no one, myself included, had given any thought to the effects of the epidural on this woman's ability to push. The baby was only eight pounds. It is possible that Melody might have pushed it out, if she had been able to push effectively.

I am disturbed by the arbitrary two-hour cutoff. Who decided, I often wonder, that second stage should only take two hours? If the first, dilating, stage can take anywhere from an hour to two days, who says the passage of the baby down the vagina should only take two hours? The concern, as I understand it, is that after two hours of maternal effort, the mother and baby both may be exhausted and further efforts risk stressing both persons. Why then are some women forced to try for longer periods of time? What would have happened if we had taken a little time to think about this, to discuss it? What would have happened if we had made sure Melody was as comfortable as possible and then let her rest for a couple of hours? The baby looked absolutely fine on the monitor and was in fact, quite healthy at birth, with excellent Apgars and blood gas results. Suppose we had backed off, let Melody rest, and then had her push without the inhibiting effects of the epidural.

It just galls me to think of how we battered and carved up this young woman's body—her abdomen, her uterus, her bladder, her rectum, her urethra—how we extended her hospital stay and her recovery time, how we made her first days and weeks with her newborn significantly more difficult, because we opted for a surgical delivery so rapidly. Each decision was made with every good intention. Mothers who push for four hours and then end up having a cesarean are never happy about the length of time taken before the decision for surgery is made. But in spite of our good intentions, we hurt this girl, and it may very well have been completely unnecessary. This kind of arbitrariness in treatment decisions really bothers me, even while I acknowledge the uncertainties of obstetrical care. The doctors weren't wrong in this case; but they weren't unquestionably right, either, and that makes Melody's injuries more difficult to accept. I know it is foolish to think one can work in any medical field and always make just the right decisions, but nonetheless I suffered over this case and my participation in it.

As I move through more years as an L&D nurse, I find such ambiguities far more difficult to accept. There are inherent problems in a residency program in a training hospital. First of all, the residents are in training, so they are going to make mistakes. That's okay, because doctors, even board-certified ones, make mistakes. But residents are inclined to be overzealous in their approach to their work. They want to do surgical procedures: they need the experience. They want to know that when they go out into private practice they will be able to perform any procedure that might be required. In addition, their approach is a pathological one: they are educated to perceive the laboring woman as a sick person, a person who is suffering a pathological disorder. But pregnancy, labor, and birth are not inherently pathological. They are normal aspects of a female's biological reproductive ability. In most cases, birth is a function of health, not illness. The woman is in the hospital not because she is sick, but for insurance, "just in case." If anything should go wrong, she's in a place where it can be corrected.

The residents' guidelines for managing a labor in a hospital are just that: guidelines, imposed externally on an internal process. The cervix doesn't know that it's supposed to dilate one centimeter every hour in a first-time mother. The uterus doesn't know that it has to expel the fetus in two hours or less. The nerves that tell the mother to push don't know that they shouldn't send those signals before the cervix is completely dilated. The uterus doesn't measure its contractions to determine if they are adequate in strength and frequency. Medical experts have arrived at all these conclusions, based on thousands of labors, years of experience, libraries of research. All this information has been distilled into a set of expectations for a normal labor progression, based on the best scientific reasoning.

But sometimes young physicians-in-training get trapped by their guidelines, their labor curves. They tend to make decisions based on the book, instead of the patient's individual needs, for a good reason: they have to justify all their decisions to their supervising advisers, just as an obstetrician must be able to justify his decisions to a peer review board or a court of law. Residents do want to do a good job for their patients, but are usually too insecure to practice obstetrics with flexibility rather than by the book. And inevitably, what they learn in their training is what they will practice as independent physicians. Their training and the technology they depend upon have the paradoxical effect of distancing them from the patients they are attempting to guide through a normal biological process.

The management of second stage in a hospital setting is a good example of this paradoxical effect. The position in which the woman pushes, the time when she is allowed to begin pushing, how long she should push, and the manner in which she actually pushes are, for me, all areas of concern and frustration.

Around the world, women trying to expel their babies will invariably assume a squatting position in which to push. It is only in Western, "civilized" countries, that women are expected to bear down in a semi-recumbent or completely supine position. The lithotomy position, in which the woman lies on her back with her legs held aloft by stirrups, was devised solely for the doctor's convenience. This position allows the attending physician to see the entire vulva, so that he can position his hands appropriately around the infant's head and apply downward and then upward pressure for the shoulders' birth; so that he can apply pressure against the perineum to prevent tears; so that he can cut the episiotomy; and so that he can repair the episiotomy. In this position, the woman is actually pushing uphill, against gravity, unless she is raised into a semi-sitting position.

The research I've studied on pushing positions seems to indicate that the lithotomy position, with the legs separated unnaturally far apart, almost guarantees the necessity of an episiotomy to prevent the tearing that would occur in already stretched tissues. Squatting simply is not conducive to management of the delivery, even though it may be the most natural position for the mother. I found myself remembering what it was like to try to empty my bowels into a bedpan while lying flat on my back after disc surgery, which wasn't natural or easy—I can tell you that!

On occasion, when I am pushing with a mother, I will attempt to get her into a squatting position. Rarely is it successful, for several reasons. One is that so many moms have epidurals. Their legs are dead weights, making it almost impossible to squat, even with assistance. Another reason is that it is difficult to squat on a bed without something to hold on to. I usually get the mother's arms around the necks of her husband and myself. Then we pull and lift her forward onto her feet, holding her weight as she bears down. This is an extremely strenuous activity, and terrible for a nurse with a bad back. Lowering and raising the mother for each push exhausts all three of us. In one hospital where I worked, the back of the bed could be raised enough so that the mother could turn around and hang onto the top of the bed while I watched her bottom from behind. This was more effective than lifting her forward.

Some nurses will have a woman squat beside the bed. I'm usually defeated in such attempts by all the wires and catheters attached to the woman, and by the lack of feeling in her legs because of an epidural. One night, with her husband's assistance with the IV pumps, monitor, and lines, I managed to walk a mother into the bathroom. She had been insisting that she needed to be on the toilet to coordinate her pushing efforts. She sat there straining, while her husband cracked jokes and I squatted in front of the toilet, peering at her vulva. She brought the baby down very nicely; I could see the head crowning. Unfortunately, we returned to her bed before the baby's head had completely passed the pubic bone. When the mother got back in bed, the baby slipped back up the vaginal canal. The obstetrician had to use a vacuum extractor to deliver the baby.

The last reason for semi-recumbent or lithotomy positions, I think is one of societal conditioning and expectations: Western mothers just don't feel dignified squatting, as though they were moving their bowels. It seems to bother them more than lying on their backs, holding back their knees, vulvas completely exposed, while they push. They believe they are supposed to give birth in a semi-recumbent position, and squatting seems gross.

Most physicians have been trained to deliver women only in the lithotomy position. I was stunned by the fury of one private attending physician when I raised the head of the bed so that his patient could push in a semi-sitting position. "Put her flat!" he yelled at me. "Put her flat. I've been in practice for twenty-five years and I know what I'm doing. Women can't push correctly unless they're flat on their backs!" I was astonished, particularly when it happened again with another of his patients before I touched her bed. I couldn't believe this guy. I wanted to ask him about all the women around the world who squat to push, but I was a good little nurse and kept my mouth shut.

I've had residents watch with fascination while I hoist a mother into a squatting position. They haven't seen it done before. Most residents don't think they can even check a cervix unless the mother is flat on her back. If I can insert a catheter through the urethra into the bladder upside down, when the mother is in a knee-chest position, surely it is possible to feel a cervix in the side-lying position! Many residents just haven't been exposed to different pushing positions. They go by the book and what they have seen.

But even established obstetricians often exhibit considerable reluctance to try something new. When birthing rooms were first offered in one of the major maternity hospitals where I did my obstetrical rotation during nursing school, the birthing rooms went unused for a couple of years by almost all of the obstetricians. Reasons cited by the physicians were several: they were too far away from the delivery room if an emergency should occur; they were too poorly lit; they encouraged too many visitors; delivering a woman in a bed, instead of on a delivery table, was too awkward and caused back problems for the doctors.

These were specious arguments. The birthing rooms were no farther away from a delivery room than the labor rooms: many a mother had been rushed down the hall from a labor room. There was no reason a mother couldn't be trundled down the same hall from a birthing room. The lighting problem was easily addressed with the use of spotlights. The number of visitors is always controlled by hospital policy. Beds that could be elevated and have their bottoms lifted away, as birthing beds can be, actually become delivery beds in a twinkling, complete with stirrups.

I believe these complaints reflected a reluctance to change habits, to be innovative. Birthing rooms, birthing beds, and even birthing chairs are beginning to be more in evidence in hospitals courting patients. Obstetricians have been forced to be more flexible as consumers demand more control over their birth experiences. Having significant others present during the delivery, even during cesareans, was not commonplace twenty years ago. Every established practice takes years of arguing, studying, and fussing about before changes occur. Policies and practices are almost written in stone in a hospital; in order to change them it has to be demonstrated that there is no medical indication why they shouldn't be changed, that there is a financial cost to not changing them, and that there is a great patient demand to do so. It also requires physicians and nurses who are willing to be innovative and flexible, qualities that are not routinely instilled in medical and nursing schools.

For instance, consider the pushing stage once again. The books tell doctors and nurses that second stage begins when the cervix is completely dilated, open to ten centimeters. The woman isn't supposed to start pushing until this is accomplished. If she does, she exerts pressure against the edges of the cervix. This may result in a swollen cervix, rendering further dilation difficult if not impossible, and may also result in lacerations or tears in the cervix. These are pretty good reasons to avoid pushing before dilation is accomplished; having to do a cesarean because the swollen cervix can't completely open or trying to repair a torn cervix aren't wonderful possibilities to contemplate. I don't have any trouble telling a mother who's only six centimeters dilated not to push. But I do have trouble with a mother who's eight or nine centimeters dilated and who has an irresistible urge to push. I am a strong believer in paying attention to the mother. If a woman says she has to push, if a woman is yelling that the baby is coming, I don't care if the doctor thinks otherwise. I can't count the number of times I've had a doctor say, "I just checked her. She's only seven (or five or four) centimeters," or "Don't let her push until she's ten."

It goes completely against my grain to tell a woman she can't push when her body is pounding its message to her. It's like telling someone not to vomit. Many women simply can't control it; the urge is undeniable, indisputable. The body says *"push"* and dammit, they are going to push. I stand over them, telling them in a loud voice to *"Blow, blow, blow!"* Supposedly, a person cannot bear down if she's forcibly blowing out air. They try so hard to obey me, but their faces scrunch up and turn red, they make grunting noises and they push in between the blows! What, I wonder, over and over again, would happen if we didn't interfere? Has anyone ever studied women who deliver precipitously to see if there is in fact a true statistical correlation between lacerated cervices and premature pushing? Is there really a correlation between cesareans and arrest of dilation due to edematous cervixes? I'm probably speaking out of ignorance here, but once again it feels like we are imposing a standard, a rule from the outside, on a physiological event that shouldn't necessarily be externally controlled.

The length of time a mother is expected to push is another area of concern. As I mentioned earlier, the guidelines call for two hours, but I have to ask again, who came up with two hours? Why not one? Why not four? I would rather ask: why not tailor the length of time to the mother's ability and to her physical stamina, based on how long, how difficult, and how painful her first stage has been? It is cruel and inhumane to make a woman push for three or more hours after she has been in labor for many hours, with no food or drink, with no rest or adequate pain relief. It is also cruel to make a woman push for several hours when she's been anesthetized with an epidural and can't coordinate her efforts. I have suffered through hours of pushing with innumerable women so handicapped. I have held the feet up and back, counted to ten, encouraged and coached and wiped the sweaty brows and goopy bottoms, all the while feeling deep inside that we're doing something wrong here. When I read *A Woman in Residence* by Michelle Harrison, I was thrilled to discover I wasn't alone with this feeling. Dr. Harrison voiced similar concerns.

Several times my suspicions have been borne out by a curious phenomenon. A woman will get an epidural. The pain of her contractions disappears. She sleeps, and her uterus keeps on contracting. We wait until she lets us know she can feel the contractions again. We pull back the sheet to check her cervix. Lo and behold! A baby's head is right there, on the perineum, pushed down by the uterine activity alone, a contraction or two away from delivery!

These women didn't have an urge to push. Their sensations were blocked by the anesthesia. But their uteri kept on doing their work, contracting and relaxing. And by God, without the mother knowing it, the uterus is strong enough to push that baby right on out, without mom doing anything to help. Now I know this doesn't happen all the time, not even frequently. Most uteri need a little assistance from the abdominal muscles to move those babies down and out, especially big babies. But maybe we ought to be more relaxed about pushing. Maybe we ought to be able to get good pain relief for the mother, so she can really rest. We can let her push after she's gotten a second wind. As long as we're monitoring the baby and it looks healthy on the monitor strip, why not get a breather for both mom and baby? If epidural anesthesia is going to be used anyway, why not put it to good use, like a nap for both patients?

Experts argue that the baby shouldn't be subjected to a lengthy time within the bony passageway out of the pelvis; that extended head compressions aren't safe for the infant. But many babies are subjected to lengthy second stages without any untoward effects. Again, I may be revealing my ignorance, but I don't know if anyone has ever researched this issue. I wonder if there is a correlation between the length of second stage and Apgars and blood gases?

The final problem I have with pushing is the way we make women do it. The customary method is for the woman to take a deep breath, hold it, and bear down as hard as she can, to the count of ten. At ten, she blows off that breath, takes another, and bears down again. She is coached to do this three times for each contraction. Everybody crowds around the bed and yells at her, "Push! *Push!* Harder! *Harder!* Give it all you've got! Come on! *Push!*" Jesus, but I hate this! Aside from the fact that usually the woman is pushing as hard as she can, I think it's outrageous to yell at her. It's assaultive and ugly. This is *not* a sports event. It isn't a boxing match or a basketball game. It's a woman trying to get her baby out. She doesn't need loud voices screaming at her. I admonished a medical student once for yelling at a mother. He was perplexed: "All the residents do it. I just figured it's like when I play basketball. I'm concentrating so hard on what I'm doing that the only way someone can give me instructions is to shout at me. I figured the mother couldn't hear me if I didn't yell at her."

I told him how it felt when I was pushing with every bit of my energy and this goddamned nurse kept poking my butt and yelling at me, "Push here, push right here!" I was enraged. I wanted to kick her in the face. *Where the fuck do you think I'm pushing, goddammit? In my nose? My ears?* I had silently fumed. I've had women tell me after their deliveries how awful it was to be yelled at, how they felt they were failing, how they thought everyone was mad at them. I've had women actually yell back, "I *am* pushing hard, damn you!" I've also had women tell me that all they focused on when they were pushing was my quiet voice in their ear, counting and encouraging them on, gently. They said they blocked out the other noises because they were too loud or distracting or disturbing.

Sometimes I admit, the quiet method doesn't work. Every once in a while, there will be a recalcitrant woman who simply will not push unless you get mean and yell at her. Often it's a young girl who has never had to work hard for something before and just wants to quit. Then sometimes it's an older woman who just refuses. She doesn't want to exert herself. She wants the staff to deliver the baby, even if it means a cesarean. She just doesn't want to give the effort. Then we have to call in a "good pusher," someone who hasn't been involved in the woman's care, who can stand at the end of the bed and shout out commands like a drill instructor!

But still, I question this. I do know of some research on the method of pushing, that tried to determine if holding the breath for more than ten seconds while straining to push affects the blood gases of the infant. As I remember, the research was inconclusive. I do think we should relax a little here. If we weren't tied inexorably to the two-hour limit, then couldn't we let the mother push more naturally? Couldn't we allow her to work with the sensations of the urge to push, bearing down for as long as she can comfortably hold her breath, pushing only twice or even four times during a contraction, whichever felt right to her? If she can't feel the contractions because of an epidural, then I can understand the need to impose an external system of three pushes per contraction. But if she does have the urge, why not back off and see how she would respond to the urge if left alone? Will she hold her breath for more than a few seconds? Will she push with little grunts or with long, sustained effort? Why not watch her and see what she does in response to her body's signals? We don't try to control the efforts of the stomach to vomit up its contents. We don't say "Stomach, you can only retch three times each minute!" We don't try to control the bowels when intestinal cramps hit us and we have to get to the toilet before we explode! Why do we try to impose these rules on a woman's body?

After several years of watching women push in the accepted, textbook manner, listening to others count and shout and scold, I began, hesitantly, to assert myself. If the mother's epidural had just been dosed when she reached ten centimeters, I urged the residents to give her a rest period to allow the anesthesia to wear off a little, so she could feel what she was doing when she pushed. Working up my courage, I also experimented with mothers who were not pushing effectively with the three-pushes-per-contraction method. If I didn't see or feel any movement of the fetus with her pushing efforts, I asked the mother exactly what she felt when she pushed. "Do you have any sensation of movement down here? Does it feel like the baby is moving? Do you feel like you are trying to move your bowels? Do you have any desire to bear down, to push?" If the mother had an urge to push, I told her to "go with what you feel. Push with the sensation. We aren't going to count. Hold your breath as long as you want, or grunt with it. Do what feels effective, okay?" Or I would instruct her, "Look, push and grunt like you would if you were moving your bowels. Little grunts, like this: *unghh, unghh!*" I would demonstrate, grunting and turning my face red. "Let me see you bulge out your rectum. If I see that I know you're pushing in the right direction."

On several occasions, this method of pushing has been highly effective. By allowing the mother to respond to her body's signals rather than imposing artificial goals on her, by working with her uterus, she is able to bring the baby down effectively. One mother followed the textbook instructions diligently, pushing in a semi-reclining position, pulling her knees back with her hands, straining to the count of ten, three times with each contraction. Only problem was, I could see she was simultaneously squeezing her anus tight, lifting her buttocks off the bed as she fought the sensations she was having.

"I feel like I'm going to poop! I can't help it! I'm sorry!" she cried.

"Hey, look! That's exactly what I want you to do. Let your rectum go. Push like you're going to the bathroom. Just like you're constipated with a watermelon in there—push it out!"

"Oh no, I couldn't do that. That would be so embarrassing!"

I gave my standard reassurance: "Listen my dear, there isn't anything a woman can secrete or ooze from her body that I haven't seen, touched, and smelled. When I see bowel movement, when I see poop, I know you're pushing in the right direction. I call it the positive poop sign." I helped this mother turn onto her left side. "Hold onto the siderail with this hand. Grab your upper knee with the other. Pull back with your hands and let your rectum go! Bulge it out. We aren't counting anymore. We're just going to help you hold up this leg. You push like you're pooping, little grunts, okay?" Her bottom relaxed, a little stool came out, wiped away gently by me, and the baby's head just descended right down the vaginal canal. The residents were astonished when I emerged from the room after just a few minutes of this experimental pushing to announce she was crowning and we were moving to the delivery room. After watching her initial, traditional pushing efforts, they had actually started filling out cesarean paperwork, so convinced they were that she wouldn't be able to push the baby down.

A similar episode reinforced my theory about pushing technique. Three residents, an intern, and a medical student, all of them female, stood gowned and masked around a patient on a delivery table. All five of them were shouting at this mother: "Push! *Push!* Harder! Get mad! *Do it!* You're not trying!

You're not pushing hard enough!" And so on. I watched for a few minutes, feeling my blood pressure rise. *This is awful,* I thought. *We're assaulting this woman. God, what a way for a baby to be born!* I wasn't the nurse in charge of this patient; I'd only come into the delivery room to assist the primary nurse, who was doing paperwork.

At the end of a yelling session, the end of a contraction, the woman fell back on the bed, exhausted and tearful. "Wait a second, here," I said firmly. I looked over my mask at each of the women standing around the bed, demanding their silence with the fiercest expression I could put into my eyes. "Do you have the urge to push?" I asked the mother. "Is there a sensation, a need to bear down?"

"Yes," she whispered.

"Okay. We're all going to be quiet now. With the next contraction, you just go with the sensation. Just push like it feels right to you. Like you're pooping or whatever. Okay? Little pushes, little grunts if that helps. Just do what your body tells you to do." The tone of my voice and the daggers in my eyes brooked no interference from anyone in the delivery room.

"Here it comes," the mother cried as she curled her body around her belly, grasping the hand grips on the bed. She grunted little grunts, pushed little pushes, maybe ten or twelve with the contraction. The five medical women stood silent, amazed to see the baby's head descend and then begin to bulge and flatten the perineal tissues. Two more contractions and we had a baby's head out. Nobody said anything except for subdued encouraging remarks, "That's it, here it comes! You're bringing the baby down!" I was gleeful! With luck those five young women learned something about effective pushing and paying attention to what the mother feels, not what the books say should be done.

Even as I worry and wonder about these problems with pushing techniques, my own personal shortcomings get in the way of really helping my patients. It's obvious by now that I don't like to challenge authority figures. All the old conditioning, the way I was brought up—to respect the doctor, to follow the rules—conflicts with what my experience and commonsense tell me. *I'm "only the nurse." I don't know as much as the doctor does.* Such thoughts are common among nurses. It is particularly difficult for me to acknowledge the truth about such attitudes; to recognize that I am qualified and experienced in my work; that flexibility is a significant attribute to bring to my work; and that my role as the patient's advocate is a legitimate one. I have to fight my own hesitancy, my insecurity about challenging authority, and work diligently to assert myself with doctors who may not be responding effectively to a patient's needs. When I am able to overcome my fears and frustration and demonstrate an alternative method of pushing, for instance, without insulting or demeaning the physicians, it feels wonderful.

Unfortunately, the longer I worked, the harder it was to generate the energy necessary for such assertiveness. Instead of just being proud of myself when I was able to be effective in my efforts, I felt like I was losing ground. The grueling hours, the intensity of the work itself, and the enormous number and variety of medical personnel I had to work with sapped my energy. Once again I tried to blame most of my frustration on the system. The problems I've outlined in these pages are real and legitimate cause for concern and frustration, but it was easier to take aim at these issues than it was to confront my own shortcomings.

Chapter Fifteen

DISENCHANTMENT

Beyond the major difficulties cited earlier, I quickly noticed, even at the beginning of my career, a number of smaller problems with nursing.

For instance, I was able to recognize a subtle pattern of behavior among hospital staff members. When the L&D unit's census, its number of patients, remained high over a period of days or weeks, the staff began to decompensate. Teamwork disappeared, hostility and irritability became commonplace. Supplies and equipment were erratically stocked and couldn't be depended upon, increasing levels of frustration and stress. Having to search for necessary items when there wasn't even time to provide adequate care was aggravating, at best. Staff members moved from general griping to specific bitch sessions and there were always one or two co-workers who were scapegoated. Malicious gossip, finger-pointing, silent treatments, and open ostracizing occurred. Almost no one was exempt from some aspect of this behavior including, to my shame, myself.

At my first job, I worked six shifts in a row on a regular basis, and at least once a month, I had a seven, eight, or nine-day run without a break. My days off were often split. Weekends off happened at best only once every four weeks, usually every five. Everyone else bore the same burden. Staff meetings rarely solved problems, they only cast blame. I grew increasingly depressed, struggling ineffectively and immaturely with the interpersonal conflicts within the group. Nursing management changed three times in four years, each time with a complete reorganization of the department and administrative upheavals. People I had grown to care about and enjoyed working with departed for other assignments, including Nick. The unit was upgraded to an obstetrical intensive-care unit, with a much needed pay raise for all of us, but staffing remained abysmal. NAACOG (the national obstetrical nursing organization) standards were blithely ignored while we nurses attempted to care for as many as four or five high-risk mothers each, instead of working at the recommended one-to-one ratio. Urgent requests for more help, for twelve-hour shifts, and more frequent days off were denied by the senior nursing administration.

Still, I had remarkable experiences with my patients. I got involved with a sixteen-year-old who had to give up her baby for adoption, after enduring a life-threatening episode of preeclampsia, an emergency cesarean, and blood transfusions. She wept with me, telling me why she knew she had to give up her baby. She expressed great anger at her previous ignorance: "They don't tell you in Sex Ed at school that you can die having a baby!"

I worked with several patients who had such severe first-trimester nausea and vomiting that they required lengthy hospitalization and even tube feeding. I fell in love with an Asian girl who spent six weeks in the hospital before giving birth to her second baby. Her first had died in her arms three days after his birth. I held her as she cried, admitting that she was unable to sleep because she was so afraid this baby would also die. She told me she sat beside the baby all night with her hand resting on it, so she could feel its breathing. I brought her books and treats from my home and admired her courage during her long stay, so far from home and family, barely able to communicate in English.

And there were always the babies, so pristine, so new, so full of potential, so gratifying after their mother's sweat and pain, after my efforts to smooth their arrival. I rejoiced in them and in their parents. A father's tears of joy touched me so profoundly once that I was high and flying, babbling away about how lovely he was, only to be rudely squelched by an exhausted resident who told me not to get mushy about it. An entry in my haphazardly kept journal reveals my growing disenchantment:

> I came home from work at 4:30 this afternoon, eleven hours after I had climbed out of bed, groggy with dreams I couldn't remember. My daughter was out with my sister and my niece, down at the convention center, watching some of the city's best performers do their thing for promotional purposes. I went last year and was awed by African dancers and a cappella singers. I knew it was a special day, but I'd had to work. I was tired and hungry and depressed. I let the dog out, went to the bathroom, put on my flannel nightie, turned on the heat for the first time this fall, and ate leftovers for dinner, reading a book about Vietnam as I ate.
>
> My daughter and sister arrived and we talked as they ate their dinner. I called my son in New Jersey, and later listened to my daughter rage about a problem at school, feeling helpless in the face of her tears and distress. I soaked in the bathtub for ten minutes and hit my bed at 7:30. I finished the book and found myself thinking about my life. I have to work tomorrow, the seventh day in a row.
>
> I don't have a social life. I don't go out. I don't talk to my out-of-town friends very often and don't have any close friends here. I work, come home, attend to the necessary aspects of home—groceries, laundry, bills, the lawn. I rent videos a couple of times a month, go to the movies once a month. That's it. I come home wasted, grab a fifteen-minute nap,

eat, try to communicate with my daughter and my sister, and read in bed. I read and read and read and remember very little of what I've read.

So, an empty life, right? Why don't I go out? Why don't I take advantage of all this city has to offer? Where are all the interesting people? Why don't I meet any eligible men? Then I realized what I had relayed to my sister in my short talk with her tonight.

Today at work, I took care of a sixteen-year-old girl, who had delivered via C/S a 35-week preemie, after developing severe preeclampsia. This girl, according to her and her father, who talked to me for thirty minutes this afternoon, had been abandoned by her mother years ago, lived with her grandparents although her father had tried to obtain custody of her, until she got pregnant, when the grandparents dumped her on her father. The father, just starting a new job, took care of her during her pregnancy, even while his second wife was going down the tubes with mental illness and multiple suicide attempts.

I listened and talked with the girl about her experience, impressed by her resilience. I listened to her father pour out his woes and anger about her pregnancy. I knew tomorrow I would have to help her deal with the adoption agency and giving up the baby.

I took care of a fortysomething woman with her first and only baby, after twelve years of marriage, two grown stepchildren and four grandchildren. She had given up hope of having a baby after years of infertility and was so overjoyed with this tiny infant, it was wonderful!

I took care of a drug addict, with a history of multiple sexual partners, recurrent pelvic inflammatory disease, current cocaine abuse, and newly discovered pubic lice. I listened to her bad-mouth the doctors, the nurses, the hospital, trying to claim she got bedbugs from the hospital, while I emptied her bedpan, her urinal, picked up her used toilet paper and tissues from the floor where she had dropped them, hung her antibiotics, changed her linens, and handled her peripads. I felt bug-ridden all day and worried about having lice. I had stroked her shoulders and legs two days before as she writhed with abdominal pain. My sympathy had cost me: now she called me by my first name, asked me to break all the rules for her, and castigated my co-workers, assuming I was her friend.

I discharged a twenty-year-old girl with her baby, sending her home with her young husband and infant to squeeze in as many days as they could together before her child died from the serious cardiac anomalies he'd been born with. I had little to offer her, except an honest look of grief, tears, and a tight hug before she left.

I spent five minutes with a former patient, a beautiful woman I had cared for a week earlier. She had endured five days of agony on tocolytics to stop premature labor, only to have a cesarean at twenty-seven weeks because she had a serious case of chorioamnionitis. Her baby was fighting for its life in the NICU and she was on the ward, using the breast-pump before going into the NICU to stroke and caress the tiny two-pound infant who was her baby. We talked and put our arms around each other and hugged for the longest time, rocking back and forth together, silent in our appreciation of each other. I had shared the most difficult experience of her life with her and was still there, on the periphery, watching her cope with this situation, ready to hold her up when it became too much to bear.

I spent thirty minutes soothing and handing tissues to a weeping postpartum day-two mother, whose hormones were wreaking havoc on her emotions while she tried to deal with an insensitive mother-in-law, a baby in the intermediate nursery on antibiotics, separation from her other two children, and a nursery staff so overworked they hadn't time to reassure her that her baby was okay.

I didn't have time to go into one room and sit down with two patients, antepartum mothers, who had been with us for more than a month, to really visit with them and get a good feel for how they were holding up through their long hospitalization. I looked at cesarean incisions, emptied bedpans, washed bloody crotches and put on clean peripads, clean sheets, clean pillowcases. I gave narcotic injections and many pills. I went through pages upon pages of documentation on all my patients and counted up the patient-care hours and available manpower hours and filled out the report for the higher-ups to shuffle around over the next twenty-four hours. I taught mothers about the changes in their bodies, about their babies' care, about hospital routines. I talked with the intern, the med students, the doctors, the nurses, the dietary lady, housekeeping. I talked to a young man who'd been sitting and sleeping and reading on the couch in the hall for two days, waiting for his sister to deliver. I went to the bathroom three times and smoked while I relieved my bladder. I ate cheese and crackers while I did paperwork. I answered the phone and tried to pay attention to the ward clerk when she droned on and on about her college courses as I tried to do charting.

I was assaulted by the dirt and grime of the ward, of our bathroom—the sinks splattered with hair, soap, and God knows what else, the floors littered with toilet paper, newspaper, dirty scrubs, used peripads. I washed my hands at least thirty times, and half the time I had to walk around with wet hands while I searched for a towel. No paper towels on the ward, no sitz baths, no washcloths, no A&D Ointment. The lids of the water pitchers don't fit. The IV poles are filthy, stinking of antibiotics. Four long-term antepartum patients don't have care plans, and two of them have been here for weeks. I walked miles of halls and answered a dozen call bells and washed three beds and made six more. It was an easy day, too.

Is it any wonder that I come home and crawl into bed with a book that I won't remember a word of next week? Is it strange that I am overcome by inertia at home and don't want to empty the dishwasher? Is it strange that I cannot think of a single thing to say to help my daughter deal with her anguish, and that I can hardly talk coherently to my faraway son? I know I make a difference to my patients and that gives me satisfaction. But I go home barren of emotion, unable to give any more, cheating my children, my sister, and myself, because there just isn't anything left. Why am I doing this?

That's next week's question. It's now 9:30 at night and I have to get up at 5:00 to go to work.

After petty fights and disagreements with my newest head nurse, I left my first job, for a promotion and work as an assistant manager at a civilian hospital. It was a painful departure, marked by my own immaturity and lack of professionalism. I had argued with this head nurse about patient care, work assignments, and malfunctioning equipment. The rapport and support I had experienced with previous bosses were impossible to achieve with this nurse. Battle lines were drawn as gossip flew. All the old problems I had asserting myself reappeared with a vengeance. Several feeble attempts to communicate effectively and directly with my boss failed to erase the bad feelings between us. The ugliness of our conflict increased as everyone on the unit added their unsolicited opinions, inciting further discontent and discord. I behaved badly, furiously defending myself and blaming others, without acknowledging that my defensiveness was inappropriate, unprofessional, and a factor contributing to the emotional storms sweeping through the unit.

It was several years before I confronted my own culpability and recognized that my exit from this job was a reenactment of the way I'd left a long-ago secretarial job, What shame I felt: Had I learned nothing in all the years since then? Had I hidden away in my housewife role to avoid emotional conflict with someone who didn't like me? How could I allow such ugly behavior to recur? Once again, twenty years later, I had allowed someone else's insecurities and hatred to embroil me in psychological warfare until, terrified by the battle, I fled in ignominious defeat.

My last day on this labor deck, my home for four years, was a nightmare: no farewell party, no acknowledgment of the effort I had made, of the fact that my heart had been completely committed to this place for so long. I embraced those nurses I cared about and, blinded by tears, stumbled off the unit. I was mortified, hurt, angry, and bitterly ashamed of my own failures.

Compared to the one I'd left at the military hospital, the labor and delivery unit at my new place of employment was huge. There were twenty labor/

birthing rooms, five delivery/operating rooms, and a large ten-bed recovery room. The nurses' station dominated the unit. A long breast-high counter with attached desk marched through the middle of the unit. Above it was a wonderful skylight, large and curved, which afforded us bright sunlight during the day and allowed me to watch the moon's progress across the skies at night. Designed as birthing rooms, we used the labor rooms as such for most normal vaginal deliveries. Though drab, most were spacious, with adjoining bathrooms. While the nurses and patients alike preferred to deliver in these rooms, a few of the doctors were uncomfortable without the technical equipment and lights available in the traditional delivery rooms, so quite a number of patients were routinely moved to the delivery rooms for their babies' births. In addition, we had a list of risk factors, such as forceps deliveries, first-time mothers, mothers with infections or preeclampsia. Any patient with a risk factor was automatically denied a birthing-room delivery.

This unit was unbelievably busy, continually taxed beyond its capacity. Each month we delivered 800 babies. The nurses routinely cared for two or three patients simultaneously. Because it was a private hospital and the physicians all had private OB/GYN practices, the majority of our patients were middle- and upper-middle class women. But the hospital also housed an OB/GYN clinic for indigent women, which was staffed by residents from a nearby university medical center. Thus, the women we cared for were a different population from the one I'd experienced in the military. Drug users, Medicare patients, non-English-speaking women, and occasional homeless women were among our population. They were with us only for labor and the birth of their babies; as soon as medically possible, usually in less than two hours, we moved them to the postpartum ward and had no further contact with them.

During my work there as assistant nurse manager, I watched with dismay as nurses in our extremely busy unit staggered through their work with little thought about or impetus to give compassionate care. As charge nurse each night, I tried to remind everyone of the significance of our work in a very simple way. When a baby was born, I drew a little figure to indicate its sex and printed its name and weight on the census board. Few staff members even noticed this attempt at personalizing the many patients we have on the unit. One nurse asked in morning report, "Who wrote that baby's name and weight on the board?"

"I did," I answered.

"Well, who cares?" she snarled. My mouth hung agape. I was unable to protest her remark, I was so shocked by it. I learned the obvious lesson that not all people feel, as I do, that it is a privilege to work with birthing mothers, to be present at such a profound event in their lives. For most, apparently, it becomes just a job.

Near the end of an exhausting twelve-hour shift one night, I walked to the recovery room to check on a patient. This woman had just delivered her first child in an emergency cesarean section because of fetal distress. I had learned the baby had a previously undiagnosed congenital cardiac anomaly that required immediate surgery, and that arrangements were being made to transfer the infant to a neonatal intensive-care unit across town. I spoke briefly to the parents. I described the transfer plans and offered the mother a private room, away from all the mothers and babies on the postpartum ward. I expressed my concern over her shock and fear, speaking straightforwardly about how difficult it must be to have this happen to her new baby. She responded to my sympathy with appropriate tears. I told her we would do anything we could to make her stay in the hospital as comfortable as possible and would keep her informed of her baby's status. I asked if she had had any opportunity to see her baby and when she said no, offered her a quick trip to the nursery before her baby was transferred. She smiled beatifically, immensely grateful for the offer, and began to ready herself for a journey down the hall, ignoring her post-op pain as she smoothed the sheet over her abdomen and asked her husband to help her sit up a bit more.

I went to the recovery nurse at the back of the room. She was sitting at the desk, finishing some charting. She'd had a busy night in which she had received and transferred several patients to the postpartum ward. Though she was still neatly attired, her blond coiffure and makeup intact, I was well aware that she was tired, but she had been able to take a break during the shift. I asked her quietly to take the patient down to the nursery for a brief visit with her baby. She looked at the clock: it was 6:00 A.M., one hour before the end of her shift.

"Oh, I don't think that's necessary. They'll bring the baby down here in the transporter before they leave the hospital."

"I know that, but she won't be able to touch the baby or have any time with it then. She needs to go to the nursery."

"Well, I don't think I can manage that. I have to finish things up here and it's getting too late."

I was angry now. I couldn't argue with her in front of the patient. There wasn't time to get into this with her out in the hall. If the mother was to have any time with her baby, it had to happen right now. Nearly exploding with anger, it didn't occur to me to use the phone. Instead, I ran down the hall to the nursery to be sure I could bring the mother on her gurney into the special care nursery. "Of course, she should see her baby!" I was told by the head nurse. "Bring her on down." I ran back to the recovery room, and with her husband's help, wheeled this mother down to the nursery. I parked her gurney as close as possible to the baby's life-support island, putting down the siderails so she could reach out and stroke her infant's body. I watched for two minutes as these parents greeted their tiny newborn, tears of joy and fear washing their faces. As I left the nursery to scramble through the last minutes of the shift before report, I struggled with my emotions.

The recovery nurse wasn't intentionally uncaring. She was tired. She worked hard. She didn't see the need to bring this little family together even briefly. To do so meant time and extra effort. She didn't feel like pushing a heavy gurney down the hall, negotiating its passage through all the equipment in the crowded nursery. She didn't want to have to chart the move and the mother's response to her baby. She thought it would be sufficient if the mother got to see the baby in the transporter. But dammit, this mother hadn't seen her baby, hadn't touched it, or had a chance to welcome it to her world. She would be separated from the baby for at least four days, recovering from her cesarean, while the baby underwent serious surgery in another hospital. Such a separation would have devastated me. I wanted her to know what her baby felt like. I wanted her to be able to touch this baby, to speak to it, to see with her own eyes how the baby was being treated by the nursery staff, to have her first questions answered. The effort required to make this brief meeting possible is the difference between competent clinical care and truly compassionate hands-on care, between a "just a job" and a commitment to excellence.

One morning, two hours past the end of my shift, I was still on the unit, trying to help with an inundation of patients. All the rooms were filled. Two cesareans and two vaginal deliveries were in progress in the four delivery rooms. Six patients sat in front of the nurses' station, waiting to be evaluated, waiting for a nonexistent room. The head nurse and I were fighting with an unreliable computer, trying to get it to take a pile of lab orders.

An obstetrician sat at the far end of the station, writing notes. He was exquisitely attired, from his designer clothes, gold bracelet, and Rolex to his handcrafted Italian loafers. Every hair on his head was perfectly in place and his handsome, tan visage was twisted with anger. There, in front of everyone, including the six patients and their husbands, he loudly and abusively excoriated the head nurse because his patient hadn't been given her IV yet. His patient was a scheduled induction, a nonemergent case! Six women sat before him, not yet evaluated, potential time bombs, and he was throwing a tantrum because his needs weren't being met, because he would be late for his office hours! He included me in his ire, pointing to me as he claimed, "There are nurses just standing around at the desk, while my patient waits for her IV!" I was rendered speechless by this outrageous, rude, insensitive behavior.

As a manager, I was continually frustrated by the administrative demands and the traffic flow, which I had to direct while on the unit. These duties prevented me from interacting with patients for any length of time. After a year on the job I was able to recognize that I had continued to grow professionally. I had been able to spend long hours juggling a thousand details and multiple personnel without once losing control on the unit. Not crying was a big step for me, since it had previously been a problem whenever I was sorely stressed. Almost every shift on this unit was sorely stressful, but I maintained control. No serious mishaps occurred while I was running the unit. I was able to use my communication skills to defuse several hazardous situations on the unit. One husband was so frightened by his wife's lengthy and painful ordeal that he became abusive, physically and verbally threatening the doctor and nurse caring for his wife, slamming his fists into the wall. I had the presence of mind to call the supervisor and then to quiet the man by listening carefully to his rage, by recognizing and acknowledging his fear and sense of helplessness, and reassuring him that we were doing all that we could to ease his wife's pain.

This man, along with other fathers, expressed the same gratitude to me: "You're the only one who has taken the time to listen to me." I was personally pleased and professionally angered: if we weren't so busy, situations like this wouldn't get out of hand. If we took the time, most conflicts and misunderstandings could be sorted out. But there wasn't enough time.

I continued to take pleasure in the families of our patients. I loved being able to walk up to a tight, tense little group of people, all anxious and tired and worried, and announce, "She's just fine! It's a beautiful baby! Come close to these doors and you can hear it yelling! Isn't that great!" I loved taking a camera from a father's hand and marshaling a family around the bed that held the mother and child, taking the first pictures in what I hoped would become a scrapbook of memories of this new little person. I loved hugging a proud mom, shaking hands with a beaming dad, and praising them both for their splendid efforts and marvelous baby.

With the nurses I had to insist on such courtesies to family members. At least once a week I had to run interference with an angry significant other and a nurse who did not want extra visitors in the room. Several nurses were always annoyed by families who tried to skirt the rules. These nurses insisted they couldn't get their work done with so many people in the room. I agreed that traffic had to be limited on the unit, that the rules were there to ensure that the patient received needed care without unnecessary distractions. But I was also aware that some nurses didn't like visitors because they didn't like being watched while they worked and/or because they didn't want to have to expend the extra effort to interact positively with anyone other than the patient. I was also aware that most of our patients were not sick. They were giving birth, not suffering from cancer or a heart attack. A new person was coming into their lives. We were there to ensure that this occurred safely, expeditiously, and comfortably. We also had the opportunity, most of the time, to shape the emotional and psychological quality of this experience. By being flexible about visiting rules, by making an extra trip to the DR to check on a patient for her family, by encouraging the family to take pictures, to hold and admire the baby, we were able to enhance a birth.

One night we had an interesting couple arrive on the unit. They were from the Middle East, and devoutly religious. It was the first baby of this arranged marriage. The father, bearded and dressed all in black, presented a list of demands to the nurse assigned to his wife. She came to me, pissed off by his attitude.

"What does he think this is, anyway? This is a Catholic hospital, for chrissake. He wants us to leave them strictly alone at specific times so they can pray. He wants to wash his hands in a special basin. He wants the crucifix off the wall. He's not supposed to stay in the room during the delivery or exams. He says only a woman can examine his wife, no male doctors. Good grief!"

I went in and talked with the couple. We negotiated his various requests. He agreed to defer to our judgment and accept interruptions if the mother's or baby's conditions so warranted. He seemed imminently reasonable to me; he just had some unusual expectations for his baby's birth. I smoothed the ruffled feathers of the nurse, ran interference, removed the crucifix, and provided the man with a chair just outside the doorway of his wife's room. His imposing demeanor and gruff manner masked a quivering mass of nerves. As his wife's labor progressed rapidly, he paced the hall, unable to sit for more than two minutes at a stretch, wringing his hands, searching my eyes questioningly every time she cried out, seeking reassurance from me that everything was all right. The nurse took care of his wife and I took care of him. When the baby was born, I pulled the curtain aside so that he could greet his son without seeing his wife's exposed bottom, and I was pleased beyond description in his exultant joy.

Because there was so little time for rejuvenating experiences such as these, I left this management job. I missed having my own patients. I detested nursing management. I was astounded by how little preparation was given to any nurse promoted into a management position. Many nurses who become managers choose to do so out of a natural desire to advance within the profession. Many others get recruited into the positions because they have demonstrated an ability to take charge.

As far as I know, there are no formal management training programs for nurse managers. There are workshops on administrative and charge nurse duties and responsibilities, but no hospital I know of prepares its managers in any systematic fashion. It's on-the-job learning, with precious little guidance from nursing administration. As a result there are any number of piss-poor head nurses out there, swinging their weight around and making life even more difficult for their harried staffs. There are many more truly devoted, well-intentioned head nurses who haven't the faintest clue how to effectively manage a unit. They need to be trained properly to manage the small business an L&D unit actually is. A nurse who is outstanding clinically isn't necessarily going to be outstanding administratively.

Fortunately, I recognized relatively quickly that management was not for me and bowed out as gracefully as I could. Enormously relieved, I moved back into a staff nurse position. Taking care of just one patient, not needing to attend to everyone else's needs and concerns—just me and my mother and baby—what pleasure!

After just three years of work, my best friend from nursing school had joined me for a week's rest at the beach. She was a labor and delivery nurse also; we spent many hours that week sharing stories of work. As we talked, it was clear that both of us were exhausted by our work. She finally told me that it shocked her to admit that she was burned out.

"I know. I am, too," I admitted.

"How can this be? To work as hard as we did to get the nursing degree and be worn out this soon? It took four years to graduate and we're exhausted after just three?"

I have struggled with this issue ever since. For more than eight years I've earned my own living by caring for women in childbirth. I have a sense of accomplishment and pride in my ability to support myself after the years of dependency upon my husband. But something has been lost along the way: my idealism, my naïveté, my eagerness, my sense of satisfaction about my work, my sense of making a contribution. Understanding this loss is difficult.

The first two years I worked were years of amazing personal and professional growth. I loved my job and enjoyed the challenge—the excitement of a busy labor deck, the chance to ease the pain and heighten the pleasure of a birth. I was learning all the time. I got along well with the doctors, most of the nurses, and all of my patients. It is a matter of pride for me that no patients or families have ever complained about me. I have a treasured collection of thank-you notes, pictures of babies, and gifts from patients. I have a heart full of memories of many women and their families whose lives I touched so briefly. I know when I go to work that I will do a good job, my patients will be well cared for, and I won't make too many mistakes. So what's the problem?

Some of it is just that I've been in the system long enough to recognize the abuses, to see the mistakes, to know when we are not doing right by our patients. Health-care workers are just like everyone else: there are good ones, bad ones, and many middle-of-the-roaders. There are people who truly care about their work and their patients, who struggle to maintain their ideals and their professional skills. There are those who hate their patients, who don't give a damn about anything but punching the clock and pulling the paycheck, who will actually go out of their way to deny a patient some small comfort, or obstruct others who are trying to do a good job. For many who have been working in health care for years, a patient has no more meaning than a sack of potatoes or a stack of books. The patient is simply the item to be dealt with in the least demanding way possible.

Some of this happens in the large medical centers or in high-volume hospitals, where it is nearly impossible to establish a true connection with patients. If several hundred women give birth each month on a particular labor deck, the patients are moved through the unit as if it were a factory assembly line. Nurses are hard-pressed to remember the faces or names of women they cared for the day before. But this can also be found in nurses and doctors on small units that are supposed to be dedicated to family-centered maternity care. Some of it happens because of chronic staffing shortages. The resultant heavy workload wrings out whatever ideals or compassion may have once existed in a nurse. But even during quiet times when the patient census is low, there are nurses who just don't give a damn.

I have watched quite a number of nurses literally drag themselves to work, shuffle and slump through their shifts, hardly say a word to their patients, dally around the nurses' station while ignoring call bells or cries of pain from their patients' rooms, and spend hours complaining bitterly about their work environment. *If they are so unhappy, why don't they leave? Why don't they look for work somewhere else?* I wondered. It took me a long time to realize that simple economics makes that difficult for many people. It's hard to leave a job where you have built up a good deal of annual leave, a retirement fund, sick leave, where you have seniority and know exactly how the unit works, how to get along with the doctors, and so on.

I wasn't like that. If I didn't feel comfortable on a unit after a period of time, I was gone. Moving from hospital to hospital helped me recognize what was important to me about a workplace. I learned, for example, that I usually preferred to work with residents rather than established private physicians; that a small unit usually meant more time to devote to patient care; that I preferred nursing in the military system rather than the civilian sector. There is a more accessible, formal chain of command for nurses in the military: if a nurse has problems with a doctor, she has nursing management to back her up. But after eight years of work I have no retirement fund, no annual or sick leave. When I worked as an agency nurse, I paid a hefty fee each month for my own medical insurance and no work meant no income. When I took a job as a staff nurse, three to six months had to pass before I had accumulated any annual or sick leave. Unless I did contract work, which left me with absolutely no job security and no benefits, my schedule was dictated by someone else and had little flexibility.

After a couple of years, I began to get wise to other problems. Nursing is a really screwed-up profession. Before the women's movement, nursing was one of the few legitimate career choices for women. In the late eighties, nursing suffered, partially because of the movement. Fewer and fewer good candidates for nursing chose that work, opting instead for newly accessible law, business, or medical schools. Educational requirements for nurses grew more rigorous: a bachelor's degree for a staff job; extra training for speciality nursing such as intensive care, cardiac care, L&D; graduate degrees for administrative or teaching positions. But despite the credentials earned, the job was and still is, in many hospitals, a menial one.

Nurses provide almost all of the hands-on patient care. They are expected to be alert, responsible, knowledgeable, and up-to-date on medical advances. In addition to attending to her physical care, they are also expected to be the patient's source of information, her advocate, and guardian of her safety. Over and above their shift hours, they are expected to contribute to the administration and management of their units—to participate in quality assurance, policy and procedure writing and reviewing, safety and continuing education, and so on. They are expected to carry out the doctor's orders safely and in a timely fashion, all the while being aware of the legal risks and limitations of their practice. Yet nursing services are not even a separate item on the patient's bill: all we do, all we give, all we contribute is lumped under hospital room and board. And until the nursing shortage of the late 1980s, pay and benefits were laughable, reflecting society's attitude toward nursing and nurses. In many places around the country, pay and benefits remain laughable. What thinking, intelligent woman would willingly choose nursing when she could go to graduate school and be a lawyer, a doctor, or a business executive?

A more indirect effect of the women's movement on nursing was the change in nurses' perceptions of their work. There has been a continuing battle among nurses over the definition of nursing. Older nurses, many of whom do not have college degrees, tend to view nursing merely as a job, and a blue-collar one at that. These women trained in a one-or two-year hospital program and worked mostly because they had to. They do not see themselves as professional colleagues with doctors, but as subservient worker bees. Their job is to carry out the orders, not to question them. They have little understanding of nursing theory, the nursing process, nursing diagnoses, or care plans. They keep up with changes in their particular field only out of necessity, when forced to by law or hospital policy.

Other nurses, often younger, have been through a baccalaureate program and are vociferous about upgrading nursing to the status of a profession, with its own policies, standards of behavior and education, body of research, and so forth. These nurses want better pay, more recognition, significant improvements in teamwork with physicians and other health-care providers, more rigorous and national standards for care, and more bargaining power. They work for legislative changes and improved research and education, making speeches, lobbying governments, holding conferences, trying to empower nurses across the nation.

In the middle of all this are the sweet young things, just graduated, who come into nursing all fired up to give hands-on care. Idealistic and filled with theory, they find themselves immediately mired down by infighting, an exhausting workload, and the stultifying, usually messy daily routines. Not surprisingly, many leave nursing within a few years, after marriage or the birth of a child of their own. While they are working, many are subjected to an insidious, subversive pressure to conform to their co-workers' expectations. They are quickly informed that extra effort is frowned upon, because it makes others look bad. Working well with doctors is frowned upon; doctors are nurses' perennial enemies. Reaching out to patients is frowned upon: after the patients are long gone, the nurses will still have to get along with their co-workers, so they shouldn't be an assertive advocate for a patient if it means change or conflict on the unit. When they attend workshops or conferences for continuing education and return to their units excited by what they have learned, older, more experienced nurses may laugh at their enthusiasm and display indifference to the information they have gleaned from the conference.

Some of this is unconscious envy, I think, and may arise out of a fear of inadequacy. Armchair analyzing, I know, but how else to explain the frequent incidents that illustrate this attitude? For instance, one quiet night most of the nurses were sitting idle at the station. A new nurse was in a labor room, "pushing" her patient. This nurse was a delightful woman, eager to learn, excelling in her orientation, working hard to carry her load. She also really cared about her patients, interacting with them in a loving manner that clearly demonstrated her concern for their welfare. We sat and listened to her loud counting, her exhortations to the woman to "push harder! Push harder! One, two, three, . . . That's it, oh that's great! You're doing such a good job!" One of the nurses with me sighed and then grinned.

"This counting!" she said with exasperation. "I've been pushing women for seventeen years and you don't hear me counting! You don't need to count. You don't need to make so much noise. Uh-uh, not me. I like it quiet in my room. None of this cheering squad business."

Did she mean to openly criticize the other nurse? Or was she just commenting on the difference in styles? Did she realize how demoralizing it would be to the other nurse if she heard these comments? Did she deliberately or unconsciously want to undermine this new nurse's self-confidence? I can't say, but I can testify that the new nurse was the one who received gifts and thank-you cards from her patients. The older nurse did her work slowly but competently, just barely meeting the performance standards of her job, never ever extending herself past what was absolutely necessary to retain her position. I never heard any of her patients thank her or praise her efforts, either.

In another situation, I was disgruntled as I listened to a nurse complain about one of our nurses' aides. "She's been around so long, she thinks she knows everything. She'll try to control the delivery room and give you a hard time about everything, but you just remember you're the R.N. and she's just an aide. That's *your* delivery room, not hers. Don't take any shit from her!"

I had had no problems with the aide. After learning how many years of experience she had, I found her to be a remarkable resource as I learned the idiosyncracies of this new hospital. Instead of being irritated by her bossiness, I continually asked her for advice and help. It only made sense to me: she knew the doctors and all the rules and she helped me enormously. I wasn't into any power games; I just wanted to accomplish each delivery as smoothly and efficiently as possible and this woman had spent years doing deliveries. She knew lots of shortcuts: she was like a reference library.

As I've said before, a significant aspect of my disillusionment is the realization that I am participating in a system that makes the act of giving birth a pathological one. In my first explorations into the mystery of childbirth, as a Lamaze instructor, I was a believer in nonintervention, in allowing a woman to labor and give birth without interference with this natural process, unless absolutely necessary. For eight years I have been working in hospitals whose very existences are premised on providing care for sick people. Every woman who comes into my unit is interfered with. Every woman gets an IV, even if she is only minutes away from delivery. Every woman is refused food and water. Every woman is tied down in her bed by monitor lines, IV lines, catheter tubes, ECG lines, and oxygen lines. Inadequate staffing and too many patients mean that I must resort to medication and regional anesthesia to ease the suffering of my patients. Only infrequently do I have the time to sit at the bedside and get a woman through her labor with just my hands, voice, and encouragement.

I think back to that counseling session with my nursing school adviser. I remember how she cautioned me on the need to compromise. I realize that I have learned to compromise with a vengeance: if a woman wants an epidural, even though she is near delivery, I don't argue anymore, I just call the anesthesiologist. If a doctor is acting like a spoiled toddler, I look the other way. If a patient on the unit has an intrauterine fetal demise I avoid her. I watch other nurses behave insensitively and hold my tongue.

All the while it gets more difficult to be honest with patients about the procedures and routines we impose on them. It's easy to explain why a woman must have a catheter in her bladder if she is going for a cesarean: the bladder must be empty and out of the way or risk getting sliced when the scalpel cuts into her lower abdomen. It's a hell of a lot harder for me to explain the necessity for an IV in a woman close to delivery or even just laboring normally. It's hard for me to watch a doctor cut an episiotomy rather than be patient enough to massage the perineal tissue to help it stretch naturally for the baby. It's hard for me to watch a woman thrash and scream as a doctor thrusts her hand and arm up inside the woman to remove a placenta that just hasn't come out fast enough for the doctor. It's hard for me to hold a woman's hand and encourage her to hang on just a little longer while a physician struggles to get a scalp blood sample from her baby, reaching up through a long cone with a little blade to cut the baby's head, while the mother lies on an upside-down bedpan, her butt up in the air, contracting and hollering. It's hard for me to tell a patient she has to suffer for a while longer because the anesthesiologist is doing rounds or another epidural. It's hard for me to stand by a delivery table and watch inexperienced residents pull and tug at a woman's vaginal tissues until they swell to hideous size, resulting in days or even weeks of ice packs, sitz baths, and pain every time she sits down or urinates.

I fight battles every day for my patients. I wade through the chain of command if necessary. I argue and cajole and plead with doctors to get concessions for my patients. I clown and play in the labor and delivery rooms, trying to get everyone to focus on the significance of this event—a new baby! a birthday!—and don't care whether my co-workers think I'm an asshole.

Once I listened to a nurse describe a birth she attended at a midwives' birthing center and I wept because it was so far removed from the births I attended. The mother soaked in a Jacuzzi; she strolled around the center on her husband's arm, her other children nearby; she cooked and ate a light lunch in the kitchen. She had no IV, no monitor. The midwives listened to the baby's heartbeat with a stethoscope, something I don't even know how to do. She gave birth in a big double bed in a sunlit room, her husband on the bed with her, her daughter reaching out for the baby as it emerged and crying out with love, "Here's my little brother! Oh, I love him, my little brother!" The family spent an hour recuperating on the big bed together, the baby quietly suckling at his mother's breast. Then they packed up and went home. No catheters, no middle of the night vital signs, no hospital food, no separation from their baby or one another.

Even as I cried over how my involvement with childbirth had become so clinical, so pathological, so medical, so unnatural, I know that quite often what we do in the hospital saves a life. A mother severely stricken with diabetes or preeclampsia can survive her illness and give birth to a healthy baby only with our help and our vigilance. A baby who might have died if his mother had tried to deliver at home, lives instead, delivered by cesarean section. A woman who could never before carry a child to term is protected and treated until the fetus is mature enough to survive. Women rarely die of childbirth anymore, because of what we do daily, because of our knowledge, technology, and clinical skills. This is a fact, something I would not argue with. I know from my own experience as an obstetrical nurse that much of what we do is significant and makes a difference to our patients. Nevertheless, I am no longer the naïve, starry-eyed, eager nurse, raring to go in there and make a difference for this patient, this birth. I have struggled to come to terms with my need for employment, my skills and successes as a L&D nurse, and my feelings of deep disenchantment.

As time passed, I grew increasingly more disillusioned. It was difficult to go to work. I had to spend ten minutes in my car psyching myself up before I could enter the hospital for my shift. I would tell myself, "It's only eight hours; you can survive eight hours." I felt disconnected from my patients and my co-workers. My work was competent, occasionally outstanding, but I didn't feel I was giving my all or getting much back. Rarely did anyone acknowledge anyone else's efforts. I tried to thank the doctors and nurses I worked with, to praise the efforts of the nurses' aides and LPNs. I tried to remain cheerful and playful, but my heart wasn't in it.

I spent twelve hours with a laboring couple one night, assisting them through a long labor. I did all the things I'd done so many times before: guarding the mother and baby by watching the monitor vigilantly; getting the mother an epidural, ice chips, clean linens; emptying her bedpan and emesis basin; wiping her mucky bottom; holding her legs up while she pushed; explaining and reassuring and encouraging. We enjoyed each other. She and her husband thanked me for my help several times through the night. After the baby was delivered, just before the end of my shift, I was cleaning up debris in the room while the doctor chatted with the new parents and did his charting. As he said his good-byes, the mother said, "Wait, Dr. X, you can't leave until we have a picture of you holding the baby. Please, we want it for the baby book!" The doctor graciously posed with baby in arms for a photo. I stood and watched.

I just couldn't get over the whole scene. I spent twelve solid hours with this couple, the doctor less than thirty minutes. He got his picture taken and heard the words "we couldn't have done it without you." It was as if I was completely invisible. I didn't care about not being included in a photograph, but I did care about how the episode made me feel. I was regarded as completely extraneous. I had provided all the care this woman received, with the exception of the physical delivery of her baby, but the doctor was rewarded with the credit. In the eyes of most people, patients and doctors alike, I'm not a professional, I'm a servant. I'm there to do the dirty work. I couldn't help but ask myself, "For this I went back to school for four years, incurred whopping debt? For this I put myself at risk of malpractice lawsuits?" It was an inconsequential event, something I wouldn't have even noticed in the early years of work. But now I was worn out and, ridiculous or not, it stung.

Then, in my sixth year of nursing, I was involved in a case that resulted in a bad outcome. The mother was having her fourth baby, but she had problems with diabetes and an intestinal disease, so she was being induced. When I took over her care, she had been in labor for more than twelve hours. The baby's monitor strip wasn't wonderful to look at: the line representing the heartbeat was pretty flat, which might have been an indication of possible stress or just a lengthy sleep cycle. I didn't look at the whole strip, just the past four or five hours' worth. At the beginning of my shift, her internal uterine monitor had come out. (This catheter, hollow and filled with water, accurately measures the direct pressure of the contraction.) The resident and I worked together to insert a new catheter. When it was inserted, clear amniotic fluid came back into the catheter, a direct indicator that there was no meconium in the fluid. If meconium had been present, the fluid would have been green, and we would have been alert to possible fetal distress.

The patient's epidural had been redosed just before we inserted the uterine catheter. Soon thereafter, the resident checked her cervix again and told her it was time to push. The doctor and I both expected a short pushing phase because this woman had already vaginally delivered three other children—an indication of a perfectly adequate pelvis. However, since she couldn't feel her legs or belly because of the epidural, the patient couldn't push effectively, so we gave her a half hour to rest. I checked her temperature and reported to the doctor that she was feverish. With a fever of 103 degrees, she probably had an infection that would pass to the baby: we knew we had to get her delivered expeditiously. We started antibiotic therapy in the IV and "pushed" her.

What should have taken only a short time lasted an hour. The resident and I worked together the entire time, holding the woman's legs for her and exhorting her to "Push! *Push!*" Finally she moved the baby down enough for forceps and we moved her to the delivery room. The pediatric residents were present because it was to be a forceps delivery.

When I try to recall the hour we spent in the delivery room, all I remember is normal confusion: two residents and an intern at the foot of the table, two pediatricians at the warmer, an aide opening equipment, another nurse in and out of the room as she brought in needed instruments. I was at the woman's head most of the time, coaching her in her pushing. What I can't explain now is why, during all that time, I wrote no notes. I had a paper record of her labor on the fetal monitor strip, but I didn't scribble anything on it to indicate when the forceps were applied, or what her vital signs were—nothing. I should have made notes but just didn't. Usually deliveries are accomplished fairly rapidly after moving the patient to the delivery room, and in my experience, most nurses do very little documentation in the DR, other than completing the standardized delivery forms. But I was in this delivery room for an hour and should have been documenting what was happening during that time.

The residents tried repeatedly to get forceps on this baby's head. They tried several different types of forceps. I remember feeling a bit concerned about how much time was going by, but I trusted the chief resident. He was a good doctor: I had never seen him make any mistakes clinically, and I just assumed he knew what he was doing. Finally the head came out, mostly through the continued pushing efforts of the mother. Behind the head came a rush of fluid—thick, pea-soup meconium with chunks of gunk in it. This is very bad stuff. If the baby breathes any of it into its lungs, meconium acts like tar and prevents adequate lung expansion and oxygenation. It can be lethal. The resident immediately suctioned the mouth and nostrils before delivering the body, to prevent aspiration of the fluid when the baby takes its first breaths. The baby was delivered and handed to the pediatricians. They used a laryngoscope to look down the throat at the vocal cords and, to everyone's dismay, saw green fluid below the cords. This is not a reassuring sign: it means some of the fluid may have been breathed in, although it doesn't necessarily guarantee the fluid has gone all the way down the bronchial tree into the lungs themselves.

The baby was not responsive to stimulation or suction. It had very low Apgars. The doctors intubated the baby and rushed it to the intensive-care nursery to be placed on a respirator. A couple of hours later, after cleaning up after the delivery, I called the nursery to check on the baby. "She's fighting for her life right now," the nursery nurse informed me. I spent some time with the parents, explaining the problems with meconium aspiration and assured them the pediatricians would keep them informed.

The next night at work, I was told the head nurse wanted to see me. I was totally unaware of the storm that had raged through the unit that day over the management of this patient. The resident who had delivered her had been roasted by his superiors. All the nurses' notes had been examined carefully and my boss gently scolded me for inadequate charting. I looked over the notes, horrified to discover that I was the only nurse in three shifts to take the woman's temperature or write anything about the baby's heart rate tracing. Even so, I only wrote that the strip looked nonreassuring; I did not write what measures were taken to improve it (oxygen, position changes, fetal scalp stimulation) or anything at all about how the doctor and I had worked in the labor and delivery rooms to get her delivered.

On paper, it looked like no one was paying any attention. I also didn't note "clear fluid" when we replaced the uterine catheter. This was critical, because the pediatricians were certain the baby had been soaking in meconium for hours before delivery but I knew from my own eyes the meconium wasn't in the fluid an hour and a half before the delivery. It is probable that the meconium was passed during the stress of having forceps applied to the baby's head, since the baby had to have inhaled it while she was still in the vaginal canal.

The realization that I had failed the resident—first with my inadequate notes and then by not pushing the resident to call his superior when he failed with the forceps—had a devastating effect on me. Here again was the old pattern: the doctor is the boss, but the nurse is expected to be vigilant and go up the chain of command when she thinks the doctor isn't performing appropriately. Residents in particular rely heavily on nurses for guidance and judgment calls, even though they have the final authority. The resident and my boss believed I had failed in my duty by not insisting or even suggesting the resident call in a superior. Even though I don't like this conflict of roles in which the figure without authority becomes the authority figure, in the past I haven't hesitated to act when I thought it necessary. I just didn't do it this time.

The resident was depending on me but I was so relaxed about his excellent clinical skills that I never thought of challenging what he was doing in the delivery room. I had let him down and it made me feel physically sick. If I'd acted differently, he might have been spared the abuse he received from his superiors. I just ached over the pain I put him through, and could hardly bear to visit the parents over the next few days because I was so stricken over what had happened to their baby. I couldn't believe how complicated the case became after the fact. In all good faith the resident and I had done our best, but it wasn't good enough, and now a little baby was battling for survival in the intensive-care nursery.

For weeks following this delivery I was tormented and obsessed by this event. I knew I had acted in good faith during those three hours. I knew I was a good nurse and that the doctors relied on my judgment. I couldn't find any rational explanation for my poor charting other than the normal lack of time, or for my lack of vigilance in the delivery room. *If only I had done . . . if only I had . . .* kept reverberating in my mind. I talked with my sister and my best friend about the case. I reviewed the events of the night repeatedly with other nurses who had been there. I cried and lost sleep and ached with guilt and anguish over this baby and the doctor's pain. Other nurses assured me I had acted in good faith. People reminded me that I was only human and that I couldn't always do this work without an occasional failure. Nothing helped.

In my heart, I knew that I was exhausted. I knew that I hadn't been vigilant enough. I knew that a year before this event I wouldn't have failed to request staff backup. A year earlier I would have been far more frantic in the delivery room as time crept on and forceps attempts failed and the mother's pushing was ineffective. I was slipping, and it absolutely terrified me. My confidence was destroyed. I went to work in fear and practiced defensively, wrote pages and pages of charting, and nagged doctors relentlessly, feeling enveloped in a cloud of anxiety and terror. I was unable to achieve any perspective about this case and continued to feel grievously at fault for failing the doctor who had come to rely on my good judgment and experience. I didn't know how I could go on, with the ever-present possibility of another bad outcome, or if I could weather this storm and survive intact as a nurse. I began to believe seriously that I needed to leave nursing.

When I started working as a labor and delivery nurse I was so innocent. I had such idealistic fantasies about enhancing the birth experience. Now, six years later, I knew better. All the frustration of being a nurse coalesced with this one case. The irregular hours, the poor pay, the immense responsibility, the legal liability, the lack of authority, the irascibility of doctors, nurses, and other hospital personnel, the needs and demands and the suffering of the patients—all had eroded the enthusiasm and love I had for my work in the first years of nursing. Now my very confidence in my own skills and judgment was demolished by one bad case, even though the baby recovered and survived with no obvious problems, going home with her parents two weeks after her birth. Still, I didn't know whether I could go on.

Chapter Sixteen

FINAL THOUGHTS

It took me a full year to recapture some of my self-confidence after the torment of that case. A number of times in the delivery room, I nearly panicked and fled. In each situation, during a seemingly normal delivery, problems such as unexpected thick meconium, or difficulties applying forceps, or a baby suddenly in need of resuscitation would give me flashbacks. Adrenaline pumped, my pulse rate and blood pressure rose as I poured sweat and panted with fear and the desire to run away. I had to consciously fight the almost overwhelming urge to just get the hell out of there! As I did what I needed to do, responding to the doctors' requests, helping with a resuscitation, pulling out equipment or bagging a baby with oxygen, I was silently praying, chanting to myself: *don't panic, keep going, you can't leave, just get through it, keep it together, keep it together.*

Before each delivery, I opened equipment for suction and resuscitation even when there wasn't any indication it would be needed, wasting costly sterile materials rather than get caught off guard. One baby's head was delivered, followed by a stream of thick meconium. I had the suction tubing ready in my hand but was so paralyzed by a flashback that I couldn't even hand it to the doctor for a few seconds, then handed it to her upside down. Every cell in my body was screeching: *GET OUT OF HERE! IT'S HAPPENING AGAIN! GET OUT OF HERE!* My documentation had never been so lengthy, detailed, and laborious. I came to work so anxious that my ability to concentrate was impaired: common obstetrical activities were sometimes completely unintelligible to me and my ability to act swiftly and respond purposefully were hindered by mental confusion. I read and reread my nursing notes, frantically searching for possible errors and omissions, unable to actually make sense of what I had written.

Only time and repeated success with patients, success I had never even thought to question before, helped ease these feelings. Very little pleasure was obtained during this period; it was all I could do just to competently meet the needs of the patients. Enjoying the process was the last thing I thought about. Not a day passed that I didn't consider quitting nursing. I forced myself to reiterate silently all the reasons why I had to keep working: my mortgage payment, groceries, the car loan, other bills, the years of education I'd invested. My physician brother listened to my story and remonstrated with me: "Susie, you've made so few mistakes in the six years you've been working. What would happen if all the good people in health care quit when something went wrong. We all make mistakes. We all suffer through heartbreaking losses that we feel somehow responsible for. But who would take care of our patients if we left? They need you!"

Yeah, yeah, I thought, *but if I left, no one would really notice, and I'm so tired of all the responsibility, the backbreaking work, the nonsensical policies, and the endless paperwork.*

After several months of this stress, along with some helpful therapy, I was able to make some positive changes. My sister Katy was going off to medical school (at age forty-six!); Rebecca was in college; and Michael was in high school, still living with his father and stepmother. I found employment at a hospital maternity center in another city. Reluctantly, Katy and I ended our six-year cohabitation. With her blessings and financial support, I moved south, bought a house all my own, and plunged into yet another job. I went through yet another orientation period, learning policies and paperwork, how patients were cared for, and the names and personalities of all the people around me. In making this move to a new home and workplace, in effect I was starting over. I had to reestablish, in new territory, that I was competent and confident. Proving that I was a good nurse to people who had no knowledge of my past successes and failures was the therapy I needed to restore my self-esteem and relieve some of the anxiety I felt about being responsible for my patients' well-being.

The hospital was a good place for me. Well funded, well staffed, and furnished with state-of-the-art equipment, the maternity center was downright luxurious when compared to my previous work environments. I walked on lush carpets past tasteful, expensively framed art. Walls were painted in muted, restful colors. I enjoyed spacious, well-designed nurses' stations. I worked in birthing rooms flooded with sunlight and/or moonlight from large picture windows. The place felt more like a hotel than a hospital.

Best of all, the nurse/patient ratio was one-to-one. I spent many hours of each shift in a birthing room with just one family to care for. For the most part, the doctors were relatively easy to work with, after they got to know me. I enjoyed my co-workers and assiduously avoided any extracurricular assignments on committees. I began to have fun again, even though I still had to sit in my car for ten minutes psyching myself up for the oncoming shift, mentally gathering myself to face whatever was to come.

One night I took care of a patient who had already been in the center for twenty-two hours. She had walked most of the night, trying to get her labor to advance from intermittent contractions to a more regular pattern. At seven in the morning she was finally admitted, after achieving one centimeter of dilation. When I walked into her room at seven that evening to begin my twelve-hour shift, she looked me up and down silently and then turned to the off-going nurse. "Is this one any good?" she asked. "I don't want anyone in here if they're not the best!" She looked back at me, "Well, *are* you any good? Do you know what you're doing?"

Oh jeez, what have I walked into here? Is the whole night going to be like this? I thought as I smiled at her and said, "Uh, yeah, of course I'm good! We don't carry any 'bads' in this place!"

What a night that woman and I had together! Ettalyn was an medical transcriptionist, so she had a lot of second-hand knowledge about medicine, but this was her first pregnancy and she knew just a little too much for her own good. When I began with her, she had just received her first dose of a narcotic to ease some of her discomfort. She was barely three centimeters and hadn't slept for two days. The narcotic made her feel good for a brief while, but she was tired and had little patience.

We got to know each other as I familiarized myself with her chart, reviewed the monitor strips, and checked her IV. As with every patient, Ettalyn's individuality had been somewhat erased when we removed her clothes to enfold her in a drab, featureless hospital gown. After so many hours, whatever makeup she might have applied before coming to the hospital had long since disappeared. A frizz of bleached blond hair framed her round face. Short of stature, she was heavy, and not only from the pregnancy. Ettalyn's bright hazel eyes revealed a woman of sharp intelligence. Tommy-Joe, her husband, was tall and beefy, with bristly brush-cut hair, squinty eyes, and big arms and belly. They warmed to me and I to them as we talked about how hungry Ettalyn was: she fantasized aloud about which foods she could have after her delivery. Her husband consumed a couple of hamburgers as the two of us talked about our favorite foods.

Within an hour, the narcotic began to wear off and Ettalyn became more uncomfortable, struggling with the contractions and begging for more pain relief. In report, I had learned from her day nurse that Ettalyn adamantly refused to even consider an epidural. I was concerned about how many doses of narcotics I could give her and what we would do when I couldn't give her anymore. If she was having this much trouble in early labor, I really dreaded the time when she would be in hard labor.

I gave her another dose of narcotics. After talking with her doctor, I decided that I was going to get to the bottom of her refusal of the epidural. When Ettalyn was comfortable, I sat next to her and asked casually, "What exactly is it about the epidural that you object to?"

"I just don't like those things," she replied.

"Well, can you tell me why?"

"I've just heard too many bad things about them. Nope, I don't want anyone playing around with my spinal column!"

"Can you tell me more specifically what you've heard? I get all kinds of misinformation about them; maybe I can clear up some of this for you," I offered. "Do you know how they're administered?"

"Yeah, I know that I probably can't push if I have one. I know I won't be able to walk afterward for up to three days. And I don't want to have a spinal headache either; I want to be able to nurse my baby right away."

Oh boy, I thought, *everybody and her sister have been telling tales about epidurals to this woman!* "Look, let me just run through this with you, okay? Used to be, years ago, that the medicine used in epidurals could make a woman's legs so numb that she couldn't move or lift or control them. Now the doses and types of medication used are so carefully measured that almost all women can still move their legs, and they absolutely can push effectively. Sometimes it takes longer because you can't feel the muscles you're using, but you can still do it. I've never, ever had a patient who couldn't walk for three days, much less a day after an epidural. Sometimes it takes a few hours to wear off, but never a day.

"Headaches are very, very rare today, too. First of all, the needle used to place the epidural doesn't even go into the spinal canal, if it's done right. Used to be, the needle they used for spinals were so big that they left a hole in the membrane that covers the canal. Spinal fluid leaked out of the hole and caused really bad headaches. But with an epidural, the needles don't penetrate the canal. The anesthetic medicine gets placed in the space around the canal, not in it."

"But I hate needles! I mean I really hate them. I'm afraid of being hurt because it's a big needle, I know it is."

"Yeah, it's a big needle, but you won't feel it because the anesthesiologist numbs the spot first with a local, using a very small needle. In fact, getting the local is usually the worst part of it. You've had locals before, haven't you? In the dentist's office, maybe? Here's what happens. First we get you into a position on your side or sitting up curled over the table. The anesthesiologist cleans your back with Betadine solution after he's felt around for the correct vertebrae. Then he gives you the local, which stings and then very rapidly goes numb. For you, the hardest part is maintaining the position while contracting! Then the doctor uses the big needle, which you can't see, to find the epidural space outside the spinal canal. When he's in the right place, he gives you a test dose while I get your blood pressure and watch your pulse. Next, he threads a really thin, flexible, plastic catheter into the epidural space, outside the canal, remember, and tapes it to your back. It gets hooked up on the other end to this little pump, just like your IV pump, only much smaller, and that keeps a continuous dose of medication running in. Your legs may tingle first and then get progressively more numb. I check your level of anesthesia by touching you with something sharp or cold from your thighs up to your breasts, and make sure that you're pain-free from your bellybutton down past your butt. You may still feel a tightening sensation in your belly with the contractions, but you won't feel the pain. We keep the medicine going until after the baby is born, so if you have an episiotomy or need some stitches, you won't feel that."

"What about the baby? Is it risky for the baby?" she asked.

"There's always some risk in any procedure done during labor and delivery, but the risks are really minimal. The most common side effect of epidurals is a possible lowering of your blood pressure, which could effect the blood flow to the baby. That's why we take your blood pressure so many times you'll hate the damned cuff, but if your pressure drops, we have medicine we can put in the IV to bring it back up. We give you extra oxygen, too, just to ensure the baby's getting enough. Other possible side effects are a level of anesthesia that goes too high, so that breathing may be affected; a rare, I mean very rare, chance of penetration into the spinal canal and a headache afterward; and sometimes an epidural doesn't work well and the patient may have an area where she still feels the pain. These are not usual or common and we can do things to correct them. That's one of the reasons I stay right here at your side through the whole of your labor, to monitor you and watch for possible problems."

"Well, I just don't know," Ettalyn mused. "I want to do this thing right, you know? I want to do natural childbirth if I can. I don't want to disappoint my husband."

"Honey, you won't disappoint me," Tommy-Joe assured her. "You're the one going through this. If you can't stand the pain, I'm not going to just sit here and watch you hurt. You get whatever you need to deal with it. That's okay with me! Seems like from what Susie's said, that it's not too bad. We didn't really know what an epidural was like," he explained to me. "Do many women get them here?"

"Most women do. Probably eighty to eighty-five percent of them do. It's real routine." I responded. "Look, if you want to try natural childbirth, I'm all for it. I used to teach Lamaze and I really like to help mothers who are motivated to try, but Ettalyn, my main concern is for you and the baby to stay healthy through this process. After that, I want having your baby to be a good experience for you. I'm not a medication-pusher but I really believe that if a woman is suffering so much from her labor that she's exhausted when the baby finally delivers, it's awfully hard to get any pleasure out of the birth. The advantage of an epidural is that you won't be wasted when it's time to push and then hold your baby. This doesn't have to be a tortuous experience, you know! Let's just take it one step at a time. I can give you more of the narcotic when you need it, and we'll see how it goes, okay?"

"Okay, I'll think about it," she answered. Shortly after this conversation, she began to get uncomfortable again. I gave her another narcotic dose, but it didn't relieve her pain. She was in active labor; a cervical check indicated she was almost five centimeters. This was slow progress, but she was dilating and the contractions were much harder to handle.

"Oh, I can't stand it, Susie! Give me some more of that stuff! Do something, anything! I can't take this!" Ettalyn was crying and yelling during the contractions, demanding relief.

"It's too soon to redose with the narcotic, Ettalyn. I just gave it to you fifteen minutes ago."

"It's not working at all, Susie! Oh, oh, this hurts, oh it's killing me! Get the epidural, let's just do it, I can't stand this!" she cried.

The anesthesiologist was called and I gathered all the supplies needed for the epidural. When he entered the room, Ettalyn started crying about how scared she was. "You're not going to hurt me, are you?" she wept. The anesthesiologist was calm, quick, and reassuring. In minutes the procedure was complete and Ettalyn felt relief.

Once again I was made aware of how little women understand about obstetrical care. This mother was in the medical field and yet had only misinformed wives' tales about epidurals. I have given my lengthy explanation of the whole process innumerable times. Each time the patient changed her mind, but I'm not sure the explanation had anything to do with the shift in attitude. I think it's probably just the pain, unexpected and unimagined in its intensity, that persuades women to ask for an epidural.

We spent the next few hours quietly. Tommy-Joe slept on the father's cot after eating something else. Ettalyn couldn't sleep so she and I had a long quiet conversation about her transcribing work. Finally she was fully dilated and ready to push. Another nurse came in and offered me a break. "You're not going anywhere!" Ettalyn hollered. "I'll never forgive you if you leave me now! I don't want someone else in this room. You're staying right here and pushing with me!"

"Okay, okay, Ettalyn! I won't go! Relax already!" I brought all the delivery equipment into the room and we got serious. Sitting on the end of the bed, holding up her feet and watching her vulva, I coached her through a couple of contractions. She was squeezing and lifting her bottom up as she pushed.

"No, wait a minute, Ettalyn," I said. "I can see you're squeezing in down here in the rectal area. You gotta let that go. Push out, don't hold in!"

"Oh I just couldn't do that, Susie! What if I fart or shit? I'd just die!"

Once again I made my little speech: "There ain't nothing a woman can squirt or ooze or leak from her body that I haven't seen, touched, and smelled. If you fart or shit, I know you're pushing in the right place. It's the positive poop sign, Ettalyn so come on, babe, and fart away!"

She laughed and got into it, pushing much more effectively than before. Finally she moved the baby down enough for me to see it if I stretched the labia and inner vaginal folds open with my fingers. Tommy-Joe got out the video camera—they wanted a record, for their eyes only, of everything! I knelt as far out of the way as I could, held open her private parts, and pointed with my finger to the baby's head, as Tommy-Joe got the camera in for a close-up. It was hilarious, all three of us talking about keeping this video hidden from the family, Tommy-Joe and I cheering Ettalyn on in her efforts, counting and grunting along with her.

Then it happened. I was leaning into her feet with my arms and hands, seated on the end of the bed between her legs. The contraction started and I was exhorting her to push, push hard. As I counted for her, I was unconsciously bearing down myself, and *poof!* out came a loud fart—and it was mine! Tommy-Joe, sitting on a rolling stool next to me, just scuttled away from me as fast as he could. Ettalyn exploded with guffaws, losing all her pushing effort, legs splaying on the bed as she and I howled with laughter, tears of mirth rolling down our faces. "Oh gosh, I'm sorry!" I sputtered. "Don't worry, Tommy-Joe, mine almost never smell!"

We doubled over and rocked with glee, all three of us. "Well, you just made it into my family's Book of the Most Embarrassing Moments," Ettalyn giggled. "You're an honorary member now!" They both went on to tell me about some of those famous moments, in between contractions. We couldn't stop giggling. I was embarrassed only for a moment. It was so funny and worked so well to relax Ettalyn that I really didn't care. We were completely comfortable with one another by now, and it also made me more human to her. The room was filled with laughter and easy congeniality, even with all her hard work. It was a good place for a baby to come into, real down-home!

An hour before I was to go off duty, Ettalyn delivered. I hadn't left the room in hours. It was a mess, even though I'd tried during the night to keep up with the trash. Dirty towels in one corner, glove wrappers on the counter, the garbage pail overflowing, a bedpan on the floor in the bathroom. Ettalyn and Tommy-Joe had occupied this room for nearly twenty-four hours and their belongings were everywhere. When we started pushing, my housekeeping efforts stopped as I focused solely on coaching her with the contractions. The charge nurse came in to assist with the delivery and started griping immediately about the mess, as she opened sterile packs of instruments and readied the warmer for the baby.

I tried unsuccessfully to ignore her. Yeah, the room was a mess, but the patient was in a great frame of mind, had pushed hard and well for more than two hours, and we were about to have a baby. What was a little mess, if the mother and father were as relaxed and cooperative and enthusiastic as these two were? All through the next forty minutes, the charge nurse muttered under her breath, criticizing everything I did: the equipment wasn't set up the way she thought it should be, I was behind in my charting *(because I can't hold up two legs and count through a push if I'm writing, goddammit!)*, and the room was a mess! My high spirits fled and I began a slow burn that lasted for days. Who was this woman to come in the room in the last few minutes and criticize me this way? I just spent eleven hours getting this woman through her labor, helping her on and off the bedpan, watching the monitors, wiping her butt, changing smelly, mucky chucks, holding an emesis basin while she vomited, changing bed linens that got vomited on, explaining and comforting and cajoling and encouraging—and writing a page of notes every damned fifteen minutes! I'd had one fifteen-minute break eight hours earlier and I had done a great job calming this woman's fears and getting her through it all.

Who was she to come in here and start passing judgment on me without having any idea whatsoever about what had transpired through the long night; how frightened this woman was of everything, of failure? Being critical of me in front of the patient, charging around the room rearranging the furniture and equipment, put an immediate damper on our relaxed happy moods. The baby was born with appropriate cheers and tears, but I was close to crying with humiliation and frustration. It made me so mad I was spitting with ire by the time I drove home.

I talked to that nurse about it the next night, trying to make her understand how her manner and her insensitivity affected me and the patient, but I didn't get through to her. She had virtually no insight into how another nurse might care for a patient effectively, if messily. She just expected me to do it the way she'd been doing it for years, efficiently, matter-of-factly, with as little emotional investment in the patient as possible. To be sure, I had to spend a little extra time catching up on my notes and I was messy, but that couple and I had a marvelous experience that night. We were comfortable with each other. I had eased a lot of Ettalyn's fear and helped make her feel good about her progress through labor.

I know now and knew then that I was overreacting to the nurse's criticism. But I couldn't help it. She pissed me off; I was too thin-skinned and too angry about the issue to let it go. I was working under someone who treated me like a child, ordering me around as if I didn't know how to do my work. I was forty-odd years old, had two college degrees and eight years of experience, a lot of it in high-risk obstetrics, and I just abhorred having someone push me around instead of according me the respect my experience and education deserved.

This was just one more in a long line of insults, all coming out of the old attitudes about nurses. We were always being told by management that we were professionals. We were expected to have college credentials and special training, to be responsible for patients' safety and well-being, while at the same time we were treated like blue-collar workers. "Professionals" do not punch a time clock. We did. Endless memos reprimanded us for trivial things that somehow consumed the attention of the administration, but actually weren't that significant in terms of patient care. I found myself carrying on the same old tired arguments in my head, fuming about how my work was routinely trivialized by people who had no concept of the effort, thought, and concern I put into my job. A pleasing interaction with a couple who responded to my care and my personality in such a positive way, a night spent tirelessly and successfully trying to ease pain and fear, ended with me in angry tears on the way home. Why was I still doing this, after eight years? Why did I let people who really didn't matter—belligerent charge nurses, rude and arrogant doctors—affect me like this?

In spite of the posh environment, these questions continued to clatter around in my thoughts; I became even more conflicted about what I was doing. Every positive feeling I had about what I did every day was countered by a negative aspect of the job. My tolerance for doctors and administrators grew thinner with each confrontational episode. Other nurses felt the same way but somehow seemed to let go of their negative emotions more easily. Many of them had just given up. They couldn't continue working if they allowed their outrage at the system's faults to surface, so most of them just shook their heads and said, "That's nursing. It's been this way forever and we aren't going to change it by complaining about it. Even if we go through official channels and write incident reports and so on, no one in management ever listens . . . why fight it?"

My anger over the way in which I felt the charge nurse had undermined my work with Ettalyn and Tommy-Joe didn't adversely affect the many normal births I assisted with in this, my last year of work. Each of those births were positive events for their parents, because of my efforts and those of the people with whom I worked. It was wonderful to have a large supportive staff that freed me from secretarial or housecleaning tasks, and I appreciated the luxurious conditions in which we labored. For the most part, the nurses I worked with were great people, supportive and caring of their patients and of one another. Gradually, I had become an accepted member of the team; I had friends at work again. I was proud of my association with this birthing center.

Every job has both blessings and curses. You have to take the bad with the good, I kept telling myself, yet I couldn't seem to maintain a balanced perception of my work. I was whining and crying and losing sleep way out of proportion to the relatively few unpleasant circumstances in my work. I truly hated how I felt—ashamed of myself, and of my groundless dissatisfaction with the work I'd chosen with such enthusiasm years earlier. What was wrong with me? I had a good job in a progressive, wealthy hospital, received good benefits, worked with good people—people I liked, respected, and enjoyed. My patients were top-of-the-line, educated, well-to-do or middle class. I didn't have to deal with drug addicts or homeless, diseased, poor patients. I could usually pick the shifts I wanted to work; since I worked three twelve-hour shifts a week, I had four other days off each week. The pay didn't match what I made as an agency nurse or as a staff nurse at a military hospital, but what the hell—this was the South, where the cost of living was lower. I really had absolutely no right to complain.

So I tried not to. I tried hard to accept my lot, to appreciate each day how privileged I was to have a good job, to be able to work with birthing families and contribute to their babies' births. I tried to remember that even if I didn't like the system, with all its faults, I still could make a difference just by doing my work well and with enthusiasm.

I found great pleasure in my new home, with its many light-pouring windows, its airy rooms stuffed with beloved houseplants. It was surrounded by flowerbeds to putter in, green lawns, and flowering trees, even a magnificent huge gardenia bush that blossomed heavily in the spring, filling my kitchen with its uniquely southern scent. Best of all were the friends I enjoyed outside the hospital. Determined to reestablish a social life, I had chosen this area because of the old friends who lived here. These dear friends from my past welcomed me with open arms, introducing me to other people who also made me feel finally at home. We spent a lot of time together, and being with people unconnected with the hospital was incredibly therapeutic.

Life was definitely improving, after too long a period of depression, loneliness, and frustration with the medical world in which I had been so deeply involved. I thought I was going to be okay—do my work, make an effort for the benefit of my patients, pick up my paycheck, and then forget about my job; enjoy my home and my friends; spread my wings a little (maybe start dating again?); find a publisher for my still unfinished book. . . . I didn't have to change the world—hell, I was worn down enough to admit I couldn't—I just had to make the best of my little corner of it. Yep, I was ready to accept the limitations in my life, to diminish my expectations (one of the developmental tasks of middle-age, according to popular theory), and find a modicum of serenity in my secure little world.

One gorgeous late May afternoon, in less than ten minutes, that hard-earned, fragile serenity was instantaneously annihilated. I had just left Rebecca at the airport; she was off to spend a week with her father before returning to be with me for part of her summer break. As I started to unlock the front door of my house, I glimpsed, through the glass panel by the door, a strange man in my bedroom. Before I had time to mentally process his presence in my house or the fact that the door was already ajar, the man rushed me. For the next four or five minutes, we fought: I was screaming, he was cursing. He was trying to pull me into the house, I was trying to get free of his grip and run. I screamed and struggled in a fury of panic, with one absolutely clear thought reverberating in my mind: *At least Rebecca's not here. I can take anything as long as my kids are safe.*

The man's brute strength finally overwhelmed me; I found myself flat on the ground, lying in the mud, smashing the flowers I had so lovingly planted a week earlier. I pleaded for my life as he stood over me, threatening to kill me. *Rape* and *death* flashed through my mind as I begged, "Please don't hurt me, please don't hurt me!" Repeating my litany as loudly as I could, I watched him trying to decide what to do with me. Abruptly, he grabbed my purse from the sidewalk where I'd dropped it in the melee and took off running. For twenty more seconds, I kept shouting "please don't hurt me," and then I bolted through my house, running faster than I've ever run in my life.

The neighbors called the cops, who arrived sooner than I thought possible, and we began the process of cleaning up after a crime. I described what happened three or four times. They dusted for prints. Nothing was missing in the house; apparently I'd interrupted my assailant only moments after he'd broken in. I went to the police station, looked at several hundred photos, helped construct a composite drawing of the guy. I called my closest friend, who joined me at the police station and later took me home with her for the night. Through all of this I alternated between near-hysterical tears, calm professional interchanges with the police, and near-euphoric laughter with my friend. Needless to say I didn't go to work that night!

The following night I slept in my own bed in my own house, defiantly: no son-of-a-bitch burglar was going to scare me away from my own home, by God! After obsessively checking the new $400 locks on my doors and taking a metal baseball bat into my bed, I actually got a good night's sleep. When I went back to work two nights after this escapade, everyone wanted to hear what happened so I repeated my story more often than I cared to, but I put in a good night's work and felt calm and in control. However, on the second night back at work, I started to shake suddenly just as I began the admission paperwork on a new patient.

Excusing myself, I sought refuge in a storage room where I stood helpless against the onslaught of my body's delayed reaction to being assaulted. Hot tears flooded my face, my sinuses and skull felt full to bursting and burned with pain. My whole body twitched and shivered uncontrollably. Still in denial, I was mortified by this development. After a few minutes, I was able to calm down enough to dry my tears and page the charge nurse. When she answered my summons, I pulled her into the storage room and, crying, asked with great embarrassment if I could go home. "I just can't seem to stop crying. I'm so sorry. I know how busy we are, but I don't think I can get it together enough to work."

"Of course you can go home, Susie," she assured me. "Jeez, to tell you the truth, I'm really relieved to see you upset. You've been so calm and controlled about this thing, we were worried about you. You have every right to be distressed, you know. It was terrible what you just went through and your tears are a good sign. Now, go on, get out of here!"

"Thanks," I mumbled. "I'm sorry about this."

"Stop apologizing, for goodness' sake! But wait, you're not going home alone! Is there someone you can stay with, someone to come get you? You want one of us to drive you home?"

I insisted I could drive myself and promised I would go to my friends for the night. I felt cold as ice driving away from the hospital, quiet and still. I felt so terribly diminished it seemed like I would just fade away. When I appeared unannounced on their doorstep, my friends wrapped me in hugs and then plied me with Scotch. I talked incessantly while they listened patiently and compassionately until I was drunk enough to stagger off to their guest room.

After the weekend off, I felt fine again, sure I was getting past the trauma of the break-in. But when I went back to work, goddammit, it happened again, completely without warning. I changed into scrubs and was walking down the hall to the report room when my tear glands when into overdrive and the shakes attacked. *God, what is the matter with me? I've got to work. How am I going to work? Jesus, I can't take this!* I made it through report, but could feel the trembling and the tears just behind my eyes. Abruptly, I went to the office of the maternity center manager. She was in, thank goodness, and listened with obvious concern as I explained this strange physiological reaction and asked if I could have some time off. She expressed amazement: "I wouldn't have even gone back into the house to get clothes, Susie! I can't believe you thought something like this wouldn't have an enormous impact on you."

After encouraging me to get some counseling, which I did, the manager gave me two weeks off. I spent the time painting, scrubbing, and gardening, consciously striving to make my house my own again. Rebecca provided me with much needed company and endearing love. At her insistence, we bought and installed an inexpensive alarm system. I ended my leave from work with a dinner for my closest friends. They gathered around me, with so much concern and love, and we made a little ceremony together. I carried smoking sage through each room, reconsecrating my home, chasing away the evil spirits, as my buddies trailed indulgently along behind me. I thought I was finally healing and returned to my job feeling strengthened and okay.

Even though I knew that some of my strange new behaviors were easy to explain, such as prowling my house at night, checking locks and windows obsessively, sleeping with the baseball bat in my arms, and feeling vulnerable in ways I'd never felt before, I figured I was doing okay. I was more angry than frightened. It made me burn with rage that some dickhead burglar could violate my beloved home so easily; that every time I walked up to my front door I went through a wave of emotions, almost as though I was having flashbacks; that I couldn't walk down the hospital corridors alone at night without feeling exposed; that I startled with fear if someone approached me from behind or too suddenly. I had lost irrevocably the wonderful pleasure I had experienced every time I had entered my house before I interrupted the burglar. I didn't even want to go home anymore. That simple awareness tore me up inside. I was okay at work, though, and thought I just needed time to dull the anger I carried around with me. Then something else happened.

After eight years of working with obstetrical patients, including quite a number of women who lost their babies, I found myself on the other side of the fence, experiencing as a family member the loss of what was to have been my first great-nephew. My niece, Michelle, was twenty-one weeks pregnant when she went in for a routine prenatal check and ultrasound. My sister Jessie, Michelle's mother, had expressed privately to me her concern about the baby because Michelle had felt very little fetal activity, far less than our sister-in-law who was also expecting her first child; she was due around the same time as Michelle and feeling her baby move a lot. So it wasn't a complete shock when Jessie called me long-distance shortly before I was mugged to tell me the ultrasound indicated a very serious problem with Michelle's baby. Over the next few days, in telephone conversations with Jessie and Michelle, along with discussions with obstetricians at work, I learned that Michelle's fetus had such severe anomalies within its little developing body that it could not sustain life after birth. Further ultrasounds, consultations with perinatologists, and tests indicated no kidney development at all, along with lung malformation and a possible cardiac defect.

The family was stricken, rallying in support of my niece and my sister, grieving over the loss of all the hopes for and pleasure in this expected child. Michelle was in the care of a remarkably sensitive obstetrical practice, physicians who explained and comforted and offered every assistance to her in making plans for the termination of the pregnancy. Michelle didn't want to continue with the pregnancy. With her husband in school full-time, she needed to be able to work without carrying this fetus any longer. She was terrified, appropriately, of going through the physical process of aborting her fetus and asked only that it be done when her mother and I could be with her.

Arranging our work schedules required no small amount of effort, but finally a date was set for Michelle to be admitted to the hospital for the termination of her pregnancy. Unfortunately, she fell into the bureaucratic abyss that has arisen from all of the social and legal controversies over abortion. Her doctors practiced in a state that did not permit therapeutic abortions after twenty-two weeks. A hospital in a neighboring state, geographically close to Michelle, was located, along with an obstetrician who would manage the termination, but would have no personal interaction with Michelle before the day of the procedure. In addition, her medical insurance did not cover most of the costs of ending her pregnancy, so she would have to assume financial responsibility for almost all of the fees incurred during the procedure. This meant that it had to be accomplished with an absolute minimum of hospital charges and as rapidly as possible.

From three states we gathered together, the women of my family, the day before Michelle was to enter the hospital. My mother, my older sister Katy, Jessie, Michelle, Rebecca, and I spent the day catching up with one another. We had lunch out, went to a movie, and spent hours sitting around Katy's living room talking, crying, sharing our love.

Michelle is petite, with a heart-shaped face and a dream-shaped body. Her huge almond-shaped brown eyes can just pull you right into their warm, sincere, liquid depths. In short, she's a knock-out. Her husband, Jonathan, is tall, slender, blonde and good-looking, with a bizarre, wry sense of humor that keeps us all laughing.

Early the next morning we all went to the hospital, an enormous inner-city affair, and checked in with the admitting office a half hour before we were required to be there. The plan was for Michelle to undergo a saline abortion, which involved having a long needle, topped by a syringe, inserted into her uterus, through which saline solution would be injected in a pocket of amniotic fluid. The saline solution would cause uterine contractions and in effect cause a miscarriage. There was no prediction of how long it would take to accomplish a labor and delivery of the fetus, but we hoped an overnight stay might be avoided, if the procedure was started early in the morning.

Thus began one of the longest waking nightmares I've ever experienced.

We waited in admitting for over two hours. Then we waited upstairs in the family waiting room of the abortion clinic for more than five hours. First we waited for the paperwork to be completed. Michelle signed consent forms: she was obliged to copy out in her own hand several paragraphs explaining what she was consenting to and that she did so agree to terminate her pregnancy without legal risk to the doctor or the hospital. She did whatever was asked her courteously and quietly, dressed in her pajamas, pale of face and emotionally numb.

We kept on waiting: for the doctor, who was at another hospital; for the ultrasound machine; for an exam room; and yet again for the doctor who was finally in-house, but not in our area yet. The nurses in the clinic were polite, but their interactions with us were the absolute bare minimum with virtually no acknowledgment of what Michelle and her family were contending with. It's possible they assumed this was just another abortion and so masked their feelings, whatever they were, in a professional cloak of silence. Her medical records were in their hands, however. I went to the clinic's office area on several occasions to inquire when we might get started, only to be blandly assured that the doctor, the ultrasound machine, the room would be available "soon." Sometime during those five hours, the physician did stick his head around the door to introduce himself (this, his first meeting with Michelle), explain some of the delay, and assure us that "it wouldn't be too long now."

At last it was finally time for Michelle to go into the small treatment room where the injection would be done. To my incredulity, they expected her to go by herself. Her husband, Jonathan, was barred from the room on the grounds that the one attending nurse couldn't be responsible for him if he were to faint or be sick. Very politely and quietly, but with vehemence, I convinced the nurses and the doctor that Michelle was not going to have a needle stuck in her belly without someone present who loved her. I argued that my presence was essential because I would be able to manage her fears and, as a professional, was unlikely to faint on them. First argument won by me, Michelle and I went into the little room.

There followed an extended, unsuccessful attempt on the doctor's part to find a pocket of amniotic fluid into which he could inject saline. Amniotic fluid is primarily produced by the fetus's kidneys; because of this baby's anomalies, there was virtually no amniotic fluid in Michelle's uterus. Michelle lay very still, rigid as stone on the table, gripping my hands and arms so tightly I bruised, her eyes as big as saucers and running with tears. She hung on to me and cried and hollered with the pain as the doctor repeatedly removed and reinserted the long needle, bringing back only blood into the syringe. She was terrified and in excruciating pain. I held her head cradled against my chest, squeezed her hands with mine, and talked to her nonstop, quietly crooning her name, trying to reassure her that it wouldn't take much longer, instructing her to hold on just a little more and don't move, telling her what he was doing, and not letting myself feel anything about how barbaric this whole thing was. The doctor and nurse were business-like and abrupt in their activities, with a minimum of exchanges between them and Michelle and me. It felt like we were alone in that room, with Michelle being tortured by two unfeeling mechanical robots. I could feel rage building up inside me as the doctor continued to poke and probe, but I stifled it, focusing on just getting Michelle through this procedure.

At length, the physician admitted defeat. He told Michelle that he was unable to find a place to safely inject the saline; therefore, she would have to go to the labor and delivery unit for a prostin-induced labor. Michelle understood what this entailed; her doctors and I had both explained it to her. I didn't understand why this procedure hadn't been the treatment of choice in the first place, given that she had so little amniotic fluid to begin with. I still don't understand, but I have a sneaking suspicion that this obstetrician hadn't bothered to examine Michelle's chart closely enough, ignoring or forgetting the absence of fluid. Michelle went to the bathroom, washed her face and pulled herself together after all the tears and pain, gathering her strength for whatever was coming next.

Forty-five minutes later, we were escorted to labor and delivery: grand-mother, mother, aunts, cousin, and husband all walking beside Michelle's wheelchair. When we arrived, the first of several negotiations began between the nursing staff and myself. They put Michelle in their exam/triage room, which was were crowded by three gurneys, a fetal monitor, and all the other equipment needed to evaluate prospective patients. The nurse announced that only one person could stay with Michelle. I courteously and persuasively contended that Michelle needed our presence, that we wouldn't be in the way, and that we would leave if another patient arrived. Out in the hallway, I privately explained to the nurse that this was not just an elective abortion of an unwanted fetus, but the termination of a nonviable but nonetheless very much loved baby. I won the argument and Jessie, Jonathan, and I were allowed to stay.

An hour or more after our arrival on L&D, Michelle had an IV started and a resident physician came in to insert the prostin gel. This gel is an effective agent for the termination of pregnancy. It softens the cervix and stimulates uterine contractions. Unfortunately, it may have several side ef-fects, such as diarrhea, nausea and vomiting, and headache. If the dosage is carefully titrated (giving the smallest dose possible to achieve the desired results), the side effects can be minimized, but most physicians routinely order additional medications to combat the side effects. What all this meant to me was that Michelle would not only have to contend with the pain of labor contractions, but the possible discomfort of these side effects. Plus, the physical ordeal she was facing was compounded by the psychological and emotional anguish of losing her baby.

Such a situation demanded every possible effort by the medical staff to minimize the physical discomfort of this procedure. I knew this. I had taken care of more women under identical circumstances than I cared to count. In a tertiary care hospital of this size, with a large number of high-risk patients, it was reasonable for me to expect that the obstetrical staff would be as knowledgeable and experienced as I. My impatience and disgust with all the previous wasted hours, the apparent indifference of the abortion clinic staff, and my anger over the cruel manner in which the saline injection had been attempted were all building up inside. Nevertheless, I continued striving to remain polite, even as I was forced to dicker for every little concession in Michelle's care, concessions I had erroneously presumed appropriate and rou-tine in a termination procedure.

The attending obstetrician stuck his head in the room briefly once again to inform us that the resident would be providing Michelle's care, but he could be reached via beeper if necessary. Chasing after the doctor, I inquired about pain relief, since I knew that once things got started Michelle was going to be in considerable pain. He said he would leave an order for his own preferred "cocktail," a combination of Demerol and something else. I asked if she could have a continuous epidural, suggesting that maintaining constant analgesia was important, to minimize the trauma of this event. "No!" he exclaimed, "I don't use epidurals for terminations!" and made a rapid exit, ending the discussion. Dismayed, I kept silent, determined to argue the point more vigorously if necessary.

After another hour of increasingly strong contractions, crying and flailing around on her gurney, Michelle was given an injection of the doctor's cocktail, the nurse explaining that it had been ordered for every six hours. Michelle had about forty-five minutes of pain-free drug-induced euphoria, giggling and asking us to tell her stories. Then, as her labor began to get more rigorous, she cried and moaned, begging for something to stop the pain. The evening shift of nurses had come on; I had once more gone through my speech about why we should be allowed to stay with Michelle and now I worked to get Michelle through the contractions. She tried, bless her heart, breathing with me or her mother and dozing or crying between contractions. I asked for the resident after a couple hours of this, pleading with him and the nurse to contact the doctor for an epidural. They stalled, promised they would try, and generally avoided Michelle's room.

The night passed in a nightmare of struggle and pain. Michelle got another dose of the pain medication, which helped only minimally. Jessie, Jonathan, and I took turns resting on the other gurneys while one of us held Michelle's hand, wiped her face, and breathed with her. At one point, she squatted on the floor, straining over a bedpan as prostin-induced diarrhea cramped her belly. She was inconsolable, crying, twisting with pain, begging for relief. I was in a fog of exhausted fury. Where were the nurses? Where was the fucking doctor? What was wrong with this place? Didn't they understand that their duty required them to get Michelle through this with a minimum of physical torture? Wasn't the emotional devastation she was undergoing enough to bear? Did they have to punish her with unnecessary pain?

Once again I pushed for an epidural, cornering the night nurse in the hallway. She was sympathetic but paralyzed by her unwillingness to buck hospital policy and call the doctor in the middle of the night. She continued to avoid our room. I was afraid that if I made a scene we would be banished from Michelle's bedside, leaving her alone in her misery.

Around 6:30 in the morning, the resident reappeared to check Michelle's cervix. She had dilated to only three centimeters. At my insistence, the resident said he would try to get another doctor from the obstetrical practice to agree to an epidural. At 7:30, a big brusque nurse bustled into the room, announced that Michelle was being moved to a labor room and that we had to choose one family member only to be with her. Yet again, I went through my spiel and convinced her to allow both Jessie and me to remain with Michelle. Jonathan left to take a nap in the waiting room, where my mother and sister Katy had camped out most of the night.

As Michelle was moved to a labor room, I took note of the census board for the unit. Only four of the twelve labor rooms held patients, all in early labor. The new attending physician for the obstetrical team appeared, a woman whose sympathy for Michelle became apparent after she listened to my still polite but now angry demand for an epidural. She agreed but we had to wait another thirty minutes for an anesthesiologist. All the while Michelle was wracked with hard uterine contractions. The epidural was finally inserted after still another delay when the anesthesiologist was called to the phone. The epidural didn't work. Michelle had some relief, but patches of her belly and groin continued to torture her during contractions. The anesthesiologist had departed for the operating room, so we were stuck with an inadequate epidural and a thoroughly wrung-out laboring mother.

I went downstairs with Jonathan around 10:30 in the morning to have a cigarette. At the elevators we heard my name being paged. We ran down the long corridor to L&D and hurried into the room to find Michelle in the throes of pushing, with Jessie supporting her shoulders. The resident delivered the tiny fetus, cut the cord, placed the baby in a sterile towel, and handed him to me. Long before the delivery, Michelle and Jonathan had asked me to examine the baby first; depending on what he looked like, I was to decide if they should see him. I described the baby and then with much verbal encouragement, placed him in Michelle's arms, as they both peered at his little face and body, bruised but only slightly misshapen from his journey out of her body.

He had a heartbeat. Hospital policy dictated that he be rushed to the neonatal intensive care unit because of that heartbeat. I handed him over to the nurse, asking her to please bring him back to his parents as soon as possible, so they could hold him until he died. I had discussed this request with every shift of nurses (three now), trying my best to convey to them that the family wanted and deserved to have this little boy with them during his brief life. Everyone knew he couldn't survive: he had no lung tissue, no kidneys—and God knows what else was missing. I asked only that we be given some time alone with him, to baptize him and say our good-byes. I didn't think he should be alone in a NICU with only strangers around him as he expired.

In the end it didn't matter. All my words fell on completely deaf, insensitive ears. After the baby was taken to the nursery and Michelle was cleaned up, I went downstairs once again for my long delayed smoke. When I returned to labor and delivery, the nurse told me we could see the baby just for a minute. His tiny blanketed form was thrust into my hands in the hallway. The family crowded into a closetlike room that held one chair and a lamp. My mother, Katy, Jessie, Jonathan, Rebecca, Jonathan's mother, and I squeezed together in this excuse for a room and passed the baby around, each of us saying good-bye, crying and holding on to one another. My heart contracted when I placed him in my mother's arms, her miniscule first great-grandchild.

Then Jonathan, standing in the doorway, said, "Here's Michelle!" To my disbelief, less than two hours after her delivery, they were moving Michelle to the postpartum unit. I stopped the gurney right there in the hallway and told the nurse we wanted to baptize the baby. She looked at me, completely at a loss. She had taken this patient out of her labor room to move her to another unit. Now here she was, stuck in the corridor with the patient and the family, who wanted to baptize the baby. I guess it didn't even occur to her to take us all to the postpartum room. I was so paralyzed with exhaustion, fury, and incredulity, it didn't occur to me, either. Someone appeared from somewhere with a beaker of sterile water and handed it to Jonathan's mother.

There we were, Michelle in her bed, her family around her, holding her baby, whose heart was still beating. There, *in the middle of the hallway,* her mother-in-law quietly baptized the baby, naming him Jason. There, *in the middle of the hallway*, with no privacy—with visitors, hospital personnel, doctors, and nurses wending their way around our group, gawking at us—we said our final good-byes to the baby. Immediately after the baptism was accomplished, Jason was whisked away from us, returned to the NICU where he died surrounded by strangers.

I was enraged. What was the big hurry to move Michelle? There were eight empty labor rooms, the unit was quiet. What would have been so wrong about giving this family a half hour alone in the labor room to be with this baby? I knew they just wanted to move her out, get her off their hands, and not have to be responsible for her anymore.

We had been awake for close to forty hours; we had stood by almost helplessly while Michelle endured an agonizing labor; now we were being denied a private time and place with her baby. I like to believe now that if I hadn't been so exhausted I would have thrown an absolute fit! I wanted in the very worst way to do as Shirley Maclaine did in *Terms of Endearment*—screeching for her daughter's pain medication—to scream and rant and compel these unfeeling, rule-bound assholes to act like compassionate human beings. But I was struck dumb. A lifetime of training—always be civil, never rock the boat, never make a scene, respect authority figures no matter how they behave—all that conditioning, coupled with my physical exhaustion and grief, completely erased the assertiveness I had developed, ever so painfully, as a nurse. My mother stood nearby, clutching her purse, wearing her public face, her expression and posture conveying her earnest desire to be proper, to act appropriately. It would never have occurred to her, I thought, how outrageous this pathetic scene was. She would have died of embarrassment if I had made a scene. (She admitted this later.) So I just stood there, defeated by it all.

I simply could not believe the total lack of concern or compassion these hospital people displayed. Here I was, a nurse who had been through similar experiences with numerous families; who had been trained in dealing with perinatal loss; who knew how little it took to minimize the physical and psychic trauma of the family and facilitate their grieving process; and I couldn't do a thing in this place to help Michelle. I could not fathom how professionals could be so heartless or so ignorant. Every hospital I had worked in, every one, had in-services and conferences on caring for patients who lose their babies. It was inconceivable to me that these nurses could work in a modern, urban, high-risk hospital and not be knowledgeable about the research, data, and education programs available on the subject of fetal loss.

Struggling with my emotions and fatigue, I did manage to convey to the postpartum staff that Michelle was to be discharged as soon as possible. I did not ask, I did not negotiate. I simply made it absolutely clear that they were to expedite Michelle's paperwork and that no delay would be tolerated. The neonatologist came into her room in the early afternoon. He told her Jason's heart had stopped and discussed the genetic studies they would do. Michelle was discharged by 4:00 that afternoon. Rebecca drove me home, praising me for all I had done. I just sat in the car stunned by the horror of it all and how little all my professional training had meant for Michelle and the family.

When I described the experience to nurse friends at work, my anger and dismay were almost palpable. They understood what I was describing and were as horrified as I was, yet none of them asked me the questions I was asking myself. Why had I been such a wimp? Where was all my assertiveness? What good did it do to have all the training and experience I had if I couldn't put it to use for a loved one? Why was it so difficult for me to insist on compassionate care for Michelle? My expertise and my insider's knowledge were the main reasons Michelle wanted me with her in the first place, to help her negotiate the twists and turns of a foreign environment during a frightening, painful event. Yes, I had protected her somewhat. She did have my hands to grasp during the saline injection attempt and her family members to provide support throughout her labor. But I'd failed her. Why didn't I *demand* an epidural at the outset of her induction? Why didn't I use my considerable communication skills to convince the doctor to allow an epidural? Why did I stand in that hallway, paralyzed and dumb, while strangers gawked at the intensely private activity of Jason's baptism?

I would never, *not ever,* allow something like this to happen to one of my patients. Eight years earlier, with only a few months of employment under my belt, for three full days I had stood up for a couple and their right to compassion, privacy, and self-determination while they dealt with the enormity of giving birth to a severely handicapped child. I had been their advocate without any self-doubt, without any hesitancy. How was it that I could act with such deliberation with strangers, only to stand defeated in a hallway eight years and a lifetime of professional experience later, allowing my family and myself to be victimized by a callous, indifferent health-care system? Even though I swore to Michelle and Jonathan that I was going to write furious letters of complaint to the hospital board, I couldn't even do that.

This event had a profound effect on me. I raged and fumed for months afterward, even when I realized the family was just glad it was over and Michelle was recovering well. They couldn't feel the shame I felt as a nurse over the callous behavior of the doctor and nurses who were supposed to care for Michelle. They couldn't understand the shame I felt about my own behavior, my own helplessness.

For the next few months, every time I tried to talk to family members about both the mugging and Michelle's experience, I met with uncomprehending resistance. My sister Katy encouraged me to "stop fixating on this, you did the best you could, get a grip!" My mother counseled me to "put it behind me" and wondered if I had some "unconscious need to be a victim." Understandably, Jessie couldn't discuss it easily with me. In fact, those family members who hadn't been with us during Michelle's hospitalization had no idea of what actually transpired. Mom's reports were sanitized versions of the truth: it had been long and uncomfortable, but Michelle was a trooper and did just fine. That was how Mom actually saw it, but privately I couldn't leave it alone.

For the next six months, I went to work and did my job, usually well. I spent long hours in the nursery, learning the details of newborn care and enjoying the babies. By volunteering for nursery duty, I was expanding my area of expertise. It felt good to be able to "float" to any assignment in the birthing center, to know I could help fill staffing needs without the anxiety I experienced years earlier when asked to work someplace other than L&D. Clinically, I was getting better and better, making myself more valuable to my employers and reinforcing my self-confidence.

Yet I was experiencing a great deal of emotional and psychological turmoil, and it continued to be triggered by even minor difficulties. At the beginning of one shift, when I received my patient in the exam room, I assessed her and called her doctor with report. "She's five centimeters, 90 percent effaced, and contracting every three minutes. Her membranes are intact and she wants an epidural. The baby looks fine." He instructed me to start an IV, move her to a room, and set up for the epidural. He'd be there in about fifteen minutes.

I started the IV without difficulty, but the fluid wouldn't flow. I checked all the stopcocks and went over the tubing three times, looking for a problem. Another nurse checked behind me. We changed all the tubing, still without results. Time was running out: the doctor was due momentarily and I hadn't even moved the patient to her room. I apologized to her, explaining I would have to stick her again to start a new IV. As I peeled off the tape, the IV began to flow. Never before had I taped an IV catheter so tightly that I cut off the flow!

Just as I started to move the patient to her room, the doctor arrived. Flustered, I explained the delay. He was pleasant about it. I called him to the room after I got the patient settled in, monitors on, vital signs taken, and epidural ready for insertion. After the physician had given her the epidural, he stood at the bedside, chatting with the couple. I had elevated the bed for his work and now quietly pressed the "down" button on the bed control panel. A loud scrunching noise interrupted all conversation. They all three looked at me. "Oops, I'm sorry," I muttered. "The waste basket is getting crunched." I pressed the "up" button as they continued their conversation. *Crash!* Now the IV pole on the rising bed was colliding with the light fixture above the bed! I blushed and apologized profusely, as the doctor and the parents stared at me, incredulous. The mother turned to the doctor and asked laughingly, "What did I get, the nurse from hell?" Everyone laughed and teased me, none of us having any idea how prophetic her label was to be!

An hour later, I did a cervical exam to check her dilation. As I pulled off the mucky glove, it snapped in my hand, splashing stringy mucus and blood all over my face! Mortified, I ducked my head and turned around, trying to avoid having the couple see my "face paint." Not fast enough! The father stared at me, horrified. I apologized some more and went into the bathroom to wash my face and cool down. Not long after that fun event, I had to empty the mother's bladder with a catheter. Almost a full liter of urine flowed out of her into the little basin between her legs. I lifted it very carefully and very deliberately set it on the floor beside the bed, intending to empty it in the toilet after I had cleaned up the mother's bottom.

Need I say more? Holding the trash from the catheter kit, I turned around from the bed and planted my foot squarely in that basin brimming with urine. *Swoosh!* Urine bathed the floor and my shoes. The father just stood there, shaking his head with disbelief. At least he didn't point out this gaffe to his wife: I know he felt sorry for me!

Not long after I mopped up the urine, my patient was fully dilated. I positioned her in the stirrups after breaking away the bottom of the bed. The baby was moving down the birth canal nicely, preceded and cushioned by a grapefruit-sized balloon of amniotic fluid—the membranes were still intact. Even though I knew that bag was going to blow, I stood between her legs and leaned forward, my face directly opposite her vulva, and told her to push. Just as she began, I stood up straight. At that very instant, *KERPOW!* A loud crack, like a firecracker or gunfire, resounded through the room as amniotic fluid shot out of her, drenching me from shoulders to knees. She yelled at the sound, and her husband jumped two feet in the air! I hollered and then just burst out laughing. "Oh, I'm sorry! I'm sorry!" the mother cried out to me.

"Are you kidding? After all the messes I've made tonight? It wasn't your fault. I knew it was going to blow, so I was an idiot to stand right here in the line of fire!" We rocked with laughter. The baby was born with no further mishaps, except I couldn't stop chuckling.

What an awful impression I must have made on that couple. It was like a Three Stooges skit, with only one stooge! When I described the night to my fellow nurses, they looked at me with horror, asking why I didn't just asked to be reassigned early in the shift. "When I start a night out like that," one of the nurses avowed, "I don't wait after one or two screw-ups. I know I'm just not gonna make it with that patient and I get me another one!" Not Susie, though. I just hung in there and made an absolute fool of myself, never thinking of how incompetent and stupid I looked.

Now I have experienced times of clumsiness: when I am very busy or rushed, it's not unusual for me to trip or bump into a doorjamb or spill something. But this night of horrors was something else entirely. Not only did I act and look like an incompetent fool, I wasn't thinking clearly enough to recognize how my behavior might cause the patient and her husband dismay or might reflect poorly on the hospital's reputation. Until that night I had never had any doubt that my patients regarded me with respect and appreciation. That I was experienced and knew what I was doing was reflected in the remarks patients had made to me over the years of work. Now for the first time I realized I this couple must have been disturbed by my behavior and might even have considered requesting another nurse. Worse, I wasn't even able to see the night as anything more than a funny story.

Emotionally, I was going down the tubes. It was increasingly difficult to go home, to walk up to my front door and unlock it. On my nights off, I couldn't sleep without looking under the beds, without all the outside lights on, without checking each room, each window, each closet, each door at least four or five times. My sleep was disturbed by nightmares and insomnia. The smallest household noises—the refrigerator's hum, the air-conditioner's fan, a creaking window—could send adrenaline rushing through my body. I'd jump up from watching a television program or taking an afternoon nap, and stomp through the house to verify my safety. Thinking more "normal" hours might improve my sleep and sagging energy levels, I even gave up my cherished night shifts. Monday through Friday, I worked the evening three-to-eleven shift.

The nightmares and insomnia just worsened. I kept getting sick—strep throat, bronchitis, belly problems—and used up the few days of leave I had accumulated. Depression fell upon me like a thick, dank fog, obscuring any clarity of thought, leaving me listless and indifferent to the daily activities I had embraced so eagerly in my new home and workplace. The flowerbeds went unplanted; even my treasured houseplants began to fail from neglect. I sought medical help, started with a new therapist, and continued my descent into the labyrinth of melancholy. Worst of all, the attacks of sudden tears and trembling I'd experienced after the mugging recurred regularly at work.

The once small irritations inherent in any job now seemed insurmountable. I finally acknowledged that I couldn't perform my duties effectively or safely. It was time to withdraw. Terrified of the implications of quitting my job, I took a medical leave-of-absence for six months, and then, reluctantly but unhesitatingly, I formally resigned.

Chapter Seventeen

THE BIRTH OF ZOE

Quitting my job was an obvious necessity. Like so many other people, I had struggled for several years to find meaning and satisfaction in my work. I had watched other nurses leave their jobs, overcome by the spirit-breaking stress of this work. They were burnt-out, exhausted.

> *I just can't listen to women in labor screaming and fighting through their labors.*
>
> *I'm tired of breaking my back, my health, trying to take care of everybody else.*
>
> *I can't deal with the politics anymore, the scrabbling for territory, for power. If I could just take care of my patients, it'd be okay, but all the other crap is just too much. I didn't become a nurse to wash down bloody beds, to empty trash, to write the same shit over and over again, to kowtow to doctors, to write policies for some stupid administrator. . . .*
>
> *I know it sounds ridiculous, but no one ever says thank-you! I spend hours with a patient, doing everything possible to provide good care. Does the doctor bother to say thanks? Does the patient bother? Maybe it shouldn't matter, maybe it should be enough to know I've done good work, maybe the paycheck is all I should focus on, but a simple thank-you is what I really want, and I just don't hear it.*
>
> *I never thought I'd get tired of L&D. When I started, I loved being involved. Now it embarrasses me to admit I just don't have any patience with my patients! I find myself just getting pissed off because they're crying or bleeding or unhappy. I don't care about them anymore and that scares me. It really scares me and makes me feel ashamed of myself.*

All of these comments came from other nurses, women I cared about and listened to empathetically, but they could be my own thoughts. By the time I had been working for three years, I was already looking for ways to handle the stress and discontent with my work. I changed jobs, hospitals. I thought if I found just the right place, I'd be happy. I talked with other nurses, finding comfort in the disillusionment and fatigue we shared. I used my computer as therapy. When I found myself frothing over with anger or drowning in regret or grief after a case at work, I was almost compelled to sit down at my computer and spew it all out. Sort of like confession—a carryover from my childhood days as a Catholic with the refreshing cleansing of the confessional booth on Friday evenings.

For a long time I thought that it was the system of care that caused me so much distress. Medical mismanagement, the abuses our patients are subjected to, the conflicts between a normal biological process and the manner in which obstetrical care has usurped that process and turned it into a nightmarish pathological event—I thought all those issues were the crux of my problem. I believed it was the system that was denying me the opportunity to fulfill my desire to truly care for women who needed my expertise.

In my fifth year of work, I thought I'd found a way to confront my anger about the abuses within the system. One morning after a particularly long, exhausting night at work, I stopped by to say hello to my old friend and mentor, Nick. I was working in another hospital; Nick was still at the military hospital, a manager of one of the nursing services. There had been a number of mornings like this one. I'd walk into his office and collapse into a chair. He would take one look at me and say, "Hard night, huh?" He'd smile at me, push back his papers and give me time, listening as I wept and complained about the doctors who were indifferent to a patient's needs, the nurses who squabbled with each other and sulked over their assignments, the failures within the hospital itself—no beds, not enough nurses, no clean blankets to wrap a newborn in, no one to run to the lab, blah, blah, blah.

This particular morning, as I drove to Nick's office, I realized that I was still hearing the cries of pain that had reverberated all night long in the large L&D unit where I worked. I knew those echoes ringing in my ears would keep me awake when I desperately needed a good day's sleep so I could go back to work that night.

Feeling sorry for myself, I poured out my heart to Nick, ending with a description of the cacophony of women in labor: "I'm so tired, Nick, of participating in a system that brutalizes women. I can't bear working in a place where I'm required to listen to women screaming in quadrophonic sound. I mean it, Nick. The sounds hurt my soul."

He leaned forward and took both of my hands in his, deep concern apparent in his face. "Then you have to find a place where there is no quadrophonic agony. You have to be working where you can keep that from happening. You also must do your writing. And you have to find an ending for it, Susie. You have to find the ending."

I wiped at the tears of exhaustion and anguish streaming down my face, nodding mutely in agreement with his words. He continued: "You need to do your writing. You need to get it out there so your voice will be heard. So women don't have to be brutalized and harmed by the system."

His words were a catalyst. Within a couple of months I had quit my management job, signed on with a nursing agency as a contract nurse, and committed myself to writing many of the pages that are found in this book. I had a mission now—a book to write—to distract me from the inner conflicts I felt about my work.

That mission and my anger about the obstetrical system of care carried me through three more years of work, three more hospitals, three more jobs, and thousands more births, before I hit the wall. Having my home invaded and being physically assaulted demolished the haven I'd created to soothe the aches and pains, both physical and emotional, of my work. My niece's pregnancy termination was the final straw. The anger, helplessness, and shame I felt during those long hours broke something inside of me. I had finally had enough.

Because of these two events, crowning all the years of work and inner turmoil, I knew finally that it wasn't just the system that I had a problem with, it was also my own personality. My own shortcomings got in the way of my work. I needed to step aside, to take a sabbatical from active employment, to rest, and to face, without flinching, my limitations. It would take time to clear my thoughts enough so that I might be able to sort out what was wrong with the system and what was wrong with me. I needed to figure out how I could alter my own behavior, how to unload all the old dysfunctional patterns, so I could discover ways in which I could do the work I loved and was good at, without giving in to the system I had come to abhor.

Quitting nursing wasn't an easy decision, even though it was clearly necessary. The exhaustion and depression that depleted me demanded a time for healing. I couldn't go on doing less than excellent work, cheating my patients and myself while I was so miserable. So I quit, knowing full well that I had financial obligations I wouldn't be able to meet. Unlike so many people who are forced to continue working because they have no other choice, I'm one of the lucky ones, blessed with family and friends who have been helping me scrape by while I pull myself together. The bills have piled up anyway; I'll be in debt for a long time, I know. But the debts are unavoidable.

I have raised my children successfully: glorious as they are and will always be to me, they are no longer my primary responsibility. Work is the heart of my life now, the defining factor of how I spend my days, how I feel about myself and the outside world, how I find meaning and fulfillment. And it has become painfully evident that I cannot shuffle through my work, denying the significance of what I do each day and how I do it. I recalled the conversation I had with my adviser years earlier, just before I graduated from nursing school. I remembered her words, echoing down the years over all the thousands of hours I'd spent as a nurse: *Your caring enhances all your interactions with your patients; it is what makes the difference between being a good clinical nurse and being an outstanding one. . . . Don't ever lose your compassion, your caring! If you find you don't care anymore, get out of nursing! Don't let yourself become jaded. Don't lose your ideals.*

I haven't lost my compassion. I haven't lost my ideals. I still care. If anything, I care too much. But I am jaded, for sure. Some time ago, listening to a Joseph Campbell audio tape, I heard him give Bill Moyers the advice he gave to young people about how to live life well. His words rocked me: "Follow your bliss." Such simple advice. So hard, sometimes, to achieve. In the early years, I had done just that. Labor and delivery nursing was my bliss. But the bliss got lost somewhere along the way. Now I am searching for it again.

And now a final story. About six months into this "sabbatical," I got a phone call from one of my half-sisters. DeeDee is sixteen years younger than me, the oldest of three daughters our father had with his second wife. I didn't know DeeDee as a child, but in the last ten years or so, we have come to know and love each other deeply. I am, as is probably apparent, very close to my "whole" sisters, Katy and Jessie, both of whom I love and respect enormously. But in DeeDee I find the sister most like myself. We share many physical, psychological, and emotional characteristics, the discovery of which has been a source of laughter and comfort.

DeeDee called me for information. The single mother of two marvelous little girls, DeeDee was pregnant with her third child. Because of this unplanned, unexpected pregnancy, which occurred in spite of meticulous contraceptive use, DeeDee had suffered a lot of emotional turmoil over the last few months. Social and familial disapproval had been nearly devastating, but this strong, independent sister of mine slugged her way through weeks of anguish and disapprobation, determined to take responsibility for another child rather than terminate the pregnancy with an abortion. Now thirty-four weeks along, DeeDee called me for advice.

Because she had no health insurance, the expense of prenatal care and hospitalization for her delivery appeared prohibitive. As a pastry chef and restaurant manager, DeeDee made a living just sufficient to meet her family's needs, but there was no way she could have this baby in the hospital without incurring a heavy debt. She wanted any advice I could offer about how to have the baby without such a debt. I told her about midwifery services, gave her suggestions for locating a midwife, and worried aloud with her about this problem. She knew how important prenatal care was and had been seeing an obstetrician faithfully, but every visit added to an already unacceptable dollar amount owed.

As we chatted, I commented casually, "Too bad you can't just have the baby at home."

"I know. That's just what I want to do. What do you think about home deliveries, Susie?"

"God, Dee, I wanted to have Michael at home in the worst way, but Frank wouldn't even consider it—too risky, you know. But seriously, see if you can find a licensed midwife who does home deliveries. I know they're out there, it's just a matter of finding them. I guess your obstetrician isn't interested in a home delivery, huh?"

"I don't even need to answer that one, do I? Even if I can find a midwife, if I have to go to the hospital because of some complication, I'm not sure if my obstetrician would take me as her patient."

"Well, see what you can do about a midwife, and then call me back, okay?"

DeeDee was, in fact, an excellent candidate for a home delivery. Her first two pregnancies had been utterly normal, completely risk-free. She had her first daughter, Sabra, in the hospital with our brother Jed coaching her through her labor, using techniques I'd taught them. The baby was healthy and beautiful and DeeDee's labor and delivery had been uneventful and without any complications. Her second daughter, Grace, arrived late and in a big rush, all ten pounds of her bursting free of DeeDee two weeks past her due date. Once again, DeeDee's labor and delivery were uneventful. She just seemed to spit out her babies with an uncommon ease.

DeeDee's history of risk-free, uncomplicated pregnancies and births, the fact that she had a pelvis adequate for a ten-pounder and the healthy normalcy of this pregnancy were all factors in deciding whether a home delivery was feasible. I knew a number of women who had delivered at home. I'd read several books about home deliveries and had long conversations with midwives about the risks and benefits. I also had enough professional experience to know what conditions were necessary to ensure the safety of the mother and baby in a home delivery. DeeDee lived around the block, literally, from a hospital with a large obstetrical unit. She was healthy and her baby was healthy. She had nutritious dietary habits and didn't smoke, drink, or do drugs. She wasn't diabetic or overweight. Her pregnancy was being monitored with regular prenatal checkups; there were normal ultrasounds and fetal heart tracings of the baby. The placenta was located high in the uterus, away from any possibility of a previa. In effect, DeeDee was a perfect candidate for a home birth.

A couple of weeks after our first phone conversation, DeeDee called me again.

"My obstetrician flatly refused to be my backup if I opt for a home birth, but I did find a midwife."

"All right! Way to go, DeeDee! That's great! Is she going to do your prenatal care? Tell me, tell me!"

"I'm going to keep on seeing the obstetrician for prenatal checks, but I've got a problem with the midwife. She says she doesn't want to be legally responsible for the birth. She'll attend it and bring supplies and stuff, but she says she doesn't want to do the actual delivery herself. She asked me if Tony [the baby's father] would feel comfortable doing the delivery if she backed him up and told him what to do!"

"Hah!' I laughed.

"Yeah, hah-hah! I wouldn't even dream of letting Tony get near me to deliver this kid!"

"Hell, I'd do it, if the midwife is really going to be there!" I declared.

"Well . . . that's exactly what I hoped you'd say! Would you really, Susie?"

Yikes, I thought, *what have I said here?* A long, intense discussion ensued. We talked and talked, until both DeeDee and I were clear in our minds about the risks, the benefits, and exactly what was expected of both of us if we did this together. I was ready, eager to do this. I'd delivered several babies myself, two of them officially under a doctor's supervision, and an uncounted number that I caught before the doctor arrived. And I couldn't count the deliveries I'd assisted with. I knew the risks and I felt pretty secure about my ability to deliver DeeDee's baby, as long as a licensed midwife was present and a hospital within immediate reach.

To be honest, I could hardly wait! Helping DeeDee was a big component of my readiness to be involved; if I could help her avoid the expense of hospitalization, that would be even better. But just to have such an ideal opportunity to participate in a home delivery, with someone I loved, was a chance I'd dreamed of ever since I'd known I'd never have my own kids at home. To be surrounded by family, those I loved the most, while bringing a new life into my world—sharing such an auspicious event with loved ones had been a recurrent fantasy through the years following Michael's birth. If I couldn't do it myself, who better to do it with than DeeDee?

So we made plans. I was eight hours away by car, living with my mother in the southern home of my adolescence. Neither of us had money for an airplane ticket, so I was going to drive up a few days before her due date. Of course, nature intervened. DeeDee called one night, eight days before she was due.

"Uh, Susie, can you get on a plane today?"

"What's the matter? Are you in labor?"

"I'm not sure, but I've been having pretty strong contractions for hours now. They feel different from what I've felt before."

Her voice was shaky, a sure indication of stress, because DeeDee usually seemed deceptively calm, almost placid. She was scared, I could tell, that I might not be there in time.

"I'll call the airlines and get back to you right away."

"Okay, thanks. I'll feel a lot better after you get here."

The next day, I was greeted at the airport by DeeDee, still pregnant, and my nieces, Sabra and Grace. Dee's contractions had stopped not long after our phone calls. For the next week, we waited. I did laundry and house-cleaning for DeeDee, whose active life and two girls left little time for such chores. I slept on the couch and got to know my nieces again after a two-year separation.

Sunday night, DeeDee began to have serious contractions once more. We scurried around her bedroom, the one room I hadn't cleaned yet, putting away clothes, toys, books, shoes. Clean sheets went on her big bed. I swept and mopped the floor while we discussed what supplies we still hadn't collected. The only thing we could think of was a box of disposable absorbent bedpads. It was quite late before the girls fell asleep. I crashed on the couch even later, leaving DeeDee trying to sleep. She was quiet but not uncomfortable.

It was 5:30 in the morning when DeeDee woke me.

"I think I'm definitely in labor. These contractions are hurting."

"How frequent are they? What do you want me to do?"

"They're three to four minutes apart, and they're strong. I'm gonna get in the tub. Maybe that'll help."

While she soaked, I called her best friend, John, who had been her coach during Grace's birth. I woke him up with instructions to go to the drugstore for chucks. Nearly incoherent, he asked, "Wait, are you telling me DeeDee's in labor?"

"John, believe me, I wouldn't be calling you at six A.M. otherwise!"

I thought I was calm, but realized I was more excited than I felt: I hadn't spoken coherently to John, either. Grace woke up and climbed into the tub with her mother. What a vision they were! A naked, silken-haired, sturdy little redhead just shy of three years and her naked, blond mother both sitting Indian-style in the water, leaning against the side of the tub. DeeDee was voluptuous, even forty weeks pregnant; her firm gravid belly swelled lavishly below her breasts. The morning light in the bathroom bathed them in a warm, buttery softness—a captivating portrait of expectant mother and child.

After a few more phone calls and another couple of hours of contractions in the bathroom, DeeDee's mother had collected Sabra and Grace to spend the day at her house. John arrived with chucks and shoelaces to tie off the umbilical cord: I still didn't know what supplies the midwife would bring. Our brother Stan drove an hour and a half to join us, excited by the prospect of attending this birth since he'd been unable to watch his own son's delivery. The baby's father, Tony, rode his bike over and arrived breathless and harried with nerves. I gave gentle instructions, largely unnecessary, to the guys about keeping the house peaceful and serene. The midwife showed up around ten in the morning. She had a delivery kit with everything we'd need for the birth.

DeeDee moved to her bed and I checked her cervix, after assuring the midwife I knew how to do so. DeeDee was only three to four centimeters dilated, but the cervix was thin and soft. She was having some bloody show. John, Stan, and Tony took turns applying pressure against the small of her back during the contractions. She was calm, breathing slowing with the contractions, complaining of back pain. Uncomfortable in bed, DeeDee moved to a rocking chair. I was moved to tears as I watched my brother lean into DeeDee, pressing his big fist against her back, his other large, loving hand stroking her hair as she rested her head on his chest, her arm wrapped around his neck. Stan murmured softly to her as she breathed at a measured pace in his embrace. It meant so much to me to be with these two siblings, sharing this time together.

The day passed quietly. DeeDee spent most of the time in the bathtub. Soaking in hot water was the most comfortable activity for her. At first she wore a T-shirt in a halfhearted attempt at modesty for the men's sake, but eventually she grew chilled around her shoulders, so we dispensed with clothing. Alternating with one another when their arms got tired, the guys each sat on the edge of the tub or knelt beside it, pushing against the small of her back. Stan washed dishes and fixed a zucchini casserole for dinner. Those of us not actively providing back pressure for DeeDee talked quietly together and read the newspaper. The midwife left for a couple of hours. Using her doptone, I listened every hour or so to the baby's heartbeat—nice and steady, in the 130s with no audible decelerations in rate before, during, or after the contractions.

We checked Dee's cervix again around 1:30. She was five to six centimeters dilated and the baby was facing her leg instead of her tailbone, so she returned to her bed for a sidelying position in hopes the baby would rotate. Tony stretched out beside her, rubbing her back and stroking her arms. It was so peaceful and quiet, I grew drowsy and had to fight a strong urge to take a nap. DeeDee wasn't happy: the contractions were painfully strong and the whole thing was just taking too long. After spitting out Grace, all ten pounds of her, in less than three hours, she expected this labor to progress rapidly. But she endured, with remarkable composure.

At 3:45 DeeDee wanted to get back in the tub. Looking tired and unhappy, she lowered herself into the water, grumpy with dismay over her pain. She couldn't find a comfortable position. She wanted to be finished. At 4:00 the midwife checked her cervix, reaching her gloved fingers down through the bathwater.

"There's just a tiny rim of cervix left here, Diedra. Push for me and let me see if I can move it back past the baby's head," she instructed.

DeeDee pushed and shouted, "Oh, that hurts! Stop it! Stop it! Take your hand out! It hurts!"

Almost immediately after the midwife withdrew her hand, DeeDee cried out, "Oh! I need to push!"

"Okay," I soothed her. "Let's get you out of the tub and into bed so you can."

She looked up at me, disgruntled. "I don't think I can get up, Susie."

"We can get you out if you want. Or we can do it here. Do you want to have the baby in the tub?"

"Yes. No. I don't know! I just can't get up. Yeah, let's do it here."

The midwife and I started spreading paper sheets out next to the tub. The bathroom was miniscule; only one person could get beside the tub. DeeDee grimaced with pain and changed her mind. "There's not enough room in here. Get me out of here."

Stan, John, and Tony hauled her dripping out of the tub, wrapped her in towels and walked her to her bed. The midwife opened her pack and laid out instruments. Under my directions, Tony climbed onto the bed and positioned himself behind DeeDee, supporting her upper body and shoulders between his legs. John sat close by her left side, Stan by her right, holding the doptone on her belly so we could hear the heartbeat. I knelt between her legs, gloved and ready to catch! She pushed. I could feel the baby's head descend against my fingers. She pushed again. I called to Stan, "Come look, you can see the head!" He peeked, eyes wide, enthralled.

DeeDee pushed again and the baby crowned. Dee cried out something about it hurting. I smoothed the perineal tissues, applying light pressure to prevent tearing. We all gently urged her on. Then there it was—head out!

"Wow, she's got her eyes wide open, DeeDee!" I suctioned the mouth and nose and felt for a cord around the neck. "There's a nuchal cord," I announced to the midwife and turned to look for clamps to tie it off. It was too tight to slip over the baby's head, so I though we'd clamp and cut it before delivering the body. But, oops, DeeDee couldn't stop pushing even though the midwife and I had asked her to. "It's coming, I can't help it, it's coming!"

Without any trouble, the baby's body just slid out into my hands.

"Turn her around, into the leg! Flex her around to the leg!" the midwife commanded. I couldn't figure out what she was saying.

"I don't understand what you mean," I sputtered as both of us turned the baby around so her head was facing Dee's pelvis. Quickly then, the midwife unwrapped the cord from around the neck, as I held the baby's body.

"One, two, three, four! Four times! It's wrapped around her four times!" We counted in unison. The midwife clamped the cord. Stan, I think, cut it. I was drying the baby off, checking reflexes, watching her color, her respirations. She was making little halfhearted cries, but looked fine. Her eyes were still open and she looked alert, very much with us. I put her on DeeDee's stomach and rested back on my heels to watch Dee and the guys greet this beautiful little girl.

"Go ahead and put her on the breast if you want to, Dee," I suggested. "It'll help to deliver the placenta."

The moments around the birth itself were so crowded with activity and emotions they're hard to remember now. I know Stan stood up to see the actual birth. We didn't have time for me to encourage DeeDee to deliver the baby's body herself, as we had discussed earlier. John reported later that he cried. Tony was in shock, blown away by the whole scene. But it was quiet and calm except for the five seconds after the baby slid out when the midwife and I weren't communicating well and trying to untangle the cord.

The baby, our Zoe, took Dee's nipple into her mouth and sucked like she'd been eating this way forever. We cleaned up the debris—only one quarter-sized bloodstain on the sheet, took pictures, got DeeDee into a clean nightgown, and talked all at once, everyone exclaiming over what we'd just accomplished and how lovely the baby was. Zoe just kept on sucking, eyes bright, skin pink, lungs clear, muscle tone firm. An absolutely marvelous little girl!

We weighed Zoe (seven pounds, six ounces) on a postal scale John had borrowed from his office. Stan buried the placenta in DeeDee's herb garden, using Grace's plastic beach shovel—the only shovel he could find! It pleased Stan, DeeDee and me to think of the placenta providing nutrients to her herbs, instead of just going up in smoke in a hospital incinerator. Except for keeping her bottom and face clean, DeeDee didn't bathe Zoe for ten days. Our father had instructed her after Sabra's birth not to bathe her for ten days: the vernix on her skin was a protective substance, and soap only dried up the natural lubricants. Grace had been bathed by nursery nurses almost immediately after birth and every day she was in the hospital. She was readmitted to the hospital two weeks after her birth for a respiratory infection. DeeDee was convinced the baths had contributed to her susceptibility to infection. So Zoe didn't get a bath until she was ten days old. Her cord came off by itself after just four days.

Zoe's birth clarified much of my thinking about the manner in which obstetrical care is provided in U.S. hospitals. The very ordinariness of her birth stands in stark contrast to the complexity of a hospital birth. Her mother labored in her own bed and bathtub in her own home. Close family members, friends, and a professional midwife assisted her as needed with her pain and her delivery. After the baby was born, she remained with her mother and family. DeeDee was up an hour after the birth to shower and eat. She had no episiotomy and no tears: her bottom hurt only because of hemorrhoids. Except for weariness, she was fully recovered by the next day. Her mother managed the older girls for the week. I ran errands, cleaned house, and did laundry. DeeDee mothered Zoe. It was routine and normal and ordinary, the baby fully incorporated into the family from the moment of her birth.

DeeDee's friend John expressed the difference most succinctly: "I have to admit when DeeDee talked about doing this at home, I wasn't real happy about it. In fact, it made me very nervous, but now I just can't imagine choosing a hospital birth over this. It was so quiet, so peaceful. No IVs, no monitors, no strange people coming and going from the room whenever they pleased. No equipment and instruments and medical stuff. It was so noisy in the hospital, even when it was supposed to be quiet."

Several years ago, I cared for a woman having her second baby. She arrived late in her labor so it was wild trying to get an IV started, monitors on, moving her to the delivery room, and positioning her in the steel stirrups. Bright lights and noise, a multitude of masked, gloved, and gowned people scurrying around opening supplies, readying the infant warmer, doctors standing between her legs yelling at her to push, her husband and I trying to help with positioning and counting. In between contractions there was a brief lull. Over my mask, I smiled at the father even though he couldn't see my smile. "Pretty hectic, huh?" I asked. She's moved so fast through this labor, it's been kinda crazy."

He looked at me and then glanced around the room at all the people and equipment, the gleaming white tile walls, the hard steel table on which his wife reclined. "This is a mind blower!" he exclaimed. "With the first baby, we uh, we had it at home with a midwife. This is so totally different I can't believe it!" "Different" doesn't begin to convey what that really means.

When I receive a normal labor patient, I know without thinking about it that I will tie her down with an IV line, two fetal monitor lines, and a blood pressure cuff. If she gets an epidural, she will have an oxygen mask, an epidural catheter in her back, ECG lines and/or a pulse oximeter line. After the epidural, she will need a bladder catheter, sometimes the indwelling type with a tube and bag to hold the collected urine. Just turning over in bed will be impossible for her without my help. She can't go to the bathroom or sit in a chair after an epidural or IV narcotics. If she is being induced, she will have another IV line attached to a heavy IV pump. There will be tape on her back, arms, legs and finger or toe. Just getting in close to the bedside can be difficult for a family member because of all this equipment.

Even though I'm the one who puts all this stuff on a woman, it drives me nuts. So much of this technical crap is just not necessary with normally laboring women. I can't bear the fact that I am participating in a system that treats a normal biological process so pathologically. On a quiet afternoon as I was driving on a long trip, I was daydreaming, thinking about all of this. I realized that most people, those who have never been involved with hospital obstetrics, have no idea what it looks and feels like to see a woman in labor thus attired. I remembered when I watched the movie *E.T.* years ago with my children. I remembered the horror and the sick feeling I had in the pit of my stomach when those government scientists took that adorable, ugly extraterrestrial in hand.

Remember how they filled the house with equipment and had his little form all tied up with lines and tubes and monitors? Remember the boy, Elliot, screaming, "You're hurting him! You're hurting him!" That's how I feel deep inside, even as I apply the lines and tubes and wires to my mothers. After Zoe's birth, my antipathy for what I'm supposed to do as an obstetrical nurse is even greater.

Why are we doing this? How is it that I have contributed to this pathological treatment of women? Me, the natural childbirth instructor, the advocate for noninterference in the birth process? Why have I capitulated to the system and become so glib at explaining rules and policies that aren't always in the patient's best interest? With every best intention, with all the most current, state-of-the-art theory and technology, we obstetrical workers have taken away the mother's dignity, her comfort, her control, all "just in case" of a medical emergency, of a malpractice suit, of breaking hospital rules, of being vulnerable to mistakes. Aside from the enormous financial cost such practice incurs, we have dehumanized one of the most significant of human events: the birth of a new being. And all of us—obstetricians, obstetrical nurses, hospital administrators, lawyers, insurance companies, and the mothers and fathers themselves—have allowed this to happen.

I wish I could end this book neatly, offering solutions to these seemingly insurmountable problems, explaining how I've come to understand my own complicities in the system and have corrected my own shortcomings. But my story isn't finished; as Nick said, I still have to find an ending for it. I know much of what happens to women giving birth in hospitals today can be changed. I know that it is possible to approximate, in the hospital, a birth like Zoe's more closely than we've achieved so far. I am searching for the right place, the appropriate forum in which I can help affect some change. I am trying to thrust aside the old learned helplessness and conflict-avoidance behaviors so I may return to this work I've loved so much and find in it once more my bliss—helping women do the work of becoming mothers.

EPILOGUE

Since this book was published, I have received a number of letters and phone calls from readers about *Hard Labor* and the subject of childbirth in this country. Many of the readers wanted to know what I have been doing since I left the hospital arena. Many asked questions about how to obtain compassionate, appropriate obstetrical care during their pregnancies. Thus this epilogue chapter.

For four years I painted house interiors, helped wealthy people pack up and move into luxurious new homes, and worked for realtors as a cleaning woman preparing houses for the market. All the while, I steadfastly refused to think about nursing, pregnant women, newborn babies, and laboring mothers.

I actually did try to return to nursing, briefly. Painting houses and helping people move paid the bills, but it was hard work and I began to long for reliable benefits and a set schedule. The first day of orientation on this new job as a labor and delivery nurse, I was sitting in a conference room in a large metropolitan hospital where my eight-week orientation was to occur. Here in this bastion of obstetrical technology and pregnancy-as-an-illness framework, I watched a film, *Gentle Birth Choices,* which depicted several nontechnical, nonmedical births that occurred at home or in a birthing center. I watched women give birth in large bathtubs, squatting over a toilet, sitting or kneeling on all fours on the floor, their families present and participating. There were no monitors, no IVs, no pain medications, no epidurals, no forceps, no sterile delivery rooms, no stirrups or masks or gowns, and no NO ADMITTANCE signs.

I loved this film. I thought the orientation leader was a real champion to show us this video at the beginning of our time together, almost as if she were throwing down a gauntlet, challenging us to remember that birth was more than a medical procedure. The nurses watching this film with me—all of them bright, accomplished, and experienced L&D nurses—gasped at the absence of technology, at the strangeness of having a baby underwater, at the extreme differences between the approach to the birthing process as depicted in the film and their own experience in hospital L&D units. After a few days, I realized that the other nurses had dismissed the film as a whimsical throw-

away, a sort of anthropological *National Geographic*–type documentary—
"Here's how the savages in East New Something give birth." The content of
the film had absolutely no bearing on their lives and work. I became known
among the group as the one who would do the water births at our new facility,
if in fact we would ever do them.

It almost goes without saying that I didn't fare well or last long in this
new job. All the reasons for leaving hospital L&D nursing years earlier were
in my face once again. A particularly inhumane delivery with a dictatorial,
insensitive male doctor tore me up, and I found myself enraged at the entire
framework of medical obstetrical care. The nurses, competent professional
women carrying heavy responsibilities and performing their duties with great
aplomb, kowtowed to this male doctor. They worked diligently to meet his
every niggling demand, while one of their own gender was brutalized and
left comfortless as she labored to birth her baby. The nurses completely ignored the mother except as the target of their physical activities; they were
busy blatantly sucking up to the doctor.

It stunned me all over again. Who's having this baby, anyway? Whose
life is being changed before our eyes? Who's bringing forth a new person
into her family and the world? Who's working hard to accomplish this act?
Why is the *doctor* the center of attention? Where has he been while the mother
has endured one contraction after another, her body sweating and toiling to
give birth? Why is his time so almighty important? Who made him God
and why do other women allow—no, *encourage*—him to play the prima donna
while a woman is birthing her baby? Where is the respect, the dignity, the
peaceful sacredness of birth in all this mechanized medical management of
birth, presided over by a supercilious, casually cruel man? How did the most
profound act of womanhood become the bailiwick of a haughty, contemp-
tuous male? Why on earth did we women relinquish our control over this
most significant female event?

It was all horrifying to me. I was utterly convinced that I didn't have
it in me in any way to continue with this job. I could not—ethically, phil-
osophically, or spiritually—be a part of a system that so blithely ignored the
fuller meaning and nature of birth. That's all there was to it. Why in the
world did I think it would be any different or easier this time around? Why
did I think I could put aside my beliefs, my ethics, my very personality,
simply to earn a regular paycheck and have reliable benefits? Who was I
kidding?

I quit the next day. I knew I might be acting precipitously, that the
work situation probably would improve if I gave it more time. But I also
knew that I could not be a part of this dehumanizing system of maternity
care. While never denying the wonders of science and research—in fact,
always paying homage to those wonders when they save a baby and/or a
mother—I could not, and will not, help to maintain the status quo of ob-

stetrical nursing "the way it's always been done." And I am too emotional and too conflicted to even attempt to change the system from within. It is my curse and my blessing that I am so hypersensitive to all the little ways in which we can ruin a baby's arrival; so now I have to accept my own failings and limitations without guilt or reproach.

I called my mother—bless her ever-loving, patient heart—and asked if I could move in with her while I figured out what I was going to do next. Three days after I quit I paid an impromptu visit to a neighborhood birthing center that had been open only a year. I truly believe that my guardian angels sent me to this place. I was fifty years old. I had no job. I was going home to my mother's, without a clue as to how I would support myself. But before I left town, something made me visit this birthing center.

Even though my visit was unannounced and unscheduled, two nurses and the midwife-director invited me into the back conference room where we sat and talked while they ate their lunches. They had read *Hard Labor* and seemed pleased to meet me. One of the nurses confessed that it had been difficult to read of my struggle because she had identified so completely with it. The midwife encouraged me to become a doula (a childbirth support person) and provided me with the registration materials for the annual Doulas of North America (DONA) conference. Then I was given a tour of the birthing center and saw with my own eyes a place where women were encouraged to do the work of birth without the mechanization and interference of the monitors, machines, and medications of hospital births, surrounded by their families and trained, compassionate professionals who respected the natural process of birth and assisted it, in the main, by keeping their hands off!

With loving hugs and warm, encouraging words, these women enfolded me literally and figuratively in their arms. They made me realize that there were options available, that there were people who held the same beliefs as I did about the sanctity of birth and the necessity of protecting the mother from invasive interventions during her travail. I left feeling hopeful and re-dedicated to the idea of pursuing work in the childbirth arena.

I moved back home. The day I unloaded the truck I drove fifty miles to attend a three-day training workshop for doulas. With this workshop, I began a period of discovery. I studied books and research articles about birth. I attended the three-day DONA conference with nearly three hundred kindred souls, talking, listening, and learning. I discovered a vast network of people and organizations around the world that has been working for the past twenty-five years to improve maternal and fetal outcomes and to return the process of childbirth to its rightful place—back to the woman and her capacity to birth her own baby.

All those years I was slaving on L&D units, feeling that uncomfortable sense of dis-ease over the things we did in the hospital to mothers and babies, there were people out in the world actively working and researching and teaching others about how distorted and dangerous the birth process has become because of technological and scientific "advances." While I had known on a gut level that the system wasn't working effectively, I hadn't had the time or the awareness to search out these "outliers."

What a joy to discover all this written evidence validating my instinctive reactions, to learn of the work being done, and to meet people who were doing it. I watched films of babies being born underwater (even a breech delivery) that stunned me with the obvious benefits of water therapy for labor pain and for the peaceful and safe arrival of new babies. I had the great good fortune to meet, chat with, and listen to two of the giants of maternal/fetal well-being research, Drs. John Kennell and Marshall Klaus, who twenty-five years ago had written the bible on the benefits of immediate and close contact between mother and baby in their book, *Parent-Infant Bonding.* Now elder statesmen in this field, they still are conducting research into the short- and long-term effects of separation of infant from mother at birth and of the use of Pitocin and other medications that may have long-lasting effects on child development and family cohesion.

I learned about the work of Michel Odent in France, a leading advocate of the instinctive wisdom of mothers in childbirth and the importance of not interfering with the process in the vast majority of births. I listened to and read the work of Marsden Wagner, of the World Health Organization, who argues cogently and effectively against the exclusion of midwifery from the arena of maternity care, making a clear case for improved outcomes, both maternal and fetal, if midwives provide care for normal, low-risk patients and obstetricians focus on the complicated high-risk pregnancies. I read Henci Goer's book, *Obstetric Myths Versus Research Realities,* which examines the existent obstetrical research and effectively puts the lie to most of the myths society holds today as fact: that hospitals are the only safe place to have a baby; that fetal monitoring is necessary; that obstetricians are the only appropriate birth attendants; that midwives are dangerous; that "natural childbirth" is something only a masochist or a New Ager would pursue; that cesarean delivery rates are high for legitimate reasons, and so forth.

And I hung up a shingle: ENLIGHTENED LABOR: CHILDBIRTH SUPPORT SERVICES. I offer my expertise to expectant mothers and their families as an experienced obstetrical nurse and a certified doula (childbirth support person or a professional labor assistant). The various labels all mean the same thing. A doula is "a woman who is experienced in childbirth who offers continuous emotional, physical and informational support to the mother before, during, and just after childbirth." This definition is provided by Marshall Klaus, John Kennell, and Phyllis Klaus, in their seminal book about doulas, *Mothering the Mother* (New York: Addison-Wesley, 1993).

The concept of the doula (the word is Greek and refers to the most significant female slave or servant of the house) is not a new one. Women have been assisting birthing women since time immemorial. Over the past century, as the place of birth moved from the home to the hospital, such assistance, once automatic, has fallen away. Women are attended by nurses, or unfamiliar professionals, rather than by family members. Within the past twenty-five years, the woman's "significant other," her husband or partner, has finally been given begrudging access to the labor and delivery rooms of hospitals. But the support, knowledge, and comfort of other women has not been universally available to laboring women. As a result, doulas have emerged to fill this gap. There are two national doula organizations: Doulas of North America (DONA) and the National Association of Childbirth Assistants (NACA). Some doulas provide only birth assistance, while others provide only postpartum and newborn care. I offer both services.

When I assist a mother through her birthing activities, my obstetrical experience and knowledge is combined with all the compassionate advocacy I can give her. When I help a mother in her home after her baby's birth, I am a surrogate grandmother, gently sharing my expertise and years of experience as a mother with women who have no extended family support and no knowledge of how to incorporate a newborn into their lives. (It is amazing how many women out there have absolutely no idea about the most basic elements of infant care. I've had clients who asked with puzzled sincerity how often to change a diaper or to bathe a baby, what to do when the baby cries, even whether it is safe to take the baby outside!) Grandmothers and aunts and neighbors used to pass along this valuable knowledge about infant care. Today, often geographically separated from their extended families, women search through books and listen to other mothers—if there are any around. But for not a few women, particularly older first-time mothers, there is no exposure to other mothers until long after those first few days at home with a demanding newborn.

I identify myself to most people as a doula, but I am actually a monitrice, which "is a labor-support person who provides the companionship and comfort of a doula but also has special obstetric training," as defined by William and Martha Sears in *The Birth Book* (Boston: Little, Brown & Company, 1994). Not only do I offer the comfort measures and support of a doula, but as a registered obstetrical nurse, I also can do cervical exams, check the mother's blood pressure, and assess the baby's heartbeat. Many doulas do not have a nursing or midwifery background and do not do any medical procedures. My background enables me to provide additional services to my clients, but I do not perform any nursing tasks when I am in the hospital with my mothers.

Specifically, what I do as a monitrice/doula is what I have always tried to do as an L&D nurse, but with significant differences. Now I contract directly with the expectant woman and her family to be her labor support person. Before her labor begins, I meet with her at least twice. In those meetings we get to know each other. I find out what her plans, hopes, and fears are for the upcoming birth, and what she expects from me. I help her create a birth plan. I discuss all the normal hospital routines, procedures, tests, equipment, and so forth with her, answering questions about why any given procedure or treatment might be used, explaining the pros and cons of these treatments, and clarifying for her what she has a choice about and what she may expect each step of the way.

My goal in these meetings and throughout our contractual relationship is not to impose on her my own belief system, but to ascertain what *she* wants this birth to be like. Then I work to help her achieve that goal. I help her know what questions to ask, provide explanations for the way things are done in the doctor's office and in the hospital, and interpret for her, as needed, the various explanations or requests the doctor or hospital staff may present to her. I am there to help her have the kind of birth she wants to have—not the kind of birth I'd like her to have, or the doctor would like her to have, or the hospital expects her to have. If she wants to "go natural," more power to her, and I do everything I can to help her do just that. If she wants an epidural as soon as possible, or an induction, or to schedule a cesarean, I help her do that. The idea is to have her come out of the whole experience with positive memories about it.

When she goes into labor, I join her at her home and help her stay at home as long as she wants, providing it is medically appropriate. Then I accompany her to the hospital, where I remain at her side *continuously* until she's given birth, bonded with her baby, and begun breast-feeding. Then I pay a few more home visits to give her an opportunity to review and remember the experience, to assist with breast-feeding and infant-care concerns, and to lavish her with praise and admiration for the work she has done to have this baby. She also gets a written narrative of the birth from me, which I address to the baby directly, writing all I can remember about the baby's birth—for the baby book!

After people ask, "Doula? What's a doula?" they want to know why it's necessary or even beneficial to have a doula. This is where it gets really interesting. Six studies have been conducted so far into the effects on the outcome of doula-attended births, detailed in Klaus, Kennell, and Klaus's *Mothering the Mother*. The results of these studies indicate that doula-attended births *decrease:*

- the cesarean rate by 50 percent;
- the length of labor by 25 percent;
- the requests for epidurals by 60 percent;
- the use of forceps and Pitocin by 40 percent; and
- the use of pain medications (narcotics) by 30 percent.

Such births also reduce the incidence of episiotomies, perineal tears, maternal fever, the amount of time a newborn may spend in the neonatal intensive care unit (NICU), and the number of septic workups on newborns. Long-term benefits of doula-attended births include improved breast-feeding; increased time spent with the baby by the mother; more positive maternal assessments of the baby's personality, competence, and health; and a decreased incidence of postpartum depression. (This information is summarized from *Mothering the Mother* and from *The Birth Book*.)

In the course of my studies, I read or heard an interesting little anecdote. (Unfortunately I can't find the reference now, but I want to share this anyway, with apologies to whoever did this research.) Laboring women at one hospital were asked if they would consent to having a female observer in their room during their labors. This observer was just that, an observer. She did nothing but sit in the corner of the room. She did not interact in any way with the mother or her partner. Amazingly enough, when compared to laboring women who did not have an observer present for their labors, the outcomes were improved for the observed mothers, and the mothers' perception of the event of birth was significantly more positive. Think about that: if just having a warm female body close at hand can make a mother feel better, how much more pleasant and intervention-free might the experience be if that warm female body was actually comforting and encouraging and supporting the mother?

The doula "mothers" the mother by providing emotional support; by keeping the mother's birth plan in mind if problems come up or if difficult decisions have to be made; by demonstrating and using comfort techniques from massage to aromatherapy to positional changes; by answering questions and explaining labor events as they occur and preparing the couple for what else is likely to happen. As the authors of *The Birth Book* describe so well, ideally the doula should be a sensitive presence, knowing when to actively assist the mother and when to retreat quietly into the shadows and leave the laboring couple alone. Probably the single most important aspect is that the doula is there for the duration. She does not leave the mother during the entire time of the labor. She is the one person other than the father or partner who is *always* there, always accessible, always supportive and comforting. She attends the mother completely and singularly.

Nurses do not remain with a mother throughout her labor. They work shifts and go home at the end of them whether their patient has delivered or not. They have more than one patient, except during the final, pushing stage of labor. They also have many other required, essential tasks they must perform before they can provide the hands-on, compassionate care every woman deserves and needs while she is in labor. Nurses have medications, charting, equipment, and the doctor's needs to attend to, and (as it must be obvious by now from the many pages of this book) these tasks place the mother, as a human being in need of emotional support and physical comfort, at the bottom of the priorities list.

People ask me, "If the father/husband/significant other is there, why do I need a doula?" In the past couple of decades, I think we've placed a heavy burden on fathers. After he attends a six-week-class series on childbirth and sees a couple of films, a father is expected to be an instant expert on birth and everything birth entails. He is supposed to give his partner physical and emotional support, act as her advocate and buffer with the hospital staff, and make sure everything stays calm and controlled. With all the expectations placed on the father, there is precious little time or thought given to the fact that this is a profound experience for him, too. He has his own emotional and psychological issues to contend with, and although he may not be going through the pain and physical stress his partner is, he may very well be just as tired and hungry and frightened as she.

Most men have never seen their wives/partners in the kind of pain and extreme exertion that birth involves. They have never helped someone onto a bedpan or wiped up vomit or seen the bloody pads that accumulate under a woman's bottom during labor. Few feel comfortable about questioning hospital routines or procedures. Most trust the hospital staff to do the appropriate things for their wives: if the staff says she needs an IV or an internal monitor or some Pitocin, it's difficult, if not impossible, for the father to challenge or question such assertions. Even if he's heard the arguments for and against various interventions, it's a whole different ball game when he's in the hospital at the bedside of a sweating, pain-racked partner, someone he loves, who's begging for relief. Many men feel overwhelmed by a sense of helplessness and fear for their partners' and their babies' well-being.

In one of the many conversations and lectures I have attended, someone pointed out that no other unit in a hospital relies so heavily on the presence of a significant other for assistance with patient care. Fathers are quite routinely asked to watch an IV bag fluid level; to call for help if there is a deceleration of the fetal heart rate on the monitor; to put their wives on the bedpan or assist them to the bathroom; to change the bloody pads beneath them. Many men have expressed to me their amazement about the amount of time they were left completely alone with their wives in the labor room. They had expected a nursing presence that simply was not there until the very end, when the baby was ready to pop out.

If a doula is present, many of the unreasonable responsibilities the hospital staff has come to expect of the father are comfortably transferred to the doula's shoulders, releasing the father from this burden so that he can concentrate on his true concerns: his wife/partner, his baby, his own emotional responses to the imminent arrival of his offspring, and his new identity as a father. Men whose wives were attended by a doula when giving birth uniformly attest to the relief they felt and the confidence that the doula's presence conferred on them. The doula and the father/partner collaborate together to assist the mother during her accouchement. It is an elegant partnership in which they surround the mother with a buffer of comfort and support so that she is free to concentrate on her birthing efforts.

Maternal satisfaction with the birth experience is closely related to the mother's sense of control over the events of her labor and birth. What is said and done to a woman in labor is remembered forever by that woman. Research into maternal satisfaction with the birth experience by the grande dame of doulas, Penny Simkin, shows that women who are treated indifferently, casually, or abusively by their caretakers have a much more negative memory of the birth, regardless of the medical facts of that birth, than women who were treated with respect, dignity, compassion, and humor. These women, even if they endured days of rigorous labor and/or had all sorts of complications, still felt the experience was a positive one, because they felt that they were involved in the decision-making process and that the people caring for them actually did care about them.

For many of my prospective clients and a growing number of hospitals and insurance companies, a final and convincing argument for professional labor support is that it is cost effective. If cesareans, epidurals, inductions and augmentations, forceps deliveries, IVs, monitoring, septic workups, and NICU care are decreased, costs are decreased. If a mother stays at home for the longest part of her labor (the latent phase), a hospital bed is not being occupied unnecessarily. If her labor is shorter and she feels better after the delivery than she would have had the doula not assisted her, she will require less care and less hospital time. Cost comparisons in my area alone indicate an average saving of $500 to $1,000 per birth if a doula attends the mother.

So now I am doing exactly what I thought I would be doing as a labor and delivery nurse those many years ago. I am helping women succeed in their birthing efforts—with my hands, my voice, my presence, and my confidence in their ability to do this work. I am not charting or starting IVs or pushing Pitocin. I am not leaving the room repeatedly to attend to someone else. I am not catering to the doctor's needs and whims. I am not required to meet hospital protocols or standards of practice. I am there just for the mother, as her assistant, her "grandmother," her masseuse, her exhorter, her promoter, her guardian angel. I give her my hands and my heart to pull on and lean against as she obeys the inexorable demands of her body and brings forth a child. It is work of great privilege and intimacy and the sharing of it with her is a precious gift.

This is not to say that my life is all peaches and cream. I live in a very conservative community in an area that is far behind much of the rest of the country in terms of obstetric care. The cesarean rate in my area is, at best, 35 percent; some obstetrical practices have a rate as high as 60 percent! Few consumers have any knowledge of the changes in obstetrical care or the options available in other parts of the country. They haven't learned to even question the interventions and medical management of the birth process to which they are subjected. Doulas, midwives, water births, and home births are rejected as New Age craziness, just as "natural childbirth" was twenty-five years ago, and is still today, by people who have no idea of the risks they take when they embrace so unquestioningly the hospital/obstetrician medical model of birth (in which birth is seen as a pathological event that must be controlled and managed aggressively to prevent further pathology). The social model of birth, which views childbirth as a normal biological process that is a natural part of a woman's reproductive life, is lost in this society's glorification of technology and science.

It is going to take a great deal of patience on my part, a lot of teaching and lecturing and demonstrating through my example—and a lot of time— to change the way women give birth where I now live. But I am not alone. There are a few women who want to maintain control over their birth process and there must be, somewhere, doctors and nurses and midwives who want to help them do just that. The Internet, bookstores and libraries, and conferences and meetings around the country are all disseminating the ideas presented in this book. There are several thousand certified and practicing doulas in the United States today, and someday in the not-too-distant future, we hope to have a doula available for every laboring woman who wants one.

To give you a final story to illustrate the contrast between the social and medical models of birth, I want to tell you about one of my doula clients. Indie is a twenty-five-year-old graduate student. Her partner, Race, is studying to be a veterinarian. Indie wanted to have her first baby at home. Her sister delivered at home with a professional midwife in attendance, but because this sister had an unfortunate and painful tear in her perineal tissue, Indie thought that a hospital delivery would be safer and make a similar complication less likely.

Like many grad students, Indie was financially very limited. She didn't qualify for Medicare but could receive free care from her university, which staffed and managed a large hospital for indigent patients. She contracted with me to be her monitrice/doula. We shared many phone calls and two home visits, getting acquainted and mapping out a mutual plan for her labor.

She wanted to stay at home as long as possible. She did not want to be separated from her baby at birth. She did not want an episiotomy, Pitocin augmentation or induction, an IV, an epidural, or narcotics. Essentially, she wanted to have as natural a birth as possible, with no medical interventions. She discussed all her plans with her physician, a resident at the clinic where she received her prenatal care. Unfortunately, she went into labor three weeks early, before she was able to get a copy of her birth plan to the L&D unit and the pediatricians at the hospital.

After a couple of phone calls over the course of one evening, it was obvious that Indie was in labor. I gathered up my doula gear and drove to Indie's at 11:30 P.M. When I arrived at her house in the dark, cool night, Race let me in. Shirtless and in shorts, his handsome face was encircled with shining, luxuriant brown curls; I didn't know that he had such beautiful hair until this moment, because he always wore it pulled back in a ponytail and hidden under a baseball cap. He was smiling and flushed with excitement. He led me to their bedroom where I found Indie naked under the comforter on her bed. Her long black hair streamed down her back. Her body was tawny and lithe, beautifully proportioned and slender but for the firm, round ball of her gravid belly. A dancer, she was in exquisite physical shape and completely at ease with her nakedness.

We talked. I palpated a couple of contractions. I tried to count the baby's heartbeat, which I could hear, but so faintly that actually getting an accurate count was difficult. Indie's beloved sister Maris arrived with a family friend, Lisa—who was absolutely hyped with excitement. Over the next few hours the four of us—Race, Maris, Lisa, and I—surrounded Indie with a quiet, gentle, loving bubble of attention. She sat for a while in a recliner, her feet on a footstool, with Race massaging her scalp and combing her hair. Maris and Lisa massaged her legs, hands, and feet. I sat opposite her, leaving her loved ones to do the actual touching as I softly and hypnotically talked her through each contraction. She had an aura around her entire being that was visible, a soft golden glow that radiated calm, peaceful attention to the work of her body. She was stunningly beautiful as she did this work. When I commented on her beauty, Race agreed with me. He was fascinated and in awe of how she looked, the sound and look of wonder in his voice and face. This was a first for him: even though he'd watched animals give birth, he'd never seen a woman have a child. He was entranced.

Over the next few hours, Indie walked, slow-danced with one or the other of us, spent some time in the tub, and lay on her side in bed. When she sat in the tub, soft candlelight bathing her in a velvety glimmer, Race kept warm wet towels around her shoulders as I sat on the floor and talked her through the contractions. Indie breathed quietly and carefully. In bed, Race lay on one side of her, stroking her back and hips. I lay on the other. As a contraction would peak, she would reach out her hands and interlace her fingers with ours, lifting our arms high and slowly swinging them in arcs to and fro. The reaching out and upward seemed to help. It was so quiet and peaceful in those small hours of the night that Race and I found ourselves drifting off in between contractions. Maris and Lisa napped in the other room.

As the contractions became more intense, at my suggestion Indie began breathing out the baby's name with each breath. Eventually, each breath was an exhalation of the word "yes." She said "yes" with such utter conviction it sounded like a prayer, a plea, and a blessing on herself and her baby all at the same time.

I checked Indie's cervix at 2:30 A.M. She was two to three centimeters dilated, 90 percent effaced, and the baby was still high in the pelvis. At five-thirty in the morning she began to get restless and expressed anxiety about her progress. She thought it was time to go to the hospital. I always pay attention when the mother says this because it usually indicates a change in the labor, an awareness on the mother's part of the imminence of birth. I checked her cervix but couldn't find it, even after sweeping my fingers pretty thoroughly around the baby's head. Not completely trusting my own ability to assess cervical status accurately, since I have been known to be mistaken (like everyone who does these exams), I told her she was either completely dilated or I just couldn't find the cervix, but I was fairly certain it was the former.

As Race and the other two women gathered bags and pillows and blankets, I stayed with Indie and talked her through a few more contractions. We loaded up in two vehicles for the thirty-minute drive to the hospital in the city. Indie crawled onto a bed of blankets and sleeping bags in the back of her sister's van. Maris drove. Race sat in the middle section, the seatback down so he could stroke Indie's legs. I lay down behind her, cocooning loosely around her from behind, lightly resting my hand on her shoulder or hip. As we drove, she alternated between a state near sleep and an intense effort to ride through the contractions. Her arm would come up like a dancer's and wave in the air, reaching for and interlacing with my fingers, and pulling against me as our arms swayed high above us. Then, as one of the contractions waned, she pulled my arm down against her, bringing my hand still interlocked with hers up under her chin so that my arm pressed against her breast. She pulled hard so that I was enfolding her in a hug, my body curled around hers, spoon fashion. I was swept with tenderness toward her as I held her close and she clung to me. It was like I had felt so many times in the past, curled around one of my children in the night, soothing them to sleep after a nightmare.

We were two warm bodies together, one in pain and distress, reaching out without a single inhibition for the comfort and consolation of the other behind her. Our bodies moved in synchrony as she rode the waves of her contractions and rested in the intervals between them. Silently, I blessed her for the simple, dignified straightforwardness of her need for physical reassurance and solace. Those few moments in such sweet shared intimacy I will never forget. We were mothers together: one who had endured a similar effort twenty years earlier and one who was on the cusp of motherhood. We were sisters sharing the ultimate in female experience. And we were mother and daughter, the one holding the other who didn't hesitate to pull the mother close for simple animal warmth and comfort.

What happened in the two hours we were in the hospital before her baby was born could not have been further removed from the peace, love, and comfort of the labor at home. Indie was separated from Race and me for almost an hour, forced to go through the hardest part of her labor without a familiar face or even a hand to hold. She endured one medical intervention after another and was subjected to fragmented, callous behavior by the medical and nursing staff.

The incredible contrast between Indie's labor at home and the hospital birth cannot be imagined. Indie achieved everything she hoped for in her labor at home. She worked through long hours of contractions, completing the entire first stage of labor and reaching ten centimeters of dilation without any of the accoutrements with which she would have been burdened at the hospital. In the soft light of candles and within the warm circle of loving care created by her partner, her sister, her friend, and her monitrice, her body opened itself to allow her baby to come forth. It was peaceful, dignified, safe, quiet, and as comfortable as possible. She directed her own activities, choosing when to change positions, how to be massaged, when to walk, and when to soak in the tub. She breathed out her love for her baby and herself with every "yes" she uttered.

At the hospital every ounce of control and autonomy was stripped from her. She had absolutely no power to insist on having a companion of her choosing at her side. She was even refused a comforting hand to hold during her contractions. Her body was stuck with needles, wrapped with lines and straps, torn apart and scraped and battered within. She ended up with a bottom that looked as if a bomb had gone off near it, and several weeks of pain every time she urinated or defecated. She birthed her baby in a room barren of any dignity, quiet, gentleness, or respect, attended by strangers so wrapped up in their "science" and technology that they couldn't begin to acknowledge the profound nature of what had just occurred. Indie and Race had become parents. A new human being had begun her life in this room, noisy with the clatter of equipment and instruments and machines; a place so sterile, white, and brightly lit it offended the eyes. The contrast between the first and second stages of her labor could not have been more profound, or more disappointing.

*   *   *

As an individual, as a nurse working within the hospital system of birth, and as a monitrice/doula working with laboring mothers as an independent consultant, I have witnessed firsthand the conflict between the medical and social models of birth. I write about it with the passion that emerges from my conviction that the medical model has all but subsumed the social and familial aspects of birth, to the detriment of the mother and baby who are the focus of all the conflict.

Once again, it is not that I disparage or discount in any way the scientific and technological expertise that protects women and their babies from the risks of complicated pregnancies or births. My argument and outrage is directed at the belief system that insists all women must be subjected to medical, technological control and intervention under the mistaken assumption that science is supreme, and that only high-tech obstetrics can be trusted to safely deliver a baby from its mother's body. This belief system completely denies the woman her rightful place at the center of the event. She becomes a thing upon which all manner of procedures and treatments and interventions are imposed. Her inherent ability as a female in the process of reproducing young to respond to the forces and urges of her body is denied, discounted, and ignored. She is told what to do and how to do it.

Unfortunately, one of the main reasons this occurs is because women have been indoctrinated with the belief that they don't know *how* to have a baby, that only a doctor and a hospital with all the high-tech scientific equipment and knowledge can guarantee them a satisfactory outcome. And, if women don't get what they expect, they take to the courts, suing the people to whom they have relinquished their responsibility for their own birth experience. Doctors and nurses practice interventionist obstetrics in a large part because of the fear of malpractice litigation. If something goes wrong in a hospital labor and delivery and the hospital staff hasn't used every technological resource available to them, the risk of liability is increased.

To the doctors and nurses who provide obstetrical care, I bow my head in humble acknowledgment of the hard work, long hours, and heavy responsibilities you bear. I thank you for your work and your commitment to the mothers and babies in your care. And I ask you to open your minds to the fact that birth is more than a medical procedure, and that it encompasses far more than just tubes and wires and needles and medicines and machines. In your hands is a whole human being gravid with another life, who deserves and demands privacy, security, safety, dignity, and compassionate respect for and belief in her own ability to perform the act of birth.

Please, I ask you physicians and nurses, don't just do things the way they've always been done. Read the "alternative press" about birth. Spend some time in dialogue with midwives and doulas and the people who are researching alternative methods of childbirth care. Attend some births in a birthing center or at home with a midwife and really observe with your own eyes how a woman can bring forth a baby without IVs, monitors, epidurals, forceps, medications, and stirrups. Become truly well rounded instead of hunkered down in a defensive attitude, denying the validity of other approaches to childbirth simply because they challenge your customs and beliefs. Work *with* your mothers instead of against them. You will find yourselves amazed by the magnificence of the process if it is allowed to progress without interference or fear or an eye on the clock. Don't assume that a labor must be accomplished by the clock: it happens as it should happen, however long that takes, and it differs with every mother, so be patient and accepting of the uniqueness and individuality of each labor.

I am not just reproaching the doctors and nurses and hospitals here. I am also berating the mothers and fathers out there who are sloppy, irresponsible consumers of obstetrical care. Having a baby is one of the most significant and profound events in a family's and a woman's life and it should not be undertaken without serious consideration of all the pros and cons of each possible permutation of treatment. We should be as serious consumers of obstetrical care as we are when we buy a house, plan a wedding, or decide to make a large investment. The experience of giving birth has short-term, immediate effects on the mother and baby: whether she has an episiotomy or a cesarean to heal from; whether she is able to bond with and breast-feed her baby successfully or is too exhausted to even care; whether the baby is subjected to a NICU for septic workups; or whether she is able to meet her baby's needs immediately after birth.

The experience also has long-term effects. Mothers who undergo a stressful, debilitating experience in which they feel they have lost control over their own bodies and their own birth process are left with lifelong psychological scars, including a diminished sense of confidence in their own bodies and their ability to be good mothers. This diminishment has a ripple effect on other aspects of their lives—their sense of self, their marriages, and their ability to take on other arduous tasks.

Long-term effects of negative birth experiences on the baby are just beginning to be researched, but there is some evidence that lengthy inductions, the overuse of Pitocin to stimulate labor, the casual use of epidurals and other medications during labor, and the high rate of cesarean and forceps/vacuum deliveries may have an impact on a child's normal development. Suspicions about their possible impact range from attention deficit disorder to hyperactivity and possibly even to autism.

Most expectant women in our society do not do the necessary work to ensure a peaceful, dignified, and safe labor and delivery and a healthy baby.

We have handed over our responsibilities for our own bodies and spirits, and that of our babies, to medical professionals without questioning any of the reasons for all the things those professionals, with the best of intentions, do to us. We have lost faith in our own bodies, in our own strength and ability to bring forth our offspring. There is a difference, after all, between *being delivered* and *giving birth*.

Uncounted generations of women have had children without IVs, monitors, epidurals, Pitocin, narcotics, forceps, episiotomies, and cesareans. Uncounted generations of women have trusted themselves and their female companions—mothers, grandmothers, sisters, and friends—to work with the labors of their bodies, to bear the pain and the long hours to safely bring forth a baby. When there are unforeseen complications, we are blessed to have the science and technology of modern obstetrics to fall back on, but we do not need to rely completely on that science and technology if it means abrogating our own responsibility to this process. And whatever the outcome, we must be accountable for our own participation in the process. We must not automatically blame the caretakers for whatever goes wrong and make ourselves victims instead of active participants in our own birth processes.

It is possible, indeed imperative, for us to combine the medical and social models of birth, to work together as a team with our doctors, midwives, nurses, and doulas for successful births—medically, emotionally, and spiritually. Within these pages I can't begin to provide a definitive list of resources or advice on how to have the best birth possible. But here are some initial suggestions:

1. *Don't wait until you are pregnant or far into your pregnancy to begin to gather information.* If you know you're going to have a baby sometime in the near future, start reading and researching now. There is a virtual library out there of books, films, and classes available to expectant or planning-to-be-expectant parents. One of the very best books, which I highly recommend to all of my clients is *A Good Birth, A Safe Birth* (Diana Korte and Roberta Scaer, Boston: The Harvard Common Press, 1992). This book walks you through all of the controversies attendant to the birth process in this country and tells you how to find the right birth attendants and the right birth place. Read this book *before* you pick a doctor or midwife or hospital. You'll be armed with the right questions to ask and know how to ask them and how to find people who will work with you to make your birth what you want it to be.

Another excellent book is *Gentle Birth Choices* (Barbara Harper, Rochester, Vermont: Healing Arts Press, 1994). It provides more information on the significance of the birth process and why it is so profoundly important to go through this process in a conscious, thoughtful, self-determining way. In addition, this book provides the most extensive list of resources with addresses, phone numbers, and brief synopses of provided services that I have found thus far. This list by itself is worth the purchase price of the book. A midwife, author, and lecturer, Ms. Harper is responsible for the film mentioned at the beginning of this chapter and is a leading authority on water births. Her belief in the transcendence of birth and the power of women to experience this transcendence shines through her words.

The Birth Book and *The Baby Book* by William and Martha Sears (physician and nurse, respectively, and parents of a whole passel of kids!) are two of my favorite books not only because of their up-to-date explanations of all the scientific obstetrical theories and practices but also because of their commonsense, practical, and compassionate approach to the issues of birth and infant care.

The Nursing Mother's Companion (Kathleen Huggins, Boston: The Harvard Common Press, 1995) is one of the best of many books on breast-feeding.

There are a number of books about the "scientific" controversies of obstetrical care. The best among them is Henci Goer's book, *Obstetric Myths Versus Research Realities: A Guide to the Medical Literature* (Westport, Connecticut: Bergin & Garvey, 1995) and *A Guide to Effective Care in Pregnancy & Childbirth* (Murray Enkin, et al., Oxford, England: Oxford University Press, 1995).

To learn more about doulas and labor support, read the book referred to earlier in this chapter, *Mothering the Mother,* and Penny Simkin's book, *The Birth Partner* (Boston: The Harvard Common Press, 1989). Ina May Gaskin's classic, *Spiritual Midwifery,* and Suzanne Arms's two books, *Immaculate Deception* and *Immaculate Deception II,* are not to be missed.

These books are just the beginning. The Internet has all sorts of chat groups, Web pages, and resources to tap into. Educate yourself and discover how marvelous the whole arena of childbirth really is.

2. *Don't assume or accept anything unless you've researched it yourself.* For instance, just because an obstetrician tells you that fetal monitoring is necessary or that the hospital is the only safe place to have a baby doesn't mean that it's necessarily true. And please, *don't listen to and be swayed by the horror stories* of your neighbors or coworkers or family. Every woman likes to tell about her birth experience, but horror stories have more impact, so what you hear will be all the bad stuff. Women who have had wonderful experiences somehow just aren't listened to as readily as those who have "been through the mill." Of course it can be difficult to stop women from telling you their horror stories, but if you are politely firm, a simple statement such as "I will only listen to

positive stories" works more often than you might expect. After all, this is your pregnancy: you don't have to be frightened or worried about what happened to someone else. When someone does tell you they've had a good experience, ask them for tips on how to assure the same for yourself.

3. *Don't hesitate to interview several doctors and midwives and to tour all the hospitals in your area before you decide where you will have your baby and who will attend you.* You are the consumer: they are providing a service and you have the right and obligation to find the right place and people for you, rather than just to acquiesce to their preferences and their convenience. Make time for these visits: it's important and will affect the final outcome. If you buy the first car on the lot, or the first house you look at, then you're stuck with what you get. Impulse shopping in obstetrical care is irresponsible and can be dangerous.

I've had women who wanted to interview several doctors but said they couldn't afford to pay for these consultation visits. This is being "penny-wise and pound-foolish." Instead of buying the latest in infant equipment, spend some of that money on finding the right doctor or midwife. Women who say they really want a midwife but their insurance doesn't cover it also amaze me. There are ways to come up with the money to retain a birth attendant who is not only professionally trained but has the same philosophical expectations of the process of birth. What is more important: a safe, satisfying, confidence-enhancing birth experience or a paid-in-full insurance bill? Why would you risk a lifetime of psychological and emotional scars just to save some money? Rely, of course, on your health insurance to cover unanticipated problems, but don't be afraid to pay the extra money for a midwife or a doula. Start saving now. Ask your family and friends to give you money for a midwife and/or a doula instead of a baby swing or a fancy stroller. I have recently learned of something called a "flexible spending account," which is offered by some insurance companies, that allows the insured to set aside pretax dollars up to a given amount to be used for approved health treatments that are not covered under regular insurance plans. This can include "alternative" treatments, such as acupuncture or doulas, as well as deductibles and copayments. Ask your insurance company or employer about this option.

4. *Don't be intimidated by the "superior knowledge" of the hospital staff or the doctor.* You can educate yourself enough to know what's appropriate in your birth experience. It is your birth and your baby and your body you're trying to protect, so it is your responsibility to insist on having

your questions answered and having your desires met, wherever medically possible.

5. *Believe in your body and your strength and your inherent ability to have a baby.* Pay attention to the magnificent changes in your body and emotions as you progress through your pregnancy and recognize that you are fulfilling the ultimate capability of womanhood. Trust your body and spirit, surround yourself with compassionate, knowledgeable support, and surrender to the process. It is glorious and uplifting and empowering: you will discover things about yourself that you never dreamed were there, and all your days will be imbued with a sense of pride and pleasure in the act of becoming a mother.

1998

ABOUT THE AUTHOR

SUSAN L. DIAMOND earned a Bachelor of Science in Nursing after spending some years as a prepared childbirth instructor. In addition to her B.S.N., Diamond holds a B.A. in English.

Diamond spent nearly a decade working on labor and delivery wards throughout the southern and eastern United States, in both military and civilian hospitals.

For the past four years, since leaving traditional medicine, Diamond has been working as a housepainter. She has recently become a faux finisher.

Safe and life-affirming childbirth remains Diamond's passion, and she has founded her own company, Enlightened Labor, to continue to bring her message to the public. Diamond is now a certified doula, offering childbirth support directly to women and their families in both home and hospital settings. At speaking engagements Diamond addresses many of the issues raised in *Hard Labor*.

Diamond has lived in Massachusetts, Indiana, Pennsylvania, Maryland, Kentucky, North Carolina, Ohio, and Texas. She now resides, with her mother, in the southern United States. Diamond has two children, Rebecca and Michael.